(For Medicine, Phamaceutical, Agriculture, Forestry and Other Related Specialties Use)

Physics

Hou Junling

Science Press
Beijing

Responsible Editors: Liu Ya Cao Liying

Published by Science Press
16 Donghuangchenggen North Street
Beijing 100717, P. R. China
Printed in Beijing

ISBN 978-7-03-054222-9

Contributors

Editor-in-chief: Hou Junling (Beijing University of Chinese Medicine)

Associate Editor-in-Chief:

Gang Jing (Liaoning University of Traditional Chinese Medicine)

Huang Hao (Fujian University of Traditional Chinese Medicine)

Guo Xiaoyu (Henan University of Chinese Medicine)

Editors:

Gao Qinghe (Liaoning University of Traditional Chinese Medicine)

Wang Li (Dalian Medical University)

Sun Ying (Beijing University of Chinese Medicine)

Ma Ji (Beijing University of Posts and Telecommunications)

Shao Jianhua (Shanghai University of Traditional Chinese Medicine)

Ye Hong (Shanghai University of Traditional Chinese Medicine)

Lin Rong (Shanghai University of Traditional Chinese Medicine)

Peng Chunhua (Shanghai University of Traditional Chinese Medicine)

Chai Ying (Zhongshan College of Dalian Medical University)

Wu Honghui (Beijing University of Chinese Medicine)

Liu Haiying (Liaoning University of Traditional Chinese Medicine)

Li Guang (Changchun University of Chinese Medicine)

Wang Qin (Guiyang University of Traditional Chinese Medicine)

Xie Renquan (Guiyang University of Traditional Chinese Medicine)

Zhang Li (Beijing University of Chinese Medicine)

Wu Ruiguang (Beijing University of Chinese Medicine)

Li Weifeng (Beijing University of Chinese Medicine)

Jin Wei (Beijing University of Aeronautics and Astronautics)

Jin Chen (Beijing University of Chinese Medicine)

Liu Wenyan (Capital Medical University)

Chen Ruixiang (Beijing University of Chinese Medicine)

Song Naiqi (Beijing University of Chinese Medicine)

Liu Xi (Beijing University of Chinese Medicine)

Wang Heyu (Liaoning University of Traditional Chinese Medicine)

Lin Duo (Fujian University of Traditional Chinese Medicine)

Yu Yun (Fujian University of Traditional Chinese Medicine)

Chen Jihong (Henan University of Chinese Medicine)

Zhang Lingshuai (Henan University of Chinese Medicine)

Introduction

According to the needs of educational reform, bilingual teaching as a teaching method is generally applied in colleges and universities, in order to help the students to take the initiative to understand the research trends of the international forefront of physics. This textbook, published by Science Press, is the English version of the fourth edition of Chinese textbook *Physics*. Professor Hou Junling from Beijing University of Chinese Medicine is the editor-in-chief, and other contributors are the in-service teachers with extensive teaching experience for many years.

We have revised and updated 13 chapters regarding the changes in mechanics of rigid bodies and elasticity of objects, fundamental of hydrodynamics, molecular physics, thermodynamics, electrostatic field and bioelectric phenomena, direct current circuit, electromagnetic phenomena, mechanical oscillations and mechanical waves, wave optics, geometrical optics, fundamental of quantum mechanics, X-rays and fundamental of nuclear physics. The main content contains the basic knowledge and fundamental theories of physics which are applied in medical colleges and universities. We insist to express laconically and refine the language, and highlight the characteristics of physics in order to help the learners to study other relative academic courses based on solid foundation of physics.

This textbook is suitable for the undergraduate students who major in traditional Chinese medicine, Chinese materia medica, acupuncture, tuina, orthopaedics and traumatology, clinical medicine, nursing, health care, rehabilitation, health management, agriculture, forestry and other related specialties in higher medical colleges and universities. It also can be used as a reference book for other health professionals and the amateurs.

Preface

Chinese Ministry of Education issued *Guiding Ideas for Improving the Quality of Undergraduate Teaching in Institutions of Higher Education* in 2001, which explicitly pointed out that to promote bilingual teaching in the universities is the general direction of educational work in the future. Bilingual teaching in general refers to the requirements about a number of elementary courses, professional basic courses and specialized courses can be taught in Chinese and English simultaneously in non-English major university curricula.

From the basic teaching principles and teaching methodologies, it is a better way to study medical physics through the bilingual teaching mode for medical students, which helps the students to obtain knowledge of physics, and greatly improves the students' ability of comprehensive language application. Also, it may provide the opportunity and foundation to study the international cutting-edge research trends of medical physics for students.

Physics course in medical colleges and universities is an interdisciplinary science that applies the basic theories and methods of physics into medicine and pharmacology. With the advances in science, technology and educational reform, the development of physics provides more scientific research methods and research means for the modernization of medical science.

This textbook is published by Science Press which is the English version of the fourth edition of Chinese textbook *Physics*, whose editor-in-chief is Professor Hou Junling from Beijing University of Chinese Medicine. This textbook was written on the basis of the requirements of Chinese Ministry of Education for the syllabus of physics in medical colleges and universities, in order to accommodate the needs of modern physics education among the higher medical colleges and universities in our country.

The writing of this textbook upholds the teaching principles of combination of theoretical property and applicability, and combination of scientificity and systematicness. There are 13 chapters in this textbook. In consideration of the characteristics of Chinese medical colleges and universities, this textbook focuses on the relevant content on medicine and pharmacy, taking physical knowledge closely related to the medicine and pharmacy as its entry to elaborate the physics science and principles, in order to improve the students' learning interest.

This textbook is available for the undergraduate students from higher medical colleges and universities, other students from adult education and distance education in all kinds of medical colleges and universities, health professionals and the amateurs. It also can be used as a reference book for other related professions.

This textbook had been written by the contributing authors from a number of medical colleges and universities, and had got the support from the leaders of those colleges and universities. I also had the benefit of translating and proofreading in some sections by Cao Wencong and Ying Zheming, students from the First Clinical College of Liaoning University of Traditional Chinese Medicine. I would like to express my heart-felt thanks to all of them. Due to the limitation of the writing ability, there might be some flaws in this textbook, and your suggestions would be appreciated.

Hou Junling

November, 2017.

Contents

Chapter 1 Mechanics of Rigid Bodies and Elasticity of Objects

The mechanical principles we've learnt in high school physice courses are mainly about the mechanics of particles. Although the objects in our study have the sizes and shapes, when the sizes and shapes of the objects are not so important for the problems discussed, we can use the ideal model of particles to represent these objects.

However, the model of particles is inappropriate in many studies. For example, when an object is rotating, the motion regularity of each point on the object is not the same, because the motion of any points is related with the size and the shape of the object, and the object can no longer be taken as a particle. In order to study the rotational motion of the object, we introduce another ideal model-**rigid body**. The so-called rigid body refers to the body with the shape completely fixed and never be deformed under the action by external forces. This is an idealized model, because under the actions by external forces, any real objects will have more or less changes in the shapes, however, when the deformation of an object is very small, it can be looked as a rigid body approximately.

1.1 Rotation of a Rigid Body

1.1.1 Translation and Rotation of a Rigid Body

1. Translation of a Rigid Body

In the motional process of a rigid body, if it is in such a moving way that the connecting line of any two points on a rigid body is always parallel to its initial position, just as the connection of *AC* shown in Figure 1-1, then this motion form is called **translation**.

By the illustration in Figure 1-1 we find that when a rigid body is in translational motion, it can be regarded as a particle (or a mass point) because the motions of any points on it are the same as the motion of its mass' center. The physical quantities which describe the motions of particles and the mechanical principles of the particles have been discussed in the study of high school physics, so it will no longer be discussed again. But the physical quantities to describe the motions of particles and the regularities on the mechanics of particles are all suitable for the translational motions of rigid bodies.

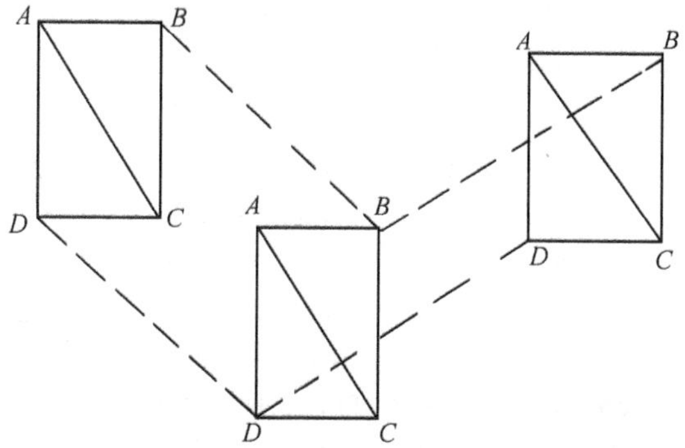

Figure 1-1 Translation of a rigid body

2. Rotation of a Rigid Body

If any points on or inside a rigid body are all performing the circular motions about a certain straight line, this kind of motion is called the rotation. And the straight line is called the rotational axis. If the axis is fixed, the rotation of the rigid body is called the rotation about a fixed axis. For example, the motion of a rotor rotating about its axis in a motor shows a rotation of this kind.

1.1.2 Description of a Rigid Body Rotating About a Fixed Axis

1. Angular Coordinate and Angular Displacement

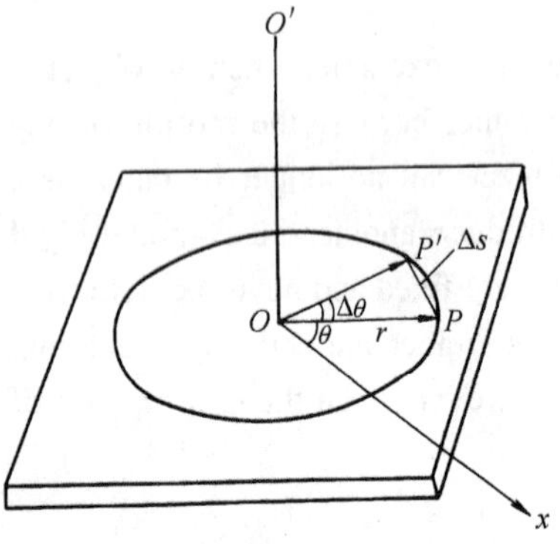

Figure 1-2 Rotation of a rigid body

To give a description of the rotation of a rigid body, we choose a plane that is perpendicular to the fixed axis as the rotational plane, as shown in Figure 1-2. OO' is the rotational axis and the coordinate axis Ox is a reference line, which is perpendicular to OO' and in the rotational plane. Now let's discuss a point P on the rotational plane, the connection line from the center O to the point P is the radius vector of OP, and the angle θ between OP and Ox is called the angular coordinate (or angular position). This quantity describes the position of the rigid body. In the process of rotation, the angular coordinate θ will change with time. Supposing in a time interval Δt, point P moves to P', the radius vector of point P scans an angle of $\Delta\theta$, which also means that the rigid body rotates the same angle of $\Delta\theta$, then we name $\Delta\theta$ as the angular displacement of a rigid body within the time interval Δt. It is a physical quantity that can describe the situation of the rotation of the rigid body. It is also a vector and its SI unit is rad.

2. Angular Velocity

The physical quantity to describe the rotational situation of a rigid body is called the angular velocity, denoted by ω. The ratio of the angular displacement $\Delta\theta = \theta_2 - \theta_1$ to the time interval $\Delta t = t_2 - t_1$ is called the average angular velocity, denoted by $\overline{\omega}$

$$\overline{\omega} = \frac{\theta_2 - \theta_1}{t_2 - t_1} = \frac{\Delta\theta}{\Delta t}$$

Instantaneous angular velocity (or called simply as angular velocity) is the limit of $\overline{\omega}$ as Δt approaches zero, that is, the derivative of θ with respect to t, and is denoted by ω

$$\omega = \lim_{\Delta t \to 0} \frac{\Delta\theta}{\Delta t} = \frac{d\theta}{dt} \tag{1-1}$$

The angular velocity is also a vector and its SI unit is rad/s.

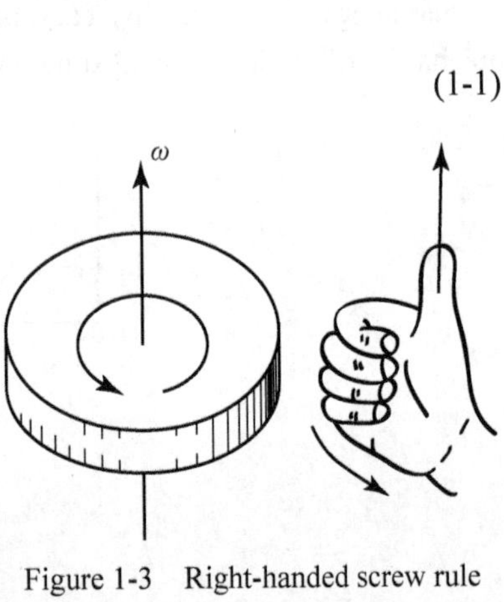

Figure 1-3 Right-handed screw rule

Angular displacement $\Delta\theta$ and angular velocity ω are both vectors, and their direction is commonly expressed by the right-handed screw rule, as shown in Figure 1-3. For example, the representation of the angular velocity vector is: Assuming a directed line segment on the rotational axis, then keep the four fingers of the right hand and the thumb being perpendicular, and let the grabbing four fingers represent the rigid body's rotation direction. The direction of the thumb represents the positive direction of the angular velocity vector, and the length of the directed line segment represents the magnitude of the angular velocity with a certain percentage.

3. Angular Acceleration

If ω_1 is the instantaneous angular velocity at time t_1, over a time interval $\Delta t = t_2 - t_1$ the instantaneous angular velocity changes to ω_2, the corresponding increment of angular velocity will be $\Delta\omega = \omega_2 - \omega_1$. We can define the average angular acceleration as the ratio of $\Delta\omega$ to Δt, denoted by $\overline{\beta}$

$$\overline{\beta} = \frac{\omega_2 - \omega_1}{t_2 - t_1} = \frac{\Delta\omega}{\Delta t}$$

The limit of the average angular acceleration as $\Delta t \to 0$ is called the instantaneous angular acceleration or the **angular acceleration** for short, denoted by β, i.e.

$$\beta = \lim_{\Delta t \to 0} \frac{\Delta\omega}{\Delta t} = \frac{d\omega}{dt} = \frac{d^2\theta}{dt^2} \tag{1-2}$$

The angular acceleration β is also a vector with the direction of $d\omega$, and its SI unit is rad/s^2.

4. Relations Between Linear Quantities and Angular Quantities

The quantities, describing the motions of particles, are commonly called the linear quantities, and the quantitie describing the rotations of rigid bodies are called the angular quantities. When a rigid body rotates about a fixed axis, every point on it moves in a circular path. For a point, its motion can also be described with the quantities which we learnt in high school physics, such as the particle's displacement, velocity, acceleration and so on. Since both the angular and the linear quantities can be used to describe the motional regularity of the rigid body, it is inevitable that there are relations between the two.

As shown in Figure 1-2, for point P on the rigid body, during a time interval Δt, the angular displacement is $\Delta\theta$, then the point reaches to point P' and the corresponding displacement is Δs. If Δt is very small, the chord length can be looked as the arc length approximately, i.e.

$$\Delta s = r \cdot \Delta\theta$$

or

$$ds = r \cdot d\theta \tag{1-3}$$

where r is the perpendicular distance from the axis to point P. According to the definition of velocity, the velocity of point P is

$$\upsilon = \lim_{\Delta t \to 0} \frac{\Delta s}{\Delta t} = \lim_{\Delta t \to 0} \frac{r \cdot \Delta\theta}{\Delta t} = r \cdot \lim_{\Delta t \to 0} \frac{\Delta\theta}{\Delta t}$$

Thus

$$\upsilon = r \cdot \omega \tag{1-4}$$

The vector formula of Equation (1-4) is

$$\boldsymbol{\upsilon} = \boldsymbol{\omega} \times \boldsymbol{r} \tag{1-5}$$

By finding the derivatives of the both sides of Equation (1-4) with respect to time we have

$$\frac{d\upsilon}{dt} = r \cdot \frac{d\omega}{dt}$$

The left side is just the tangential component of the particle's acceleration, expressed by a_t, and $\frac{d\omega}{dt}$ is the angular acceleration of the rigid body, so, there will be

$$a_t = r \cdot \beta \tag{1-6}$$

On the other hand, the centripetal acceleration is $a_n = \upsilon^2 / r$, i.e., $a_n = r\omega^2$, so the integrated acceleration of any point on the rigid body is $\boldsymbol{a} = \boldsymbol{a}_t + \boldsymbol{a}_n$ and its magnitude is

$$a = \sqrt{a_n^2 + a_t^2} \tag{1-7}$$

1.2 Rotational Kinetic Energy and Moment of Inertia

1.2.1 Kinetic Energy of a Rigid Body in Rotation

For a rigid body rotating about a fixed axis, we can consider it as the one that being composed of numerous little mass elements with the mass of Δm_1, Δm_2, $\cdots$, Δm_n, and the distances from these elements to the axis are respectively r_1, r_2, $\cdots$, r_n; any elements rotating about the axis have the same angular velocity of ω, but these elements have different linear velocities of v_1, v_2, $\cdots$, v_n. The kinetic energy of the rigid body is the sum of the kinetic energies of all these mass elements, i.e.

$$E_k = \frac{1}{2}\Delta m_1 v_1^2 + \frac{1}{2}\Delta m_2 v_2^2 + \cdots + \frac{1}{2}\Delta m_n v_n{}^2 = \sum \frac{1}{2}\Delta m_i v_i^2 = \sum \frac{1}{2}\Delta m_i r_i^2 \omega^2 = \frac{1}{2}(\sum \Delta m_i r_i^2)\ \omega^2 \tag{1-8}$$

1.2.2 Moment of Inertia

The quantity $\sum \Delta m_i r_i^2$ in Equation (1-8), denoted by I, is called the **moment of inertia** (or the rotational inertia) of the rigid body about this axis, therefore, the rotational kinetic energy E_k of a rigid body is

$$E_k = \frac{1}{2} I \omega^2 \tag{1-9}$$

To compare Equation (1-9) with the expression of the kinetic energy of a particle $\frac{1}{2}mv^2$, we can find that ω corresponds to v in particle mechanics, and I corresponds to the mass of a particle m. We all know that, m is the physical quantity to express the inertia of a particle in motion, similarly, I is the physical quantity to express the inertia of a rigid body in the rotation about some axis. The calculation formula of the rotational inertia is

$$I = \sum \Delta m_i r_i^2 \tag{1-10}$$

If the mass distribution of a rigid body is continous, its moment of inertia is rewritten as the integral form.

$$I = \int r^2 \mathrm{d}m = \int r^2 \cdot \rho \mathrm{d}V \tag{1-11}$$

Where $\mathrm{d}V$ represents the volume element corresponding to $\mathrm{d}m$; ρ represents the density of the rigid body at the point where the volume element $\mathrm{d}V$ exists; and r represents the distance between the volume element and the axis. The unit of the moment of inertia is $\mathrm{kg \cdot m^2}$.

The moment of inertia of a rigid body not only depends on the total mass of the rigid body, but also on the shape, the size and the mass distribution of every part of the rigid body. For a certain object, the moment of inertia will be different if the position of the axis changes.

As shown in Figure 1-4, there is a uniform rod with the mass of m, the length of l, and the cross-sectional area of S; and the axis is perpendicular to the rod.

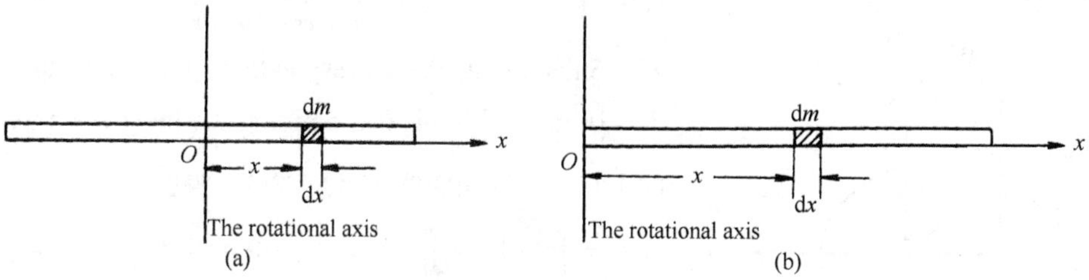

Figure 1-4 Axis at different positions

If the axis passes through the center, then the moment of inertia is

$$I=\int x^2\cdot \mathrm{d}m=\int x^2\cdot\rho\cdot S\cdot \mathrm{d}x=\int_{-\frac{l}{2}}^{\frac{l}{2}} x^2\cdot\frac{m}{S\cdot l}\cdot S\cdot \mathrm{d}x=\frac{1}{12}ml^2$$

If the axis is at one end of the rod, then the moment of inertia is

$$I=\int x^2\cdot \mathrm{d}m=\int x^2\cdot\rho\cdot S\cdot \mathrm{d}x=\int_0^l x^2\cdot\frac{m}{S\cdot l}\cdot S\cdot \mathrm{d}x=\frac{1}{3}ml^2$$

For the rigid bodies with relatively simple geometric shapes, and uniform or regular densities, their rotational inertia can be calculated with mathematical methods; otherwise, their rotational inertia should be determined by experiments. Table 1-1 presents the rotational inertia of several objects with special shapes about the fixed axes for reference.

Table 1-1 Moments of inertia of several objects with special shapes

Thin ring	Thin disc	Solid cylinder
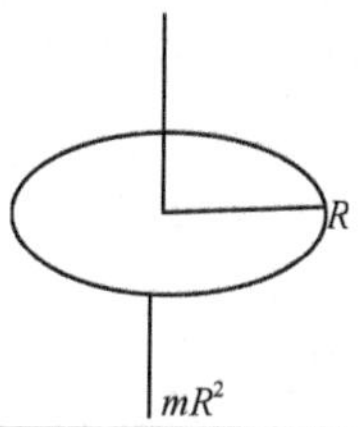	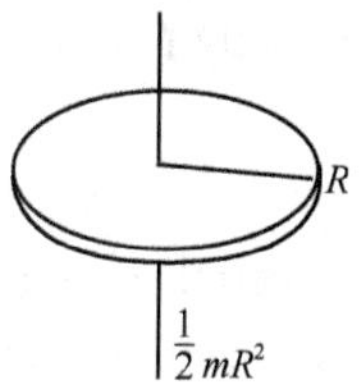	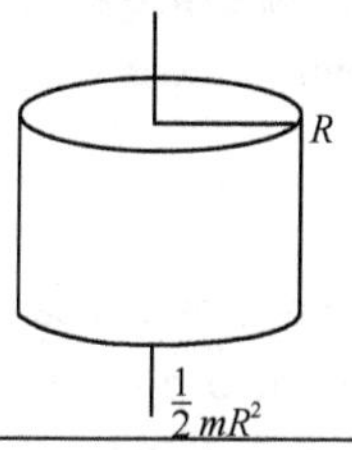
mR^2	$\frac{1}{2}mR^2$	$\frac{1}{2}mR^2$
Uniform fine rod	**Uniform fine rod**	**Sphere**
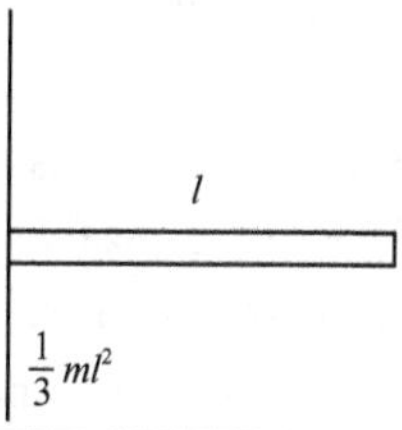	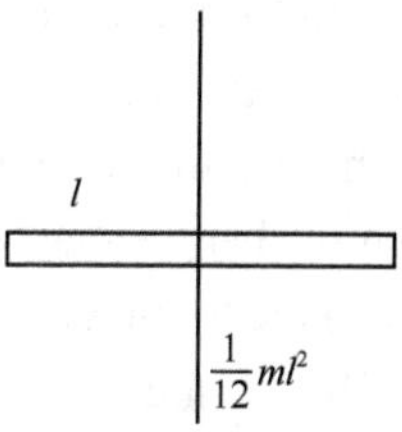	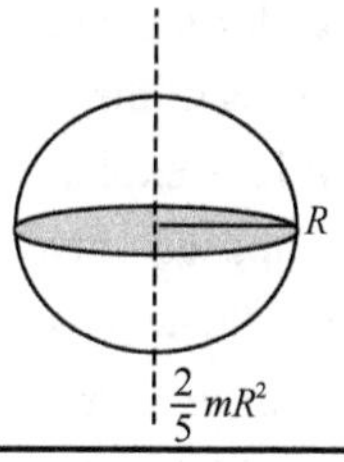
$\frac{1}{3}ml^2$	$\frac{1}{12}ml^2$	$\frac{2}{5}mR^2$

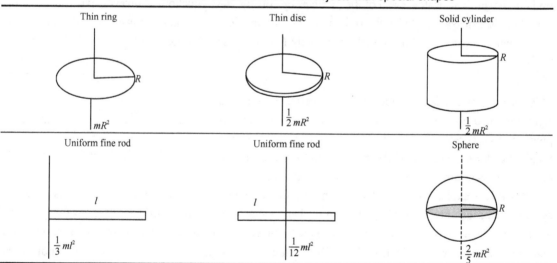

Example 1-1 Figure 1-5 shows a uniform plate disc with mass m and radius R. Determine its moment of inertia about the perpendicular axis through the center.

Solution: Let's assume a mass element of dm as a fine ring with the width of dr, at the distance of r from the center. If the surface density of the disc, i.e., the mass per unit area is σ, we have $\sigma=\frac{m}{\pi R^2}$, and the mass of the mass element is

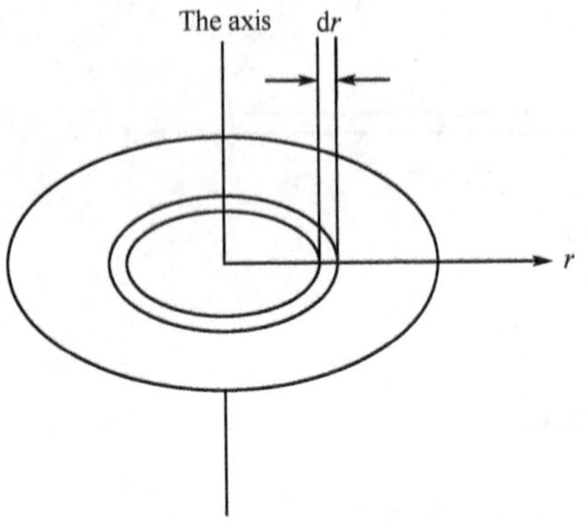

Figure 1-5 Rotation of uniform plate disc

$$dm = \sigma \cdot 2\pi r \cdot dr$$

Substituting the corresponding quantity in the equation $I = \int r^2 dm$ with this dm, defining the integral limits of r and performing the appropriate integral, we get

$$I = \int r^2 \cdot dm = \int_0^R r^2 \cdot \sigma \cdot 2\pi r \cdot dr = 2\pi\sigma \int_0^R r^3 \cdot dr = \frac{1}{2} mR^2$$

That is to say, the moment of inertia of this disc about the axis is $\frac{1}{2} mR^2$.

1.2.3 Determination of the Coordinate of the Mass Center

If a rigid body is considered as the one composed of particles, Newton's second law can be written for one of the particles, i.e.

$$m_i \boldsymbol{a}_i = \boldsymbol{f}_i + \boldsymbol{F}_i \tag{1-12}$$

where m_i is the mass of the particle i; $\boldsymbol{a}_i$ is its acceleration; $\boldsymbol{F}_i$ is the integrated external force on it; $\boldsymbol{f}_i$ is the internal force exerted by all the other particles. Obviously, the number of this kind of equations should be equal to the number of the particles. The number of the equations is so numerous that it is too difficult to find out the motional states for all of the particles by solving these equations. However, experiments show that, there is a special point C in the rigid body, the acceleration $\boldsymbol{a}_C$ at that point is equal to the ratio of the vector sum of the external forces on the rigid body $\boldsymbol{F}$ to the mass of the rigid body m, i.e.

$$\boldsymbol{a}_C = \frac{\boldsymbol{F}}{m} \tag{1-13}$$

This means that we can consider that the overall mass of the rigid body and all the external forces are concentrated in this point, and its acceleration can be determined by the motional regularities for a particle. And the special point is known as the center of mass of the rigid body (or center of mass for short).

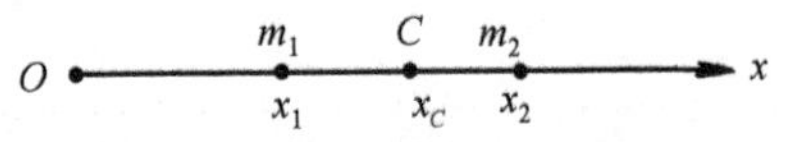

Figure 1-6 Center of mass of two particles

Now, let's explain how to determine the position of the center of mass. First, let's discuss a particle system composed of two particles, and assume that the masses of the two particles are respectively m_1 and m_2, the coordinate axis Ox is along the the connect-line of the two particles, the coordinate of m_1 is x_1, the coordinate of m_2 is x_2, as shown in Figure 1-6. If the center of mass is at point C, x_C—the coordinate of point C should satisfy the following formula.

$$m_1(x_C - x_1) = m_2(x_2 - x_C)$$

Then

$$x_C = \frac{m_1 x_1 + m_2 x_2}{m_1 + m_2}$$

For the particle system composed of three particles, we can use the above method to determine the center of mass for any two particles, and take this center of mass as a new particle, then find out the center of mass for the new particle and the third particle with the same method. The center of mass determined finally should be the center of mass for the particle system composed of three particles. According to the above principle, for the system of many particles, the position of its center of mass can be determined by the following three formulae.

$$x_C = \frac{\sum m_i x_i}{\sum m_i} \tag{1-14}$$

$$y_C = \frac{\sum m_i y_i}{\sum m_i} \tag{1-15}$$

$$z_C = \frac{\sum m_i z_i}{\sum m_i} \tag{1-16}$$

1.2.4 Parallel Axis Theorem and Perpendicular Axis Theorem

When calculating the rotational inertia of a rigid body, we often use the parallel axis theorem and the perpendicular axis theorem.

1. Parallel Axis Theorem

For the same rigid body, the moments of inertia about different axes are different. Suppose there are two rotational axes, as shown in Figure 1-7, one is Cz which is through the mass center C and the other one is axis Oz' which is parallel to Cz. We can choose the coordinate systems $Cxyz$ and $Ox'y'z'$, and keep the axis Cy overlapped with the axis Oy', the distance between axis Cz and axis Oz' being d. If the distances from the mass element Δm_i to axis Cz and axis Oz' are respectively r_i and r_i', and the coordinates of the mass element Δm_i in $Cxyz$ and $Ox'y'z'$ coordinate systems are respectively (x_i, y_i, z_i) and (x_i', y_i', z_i'), then the moment of inertia to axis Cz and the moment to axis Oz' of the rigid body are

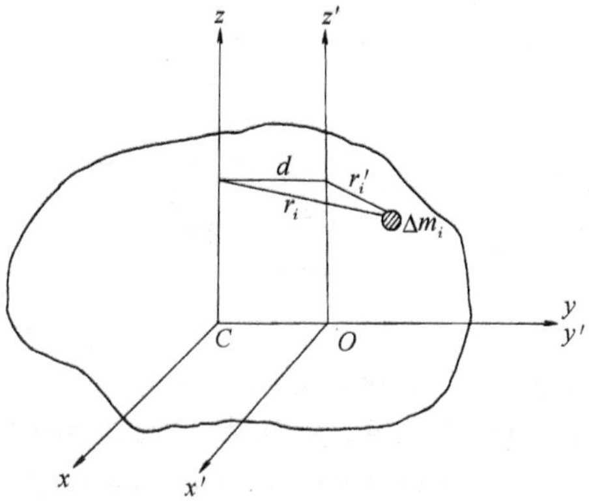

Figure 1-7 Parallel axis theorem

$$I_{Cz} = \sum \Delta m_i r_i^2 = \sum \Delta m_i (x_i^2 + y_i^2)$$

$$I_{Oz'} = \sum \Delta m_i r_i'^2 = \sum \Delta m_i (x_i'^2 + y_i'^2)$$

The coordinates of the mass element Δm_i in the two coordinate systems have the following relationships.

$$x_i' = x_i$$

$$y_i' = y_i - d$$

$$z_i' = z_i$$

Substitute these into the expression of $I_{Oz'}$, and we can obtain

$$I_{Oz'} = \sum \Delta m_i [x_i^2 + (y_i - d)^2] = \sum \Delta m_i (x_i^2 + y_i^2) + d^2 \sum \Delta m_i - 2d \sum \Delta m_i y_i$$

According to the formula of the center of mass Equation (1-15), we know that

$$\sum \Delta m_i y_i = y_C \cdot \sum \Delta m_i$$

and y_C is the coordinate of the center of mass of the rigid body. Now if we assume the coordinate for the center of mass of the rigid body in the $Cxyz$ system to be $(0, 0, 0)$, which means it is overlapped with the origin point, then we will find $y_C = 0$, i.e., $\sum \Delta m_i y_i = 0$. We can also determine

$I_{Cz} = \sum \Delta m_i (x_i^2 + y_i^2)$,

then

$$I_{Oz'} = I_{Cz} + md^2 \tag{1-17}$$

As shown in Equation (1-17), the moment of inertia for a rigid body about any rotating axis is equal to its moment of inertia about the axis through its center of mass and parallel to that rotating axis added by the product of the mass of the rigid body and the square of the distance between these two axes. This conclusion is called the **parallel axis theorem**.

2. Perpendicular Axis Theorem

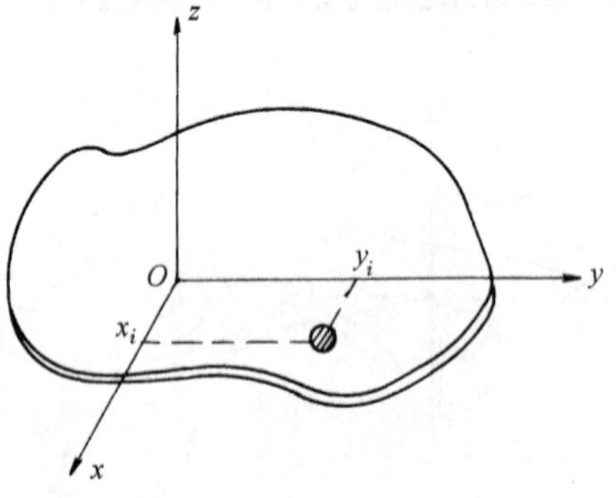

Figure 1-8 Perpendicular axis theorem

Suppose there is a thin plate, and the axis Oz of a coordinate system $Oxyz$ is perpendicular to it, the axes Ox and Oy are also in the plane of it, meanwhile, these three axes intersect at point O, which is shown in Figure 1-8.

The moment of inertia of the thin plate about axis Oz is

$$I_{Oz} = \sum \Delta m_i (x_i^2 + y_i^2) = \sum \Delta m_i x_i^2 + \sum \Delta m_i y_i^2 = I_{Ox} + I_{Oy} \tag{1-18}$$

As expressed in Equation (1-18), the moment of inertia for a thin plate about the axis Oz, which is perpendicular to it, equals to the sum of the two moments of inertia about the two axes Ox and Oy, which are perpendicular to each other in the plane of the plate and intersecting perpendicularly with this axis Oz at a point O. This conclusion is called the **perpendicular axis theorem**.

Example 1-2 A thin disc with a mass of m and a radius of R rotates about an axis, which passes through point A (A is on the edge of the disc) and is perpendicular to the plane of the disc, as shown in Figure 1-9. Find out the moment of inertia of the disc about the axis.

Solution: We know that the moment of inertia for a disc with the mass of m and with the radius of R about the axis through its center of mass is

$$I_C = \frac{1}{2}mR^2$$

According to the parallel axis theorem, we have

$$I_A = I_C + mR^2 = \frac{1}{2}mR^2 + mR^2 = \frac{3}{2}mR^2$$

Example 1-3 Try to find out the moment of inertia I_P of a thin disc with the mass of m and the radius of R, which rotates about an axis OP through its diameter, as shown in Figure 1-10.

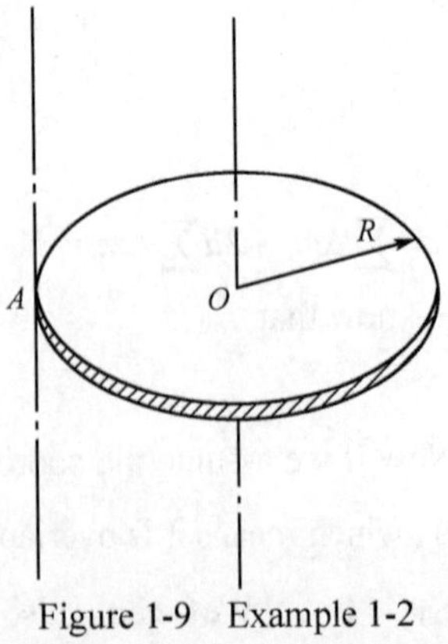

Figure 1-9 Example 1-2

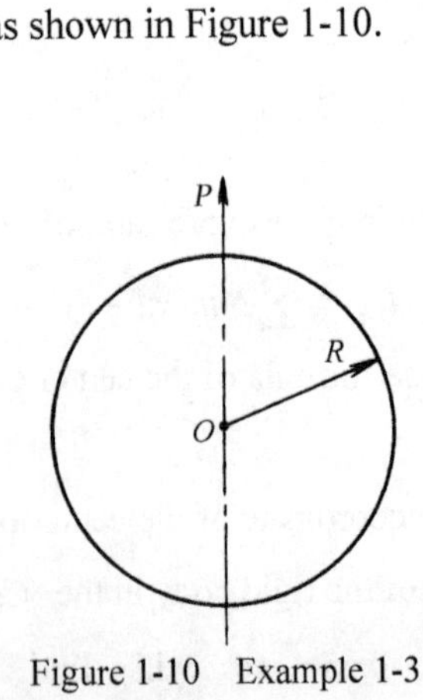

Figure 1-10 Example 1-3

Solution: As we know, $I_O = \frac{1}{2}mR^2$ is the moment of inertia of the disc, rotating about the axis through its center and perpendicular to it. By applying the perpendicular axis theorem to this question, we have

$$I_O = 2I_p$$

Then

$$I_p = \frac{1}{2}I_O = \frac{1}{4}mR^2$$

1.3 Law of Rotation

1.3.1 Torque

For a rigid body with a fixed rotational axis, under the action of external force, the change of its rotational state is dependent not only on the magnitude and the direction of the external force but also on the position of its acting point. Then we need to adopt the concept of torque.

If the external force on the rigid body, i.e., $\boldsymbol{F}$ is on the plane perpendicular to the rotation axis OO', as shown in Figure 1-11, the perpendicular distance between the acting line of force and the axis, i.e., d is defined as the arm of the force. The product of the force and force arm is called the **torque** (or the moment of force), denoted by $\boldsymbol{M}$, i.e.

$$M = Fd \tag{1-19}$$

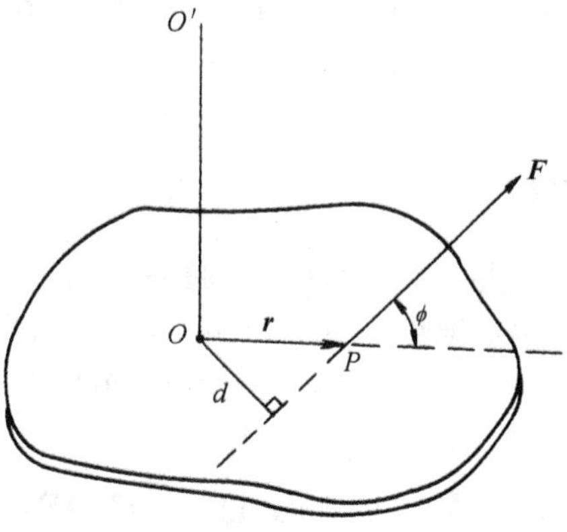

Figure 1-11 Torque

If the acting point of the force is P, and the position vector of point P is $\boldsymbol{r}$, with the presentation in the graph we can get $d = r \cdot \sin\phi$; ϕ is the angle between vector $\boldsymbol{F}$ and vector $\boldsymbol{r}$, so that Equation (1-19) can be written as

$$M = Fd = F \cdot r \sin\phi \tag{1-20}$$

We can also define the direction of the torque with the right-handed screw rule, and write its vector expression as

$$\boldsymbol{M} = \boldsymbol{r} \times \boldsymbol{F} \tag{1-21}$$

Equation (1-21) shows that, the direction of the torque vector can be determined as follows: When the fingers of the right hand curl from the direction of $\boldsymbol{r}$ to the direction of force $\boldsymbol{F}$ via the angle less than 180°, then, the direction pointed by the thumb is the direction of the torque. The unit of the torque is N · m. If the force is not on the plane perpendicular to the axis, it must be decomposed into two components perpendicularly: one is parallel with the $\boldsymbol{r}$ axis; the other is perpendicular to the axis. The former can not make the rigid body rotate, while the latter does.

1.3.2 Law of Rotation

First, let's discuss the work done by the torque. As shown in Figure 1-12, under the action of the force $\boldsymbol{F}$, a rigid body is rotating about the axis OO'. During a time interval dt, the rigid body rotates an anglar displacement of dθ about the axis, the displacement of the acting point of the force is d$s = r \cdot$ dθ,

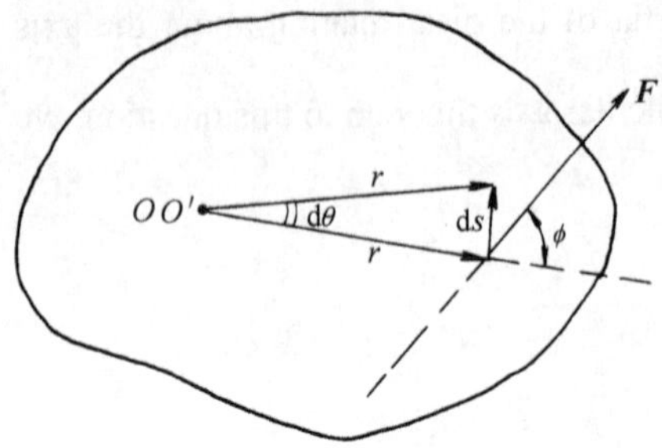

Figure 1-12 The work done by a torque

and the work element done by the force $\boldsymbol{F}$ will be

$$dA = F \cdot \sin\phi \cdot ds = F \cdot \sin\phi \cdot r \cdot d\theta$$

There fore, according to Equation (1-20), $F \cdot \sin\phi \cdot r$ is just the physical quantity M, i.e.

$$F \cdot \sin\phi \cdot r = M$$

So, the work element done by the torque is rewritten as

$$dA = M \cdot d\theta \tag{1-22}$$

By applying the work-energy principle, we know that, the work done by the torque on a rigid body is equal to the increment of the rotational kinetic energy of the rigid body. So we obtain

$$M \cdot d\theta = d\left(\frac{1}{2} I\omega^2\right)$$

For a rigid body, its moment of inertia I is a constant, then

$$M \cdot d\theta = I\omega \cdot d\omega$$

If the two sides of the above equation are divided by the time interval dt, it becomes

$$M\frac{d\theta}{dt} = I\omega\frac{d\omega}{dt}$$

i.e.,

$$M = I\beta \tag{1-23}$$

Equation (1-23) indicates that, the angular acceleration of a rotating rigid body is directly proportional to the torque acting on it, and inversely proportional to its moment of inertia. This conclusion is called the **law of rotation**.

1.4 Law of Conservation of Angular Momentum

1.4.1 Angular Momentum

1. Angular Momentum of a Particle

When studying motions of some objects, we often encounter the cases that particles rotate about a certain point or a certain axis. For example, the electrons inside an atom rotate around the nucleus; the earth turns around the sun and so on. If the mass of a particle is m, the velocity is $\boldsymbol{v}$, its momentum should be $\boldsymbol{p} = m\boldsymbol{v}$; and if the position vector of the particle relative to a fixed point of O is $\boldsymbol{r}$, as shown in Figure 1-13, the definition of the angular momentum of the particle with respect to point O is expressed as the following.

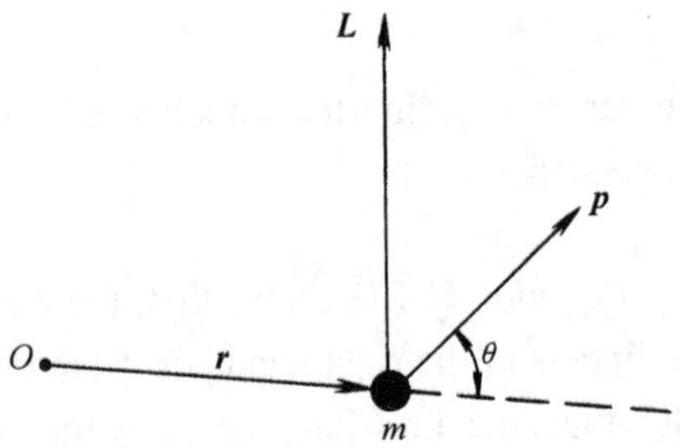

Figure 1-13 Determination of the angular momentum of a particle

$$\boldsymbol{L} = \boldsymbol{r} \times \boldsymbol{p} = \boldsymbol{r} \times m\boldsymbol{v} \tag{1-24}$$

where $\boldsymbol{L}$ is perpendicular to the plane on which $\boldsymbol{r}$ and $\boldsymbol{p}$ exist, and its direction can be determined by the right-handed rule, i.e., when the fingers of the right-hand curl from the direction of $\boldsymbol{r}$ to the direction of momentum $\boldsymbol{p}$ via the angle less than 180°, then, the direction of the thumb is the direction of $\boldsymbol{L}$. The unit of the angular momentum is $kg \cdot m^2/s$.

2. Angular Momentum of a Rigid Body About a Fixed Axis

If a rigid body rotates about a fixed axis, which is shown as the axis Oz in Figure 1-14, when we consider the moment of inertia of the rigid body, we can assume that it is decomposed into many mass elements, the mass of the i th mass moment is Δm_i, and the perpendicular distance from Δm_i to the axis Oz is r_i. If the angular velocity of the rigid body is ω, the angular momentum of ith element with respect to the axis Oz can be determined with Equation (1-24).

$$L_i = \Delta m_i \cdot r_i \cdot v_i = \Delta m_i \cdot r_i^2 \cdot \omega$$

So, the angular momentum of the total rigid body, i.e., the sum of all the angular momentum of the whole mass elements rotating about the axis Oz is

$$L_{Oz} = \sum L_i = \sum \Delta m_i \cdot r_i^2 \cdot \omega = \omega \sum \Delta m_i \cdot r_i^2$$

where $I = \sum \Delta m_i \cdot r_i^2$ is just the moment of inertia of the rigid body.

So, we have

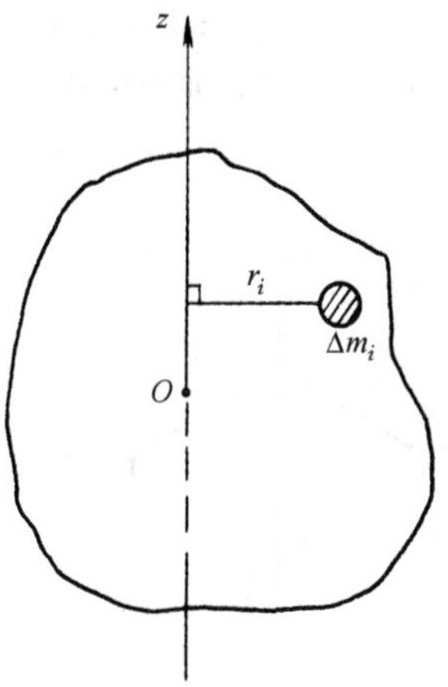

Figure 1-14 Determination of the angular momentum of a rigid body

$$L_{Oz} = I\omega \tag{1-25}$$

1.4.2 Theorem of Angular Momentum

According to the law of rotation we have

$$M = I\beta = I\frac{d\omega}{dt} = \frac{d(I\omega)}{dt}$$

where the product of the moment of inertia and the angular velocity of a rigid body $I\omega$ is just its angular momentum L, so we obtain

$$M = \frac{dL}{dt} \tag{1-26}$$

Equation (1-26) shows that the time ratio of change of a rigid body's angular momentum about a given axis or a point is equal to the magnitude of the resultant torque about the same axis or point. This conclusion is called the **theorem of angular momentum**.

Equation (1-26) can be rewritten as

$$M \cdot dt = dL$$

where $M \cdot dt$ is called the **moment of impulse** acting on the rigid body. So the theorem of angular momentum also can be described as the moment of impulse, acting on a rotating rigid body, is equal to the increment of the angular momentum of the rigid body in the time interval dt.

During a period of time from time moment t_0 to time moment t, if the angular velocity of the rigid body changes from ω_0 to ω, we can get

$$\int_{t_0}^{t} M \cdot dt = \int_{t_0}^{t} dL = L - L_0 = I\omega - I\omega_0 \tag{1-27}$$

The moment of impulse is a vector, and its direction is the same as the direction of the torque vector; the moment of impulse represents the cumulative effect of the torque with time. The unit of the moment of impulse is N · m · s.

1.4.3 Law of Conservation of Angular Momentum

According to the theorem of angular momentum, we know that if the resultant external torque acting on the rigid body is zero (i.e. $M = 0$), then $dL = 0$. That is

$$L = I\omega = \text{constant} \tag{1-28}$$

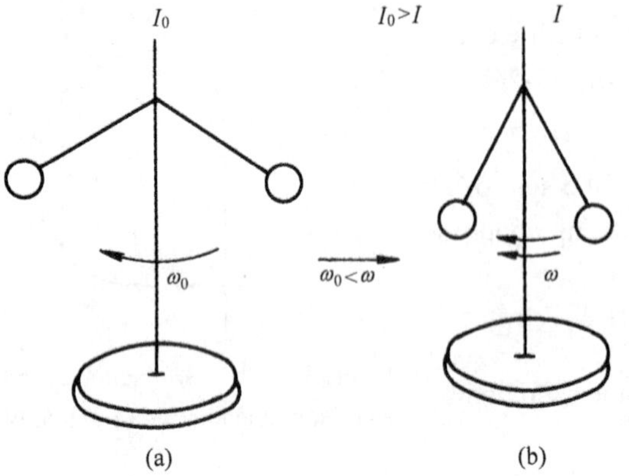

Figure 1-15 Demonstration of the conservation of angular momentum

Equation (1-28) shows that, if the resultant external torque acting on a rigid body is zero, the angular momentum of the rigid body will keep constant. This conclusion is called the **law of conservation of angular momentum**.

Figure 1-15 is the diagram of a two-particle system. Figure 1-15(a) shows the initial state of the system and its angular momentum is $I_0\omega_0$; Figure 1-15(b) shows the state when the distance from the axis to the particles is shortened, i.e., $I < I_0$. According to the law of conservation of angular momentum, we know that the angular velocity corresponding to Figure 1-15(b) is larger than that to Figure 1-15(a), i.e., $\omega > \omega_0$.

The law of conservation of angular momentum is the mechanical basis to analyze the rotations of human bodies. For example, a figure skater often stretches out his arms and spins with a certain angular velocity first; when he puts his arms back, we can see that, the angular velocity of the skater will increase, so the special tricks will be performed. This case shows that in the condition of the angular momentum being conserved, if the moment of inertia lessens (as the arms being put back), the angular velocity must enlarge.

1.5 Motion of the Gyroscope

If a static gyroscope is put at a fixed supporting point O, because the mass center of the gyroscope is at point C (higher than point O), and there is the torque of the gravity mg to the point O (i.e. the torque of M), the gyroscope will topple over under the action of the torque M. But, if the gyroscope is spinning rapidly about its symmetry axis with a large angular velocity of ω, it can be seen that, the the gyroscope will not topple over under the action of the torque M, and besides the spinning motion of the gyroscope, the symmetry axis of the gyroscope will slowly rotate about the vertical axis Oz with a very low angular velocity Ω. This kind of motion of a gyroscope is called the **precession**. Now let's make a quantitative analysis for the precession.

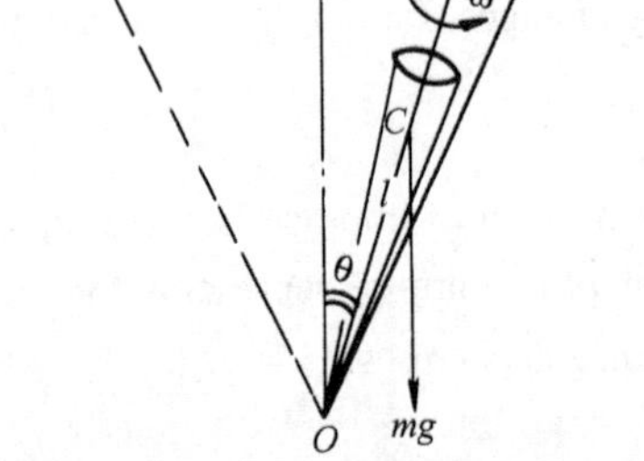

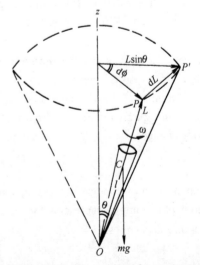

Figure 1-16 The motion of a gyroscope

As shown in Figure 1-16, a gyroscope is spinning with a large angular velocity ω about its symmetrical axis. If the angle between the rotation axis of the gyroscope and the vertical axis

Oz is θ, the distance from the mass center of the gyroscope C to point O is l, the magnitude of the gravitational torque M on the gyroscope can be expressed as

$$M = mgl \cdot \sin\theta$$

According to the theorem of angular momentum, after a time interval dt, the torque M will cause a change of the angular momentum of the gyroscope. If the changed amount of the angular momentum is dL, the endpoint of the gyroscope's angular momentum L moves from P to P', the corresponding expression of the theorem of angular momentum will be

$$\mathrm{d}L = M \cdot \mathrm{d}t$$

Because point P is performing a circular motion along a circle with the radius of $L \cdot \sin\theta$, according to the relationship between the anglar quantities and the linear quantities, we know that

$$\mathrm{d}L = L \cdot \sin\theta \cdot \mathrm{d}\phi$$

where dϕ is the central angle corresponding to dL. Substituting the expression of the theorem of angular momentum with the result of the above formula, we have

$$M \cdot \mathrm{d}t = L \cdot \sin\theta \cdot \mathrm{d}\phi$$

That is,

$$M = L \cdot \sin\theta \cdot \frac{\mathrm{d}\phi}{\mathrm{d}t}$$

where $\frac{\mathrm{d}\phi}{\mathrm{d}t}$ represents the rotational angular velocity of the gyroscope's spinning axis about the vertical axis, which is called the angular velocity of precession, denoted by Ω; the above formula can be rewritten as

$$M = L \cdot \sin\theta \cdot \Omega$$

For $M = mgl \cdot \sin\theta$, combining this relationship with the above formula, we have

$$\Omega = \frac{mgl}{L} = \frac{mgl}{I\omega} \qquad (1\text{-}29)$$

By applying the regularity of gyroscope's motion we can explain the phenomenon of nuclear magnetic resonance of matter, so as to analyze the structure of matter better. In recent years, the theory nuclear magnetic resonance is widely used in the fields of medical diagnosis and druggery analysis.

1.6 Elasticity of Objects and Mechanical Properties of Bone Material

1.6.1 Strain, Stress and Elastic Modulus

Under the action of the external force, an object will have a change in the shape and size, known as the deformation. In the range under the elastic limit, if the external force is withdrawn, the object's shape and size can be rehabilitated, the corresponding deformation is called **elastic deformation**. If the force is too large, the deformation of the object is beyond its elastic limit, and the object cannot be rehabilitated, the corresponding deformation is called **plastic deformation**. This section will mainly introduce the conceptions such as strain, stress and elastic modulus correlative with the elastic deformation of an object.

1. Normal Strain and Normal Stress

Whenever an object is stretched (or compressed), its length will change. As shown in Figure 1-17,

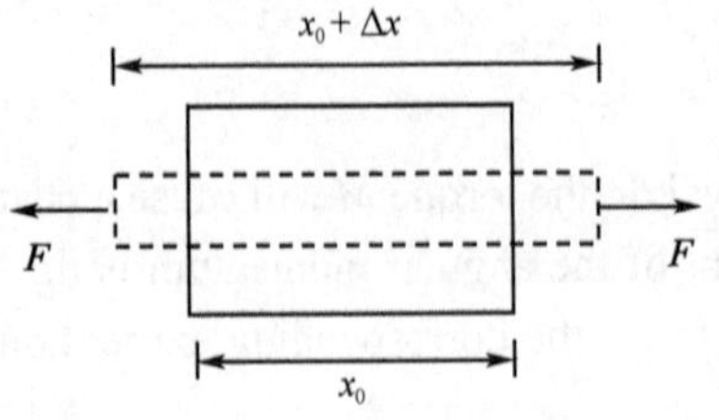

Figure 1-17 Deformation under the tension

for a homogeneous rod with the length of x_0, if both of its ends are stretched by a tension with the magnitude of F, the rod will get an elongation of Δx under the tension. In order to express the stretched (or compressed) variation of length, we introduce a dimensionless physical quantity, which is called as **tensile strain**, denoted by ε.

$$\varepsilon = \frac{\Delta x}{x_0} \tag{1-30}$$

When stretched (or compressed), an object will become elongated (shortened), meanwhile, on any cross section with the area of S inside the object a tension (or compression) force will generate. The internal force on a unit area is known as the **tensile stress** (or **compressive stress**), denoted by σ.

$$\sigma = \frac{F}{S} \tag{1-31}$$

The unit of σ is N/m^2. The direction of the tensile stress (or compressive stress) is perpendicular to the cross section of the object. The tensile stress and compressive stress are both called the **normal stress**, and the corresponding strain is called the **normal strain**.

Experiments show that, when an object has a tension or compression deformation, in a certain elastic limit range, the stress is proportional to the strain, following Hooke's law, i.e.

$$\sigma = E\varepsilon \tag{1-32}$$

where the proportional coefficient E is called the **modulus of elasticity** of the material, also called **Young's modulus**, whose value is determined by the material itself, and its unit is N/m^2. In a certain elastic limit range, it is equal to the stress corresponding to a unit strain. It can be used to express the ability for the material to resist the deformation.

Taking Equation (1-30) and Equation (1-31) into Equation (1-32), we can get the expression to Young's modulus

$$E = \frac{\sigma}{\varepsilon} = \frac{\frac{F}{S}}{\frac{\Delta x}{x_0}} = \frac{F x_0}{S \Delta x} \tag{1-33}$$

Therefore, if the other parameters have been measured by experiments, Young's modulus of the material can be calculated by Equation (1-33), so the mechanical properties of the material could be determined.

When the deformation exceeds the elastic range for some material, if the tension is increased continuously, it will cause the material fractured, and the corresponding tensile stress is called **tensile strength** of the material; if in the case of a compression fracture, the corresponding compressive stress is called **compressive strength**. These two physical quantities are also important indexes for judging the properties of mechanics of materials for test pieces.

2. Shear Strain and Shear Stress

When a pair of near forces with the same magnitude and opposite direction acts parallel on the upside and underside of an object, there will be a deformation corresponded, it is called the **shear deformation**. As shown in Figure 1-18, the underside of a blocky object is fixed on the surface of a table-board; and a parallel force $\boldsymbol{F}$ is applied on the upside of the object. It is clear that, the underside will be acted by a force of $\boldsymbol{F}'$ with the same magnitude and opposite direction from the table-board. So, the two sides of the object will have a relative displacement under the action of this pair of forces $\boldsymbol{F}$ and $\boldsymbol{F}'$. Suppose the relative displacement of the upside and underside is Δx and the vertical distance is d, the ratio

$\frac{\Delta x}{d}$ can represent the degree of the shear deformation, which is called **shear strain** (or **tangential strain**), denoted by γ.

$$\gamma = \frac{\Delta x}{d} = \tan\varphi \tag{1-34}$$

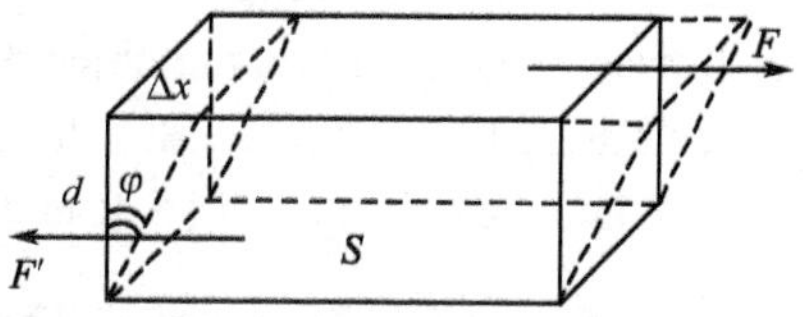

Figure 1-18 The shear deformation

In practice, φ is generally very small, then Equation (1-34) can be rewritten approximately as $\gamma \approx \varphi$. The shear strain is a dimensionless quantity.

When a shear deformation happens, an object is divided into two parts by any cross section parallel to the upside and underside. Because there is a tangential internal force between the two parts and the magnitude of the force is equal to external force, so, there will be a relative displacement between the two parts. The ratio of the tangential internal F and the area S are called the **shear stress** (or **tangential stress**), denoted by τ, and its unit is N/m^2.

$$\tau = \frac{F}{S} \tag{1-35}$$

Experiments show that, when an object has a shear deformation, in a certain range of elasticity, the shear stress is proportional to the shear strain, i.e.

$$\tau = G\gamma \tag{1-36}$$

where G is called the shear modulus.

By using Equation (1-34), Equation (1-35) and Equation (1-36), we can get the expression of the shear modulus.

$$G = \frac{\tau}{\gamma} = \frac{\frac{F}{S}}{\frac{\Delta x}{d}} = \frac{Fd}{S\Delta x} \tag{1-37}$$

3. Volumetric Strain and Volumetric Stress

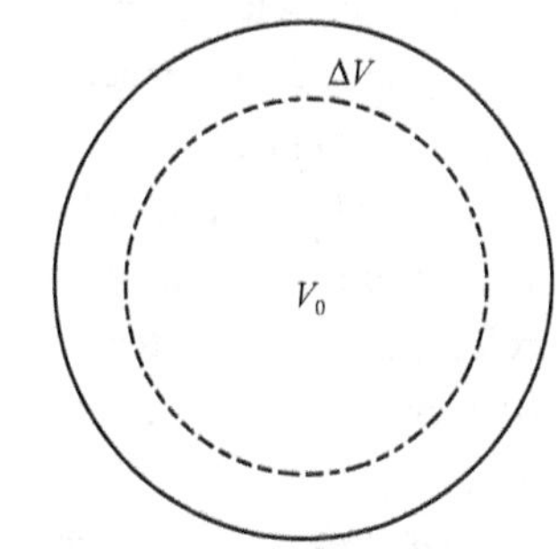

Figure 1-19 Under a pressure, the volume changes but the shape doesn't

When an object is acted by pressure, its volume has a change, but its shape does not, as shown in Figure 1-19. The ratio of volume change ΔV and the original volume V_0 is called the **volumetric strain** (or **bulk strain**), denoted by θ, i.e.

$$\theta = \frac{\Delta V}{V_0} \tag{1-38}$$

The stress for the change of the volume is expressed with the pressure P; this pressure is also called the **volumetric stress**.

Experiments show that, when an object has a volumetric strain, in a certain elastic range the pressure is proportional to the corresponding volumetric strain, i.e.

$$P = -K\theta \tag{1-39}$$

The negative sign in Equation (1-39) expresses that when the pressure increases the volume will shrink; the proportional coefficient K is called the **bulk modulus**. In the general applications, the reciprocal of the bulk modulus is usually called the **modulus of compressibility**. By combining Equation (1-38) and Equation (1-39), we can get the formula for calculating the bulk modulus.

$$K = -\frac{P}{\Delta V}V_0 \tag{1-40}$$

In conclusion, the strain can express the relative deformation of an object; while, the stress reflects the stressed situation inside the object when deformation occurs, and it refers to the internal force acting on a unit area. In most cases, the stresses at different points on the same cross section of an object are different, and the object can also be under the actions of the shear stress and the normal stress.

1.6.2 Mechanical Properties of Bone Materials

The human skeletal system is the body's framework, and its main functions are: to support body weight, to keep body form, to complete motions, and to protect visceral organs. The bones at different parts inside a body have different functions; among them, the most representative ones are cartilages and tubular bones.

Cartilages are indispensable in the skeletal system, and the functions are dependent on the positions. For example, the functions of the cartilage pads between the vertebrae of a spine are: to make the spine possesses flexibility and elasticity; to play a role of buffering in motions especially in jumping motions, just like springs, and then reduce the shake to the brain; and to assist the spine for all kinds of motions in a certain range. Another example, the cartilage in the front end of a rib enables the rib to meet the changing request for the respiratory motion. In addition, articular cartilages can provide lubricating on the joint surfaces, so, the articular surfaces can slide relatively with the minimal friction and wear.

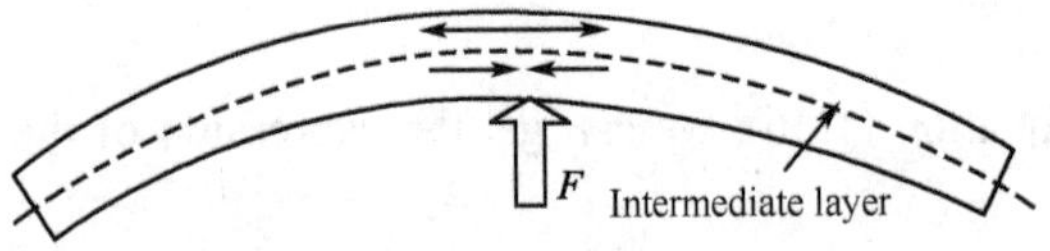

Figure 1-20 A bended beam

Tubular bones are formed in the process of biological evolution according to the mechanical requirements. The bones such as the femur, tibia, and so on, belong to the tubular bones. Figure 1-20 is a diagram of a bended beam affected by the action of a load; if divide it into several layers, an **intermediate layer** with zero stress can be found. All the layers above it are stretched to undergo tensile stresses; and the layers below it are compressed to undergo compressive stresses; thus, the intermediate layer and the layers near it will undergo the smallest stress acted, so these layers are not essential. This is the mechanical basis of the formation of tubular bones. The central part of a tubular bone is a cavity. The layered structure of a tubular bone is very clever; the outer layer is the periosteum with the excellent tenacity. Layers by layers towards the interior are compact bone, cancellous bone and bone marrow cavity. The materials with the higher density and higher strength are arranged at the area undergoing the higher stress. This structural manner of tubular bones can not only reduce the bones' weight, but also make the bones have higher strengths to bear stresses. What's more, the two ends of this kind of bone are more bulky than central section. Therefore, the contact area of the joint is enlarged, and the corresponding pressure can be reduced. All in all, human skeleton is a good stress-bearing structure with the reasonability in the cross section and the shape.

Under the actions of external forces the bone material will generate internal stresses. By doing the tensile test with a fresh femur, which is just acquired from anatomical operation, we can measure the relationship between the tensile strain and the tensile stress. As shown in Figure 1-21, the relationship between stress and strain is nonlinear; with the increase of the stress, the degree of nonlinearity increases; when the stress is about 120×10^6 N/m^2, the femoral test piece is fractured. The tests of mechanics of materials show that, the density of the bone is small er than the steel's and the granite's, but its tensile strength is about 1/4 of the steel's, and its compressive strength is close to the granite's.

The bone materials have the anisotropic mechanical properties. Under the action of the load in different directions, a test piece of bone shows different strengths, as shown in Figure 1-22 (the black short lines express the tensile directions). It can be seen from the graph that when the load is in the direction along longitudinal axis, the test piece has the maximum strength; while, in the horizontal direction, the strength is minimum; so the bones' ability to resist shearing is weaker than the ability to resist stretching or compressing.

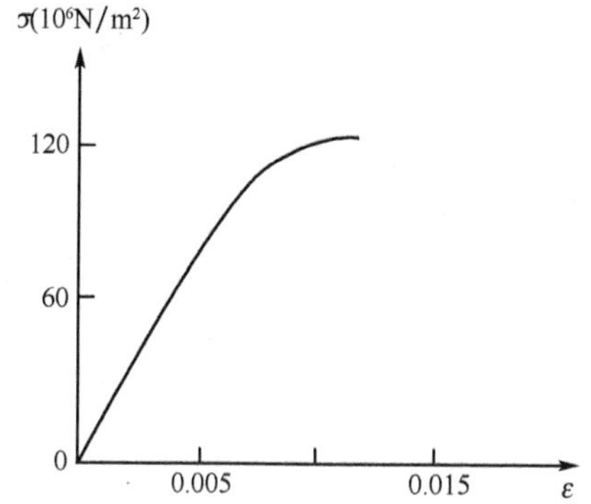

Figure 1-21 Tensile strain curve of thigh bone

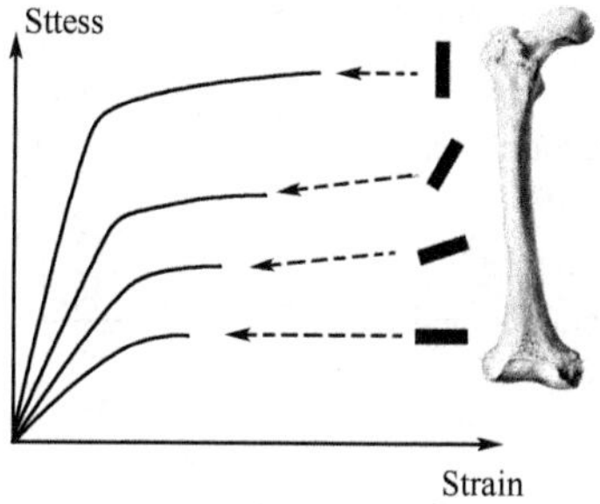

Figure 1-22 Strengths of thigh bone in different directions

The bones in human skeletal system may be stressed with various forms; according to directions of the external forces and the external torques, the cases can be divided into the following five types.

(1) Stretching: The loads exerted outwardly on a bone's surface or at the two ends along the main axis of the bone (such as the load of the body weight on the bones when the body is pended).

(2) Compressing: Couples of loads with the same magnitude and the opposite directions exerted at the two ends of a bone (such as the compressing loads on human bones when he is performing weight lifting).

(3) Bending: The loads exerted on the bone to make its main axis bend.

(4) Shearing: The loads exerted on the bone are parallel to the cross section of the bone.

(5) Twisting: The loads on the bone to make the bone twist around its main axis.

The mentions listed above are only several simple cases of loads withstood by human bones; in the routine lives, the loads exerted on human bones are often the integrated effects of those loading types.

A Brief Summarization of This Chapter

(1) Mechanics of Rigid Bodies

1) Angular velocity: $\omega = \lim_{\Delta t \to 0} \frac{\Delta\theta}{\Delta t} = \frac{d\theta}{dt}$

2) Angular acceleration: $\beta = \lim_{\Delta t \to 0} \frac{\Delta\omega}{\Delta t} = \frac{d\omega}{dt} = \frac{d^2\theta}{dt^2}$

3) Moment of inertia of a rigid body about a fixed axis: $I = \sum \Delta m_i r_i^2$ or $I = \int r^2 dm = \int r^2 \rho dV$

4) Rotational kinetic energy of a rigid body: $E_R = \frac{1}{2} I\omega^2$

5) Definition of the torque vector: $\boldsymbol{M} = \boldsymbol{r} \times \boldsymbol{F}$

6) Law of rotation: $M = I\beta$

7) Angular momentum: $L = I\omega$

8) The law of conservation of angular momentum $L = I\omega =$ constant, i.e., if the net external torque acting on a rigid body is kept as zero during a time period, the angular momentum of the rigid body will remain constant.

9) Formula for calculating the angular velocity of the procession of a gyroscope: $\Omega = \frac{mgl}{L} = \frac{mgl}{I\omega}$

(2) Elasticity of Objects

1) Normal strain: $\varepsilon = \frac{\Delta x}{x_0}$

2) Normal stress: $\sigma = \frac{F}{S}$

3) Young's modulus: $E = \frac{\sigma}{\varepsilon} = \frac{\frac{F}{S}}{\frac{\Delta x}{x_0}} = \frac{Fx_0}{S\Delta x}$

4) Shear strain: $\gamma = \frac{\Delta x}{d} = \tan\varphi$

5) Shear stress: $\tau = \frac{F}{S}$

6) Shear modulus: $G = \frac{\tau}{\gamma} = \frac{\frac{F}{S}}{\frac{\Delta x}{d}} = \frac{Fd}{S\Delta x}$

7) Volumetric strain: $\theta = \frac{\Delta V}{V_0}$

8) Bulk modulus: $K = -\frac{P}{\Delta V} V_0$

Exercises 1

1-1. A flywheel is accelerated in rotating. To the two particles with different radiuses on the flywheel, have they gotten the same tangential acceleration and the same normal acceleration or not?

1-2. A wheel starts to rotate from stationary with a constant angular acceleration. After 20 s, its angular velocity reaches to 60 rad/s. Please determine the angular acceleration of the wheel at that moment and the angle which the wheel has turned in this 20 s.

1-3. A motor rotor starts to rotate from stationary. After 30 s, the rotor's rotating speed increased to 250 r/s. If the diameter of the rotor is 0.04 m, find the velocity and the acceleration at a point on the surface of the rotor when t=30 s.

1-4. Determine the rotational inertia of a uniform fine rod with the mass of m and length of L about the axis in the following cases:

(1) The axis is through the center of the rod and perpendicular to the rod;

(2) The axis is through one end of the rod and perpendicular to the rod;

(3) The axis is through the center of the rod and making an angle with the rod.

1-5. In a diatomic molecule, the distance between the two atoms is r, and their masses are respectively m_1 and m_2, they can rotate about the axis, which is through the mass center of the molecule and perpendicular to the connecting line of the two atoms shaft. Find the moment of inertia of the diatomic molecule.

1-6. A grinding wheel has a diameter of 0.2 m, the thickness of 0.025 m, and the density of 24 g/cm^3. Determine

(1) The moment of inertia of the wheel;

(2) The rotational kinetic energy of the wheel when its rotating speed is 2940 r/min (the grinding wheel can be regarded as a solid disk here).

1-7. A flywheel with the diameter of 0.3 m and mass of 5 kg can rotate about the axis, which is through the mass center and perpendicular to the surface of the flywheel. Now, a rope is winded around the edge of the flywheel and the end of the rope is pulled by a constant force so that the flywheel is uniformly accelerated from stationary state. After 0.5 s, the rotating speed reaches to 10 r/s (assume that the flywheel can be regarded as a solid cylinder). Determine

(1) The angular acceleration of the flywheel;

(2) The number of rotations the flywheel turned within this interval of 0.5 s;

(3) The work done by the force on the rope within this 0.5 s.

1-8. A disc with the radius of 1.0 m and the mass of 10 kg can rotate about the axis, which is through the mass center and perpendicular to the surface of the disc. It is assumed that, in the beginning the angular velocity of the disc is 10 rad/s; now, an object (particle) with the mass of 2.0 kg is put on the edge of the disc, and at this time, what is the angular velocity?

1-9. A disc with the radius of $R = 0.5$ m and the moment of inertia of $I = 20$ kg·m^2 can rotate about the axis, which is through the mass center and perpendicular to the surface of the disc. In the beginning the disc is stationary, if a constant force with the magnitude of $F = 100$ N is put at the edge of the disk along the tangential direction of the edge. Determine

(1) The angular acceleration of the disk;

(2) The linear velocity of a point at the edge of the disc at the end of the 10th s.

1-10. A uniform fine rod AB with the mass of m and the length of L can rotate in the vertical plane about a smooth horizontal axis. The distance from the axis to the end A is $L/3$. Now, the rod begins to rotate about the axis from the horizontal position and the stationary state. Determine

(1) the angular acceleration of the rod when it is at the horizontal position to start the rotation;

(2) the angular velocity and the angular acceleration of the rod when it rotates to the vertical position.

1-11. A fine rod with the length of $2l$ and the mass of M is put on a smooth horizontal plane. The rod can rotate about the axis, which is through the mass center of the rod and perpendicular to the horizontal plane. The bearing is smooth. Now, a bullet with the mass of m and the velocity of v_0 along the horizontal direction is perpendicularly shot inside the endpoint of the rod. Determine the angular velocity of the rod and the bullet about the axis.

1-12. The femur is the main bone of the thigh bone. The minimum cross-sectional area of femur of a normal adult is 6×10^{-4} m^2. What is the biggest compressing load over which the femur will be fractured? How many times heavier is this load than the body weight of 70 kg (the compressive strength of the femur is 17×10^7 N/m^2) ?

1-13. Suppose that one of the femurs of someone's legs has the length of 50 cm and the average cross-sectional area is 4 cm^2. When the two legs are supporting the body weight of 60 kg, what is the shortened length of leg's femur? What is the percentage of this shortened length to the original length (when compressed, the Young's modulus of the bone is approximately 10^{10} N/m^2) ?

Chapter 2 Fundamentals of Hydrodynamics

Generally, all of the matters in the natural world exist in three states: solids, liquids and gases. A liquid matter or a gaseous matter is commonly named as **fluid**.

Hydromechanics is the study to reveal the motion laws of fluids, which includes **hydrostatics** and **hydrodynamics**. Hydrostatics is the study of mechanical laws of fluids in the stationary state, and it has been discussed in high school physics. Hydrodynamics is a subject to study the motion laws of flowing fluids and the interactions between flowing fluids and the adjacent other objects. Many activities inside organisms such as the circulations of blood and lymph, nutrient transporting process, the excreting process of waste and the process of respiration are all closely related to the motions of fluids.

In this chapter, we will discuss some basic laws of hydrodynamics. And the key point is focused on the basic motion laws of the incompressible fluids. Meanwhile, some applications of the laws of hydromechanics in medicine will also be introduced.

2.1 Steady Flow of the Ideal Fluid

2.1.1 Ideal Fluid

In the case that a fluid is under the action of an external force, it is clear that one portion of the fluid will have a relative motion to the other portion easily. That is the most basic characteristic of a fluid called the **fluidity**.

Inside an actual fluid, the flow velocities of different portions are not necessarily the same. Along the tangential direction of the interface of two adjacent flow layers with different velocities, there exists a friction—the internal friction. The internal friction hinders the relative sliding between flow layers. This property of fluids is called the **viscosity**. All of the actual fluids have the viscosity.

Although the actual fluids always have the viscosity more or less, but for some liquids such as water and ethanol, their viscosities are very low; for gases, their viscosities are lower. In many studies, such viscosities have little effect on the motions of fluids. Therefore, in the discussion of the flow of these fluids, their viscosities are ignored, and they are regarded as non-viscous fluids.

The actual fluids are all compressible. The compressibility of liquids is very small; therefore, the compressibility of liquids can generally be ignored. For gases, although the compressibility is very significant, under the condition that gases can flow, a very small pressure difference enables the gases to flow rapidly, and causes little change in their density. Hence, the compressibility of gases can also be ignored.

In the study of physics, in order to highlight the main characteristics of the objects researched and to simplify the problems, the ideal models are commonly used to replace the actual objects for analyzing. In many practical problems of hydromechanics, compressibility and viscosity are only secondary factors to affect the motion of a fluid; the fluidity is the main factor to determine the motion of the fluid. Here, we use an ideal model—the **ideal fluid** to replace the actual fluid for analyzing; and then, we derive some basic motion laws of the ideal fluid. **The so-called ideal fluid is a fluid which is absolutely incompressible and is completely free of viscous.**

For the model of ideal fluid as the object studied, its compressibility and viscosity are neglected and its fluidity is highlighted. It is a kind of scientific abstract for the study of the motions of the fluids which have smaller compressibility and lower viscosity.

2.1.2 Steady Flow

In general situations, when a fluid is flowing, the particles of the fluid, flowing through any points in the space, have different velocities and the velocities at any points will also vary with time. The flowing form, in which the velocities change with time, is called the unsteady flow. If at any certain point in the space, the flow velocity does not change with time, or to say, at some moment everywhere in the fluid, the flowing velocities may be different, but for the particles of the fluid flowing through any given point in the space the velocity is fixed and does not change with time, we deem that the flowing form is stable. This flow is called the **steady flow**.

To describe the motion of the fluid visually, let's introduce the concept of **streamlines**. Streamlines are such a cluster of imaginary curves that the tangential direction at any point on a curve is in the same direction of the velocity of fluid mass elements through the point. As shown in Figure 2-1, although there are different velocities as the fluid flows through the three points A, B and C, at any time the velocity of the fluid flowing through point A is always $\boldsymbol{v}_A$, the velocity flowing through point B is always $\boldsymbol{v}_B$, and the velocity flowing through point C is always $\boldsymbol{v}_C$. Hence, when the fluid is performing a steady flow, the shapes of the streamlines will not change with time. Meanwhile, the streamlines coincide with the trajectories of fluid mass elements. When the fluid is performing an unsteady flow, because all the velocities of the mass elements flowing through any points will change with time, for different time there will be different streamlines, the streamlines and the trajectories of fluid mass elements are no longer coincided.

The density of the streamlines can reflect the magnitude of flowing velocity of the fluid: on the one hand, where the streamlines are intensive, the velocity is higher at that place; on the other hand, where the streamlines are sparse, the velocity is lower. Assume to draw a small section in the flowing fluid and draw a series of streamlines through the points on the periphery, the tubular region surrounded by these streamlines is called the **flow tube**, as shown in Figure 2-2.

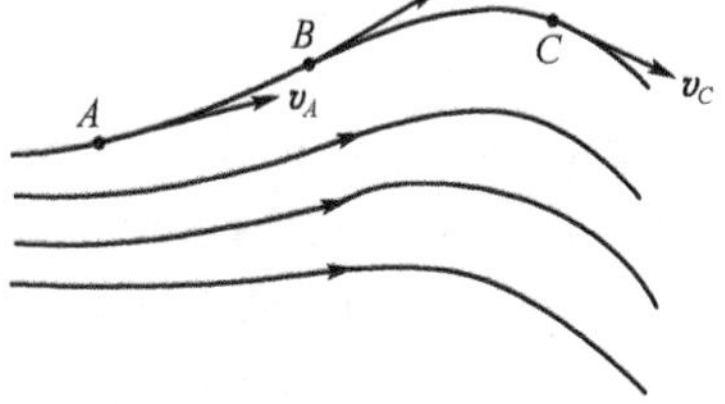

Figure 2-1 Streamlines

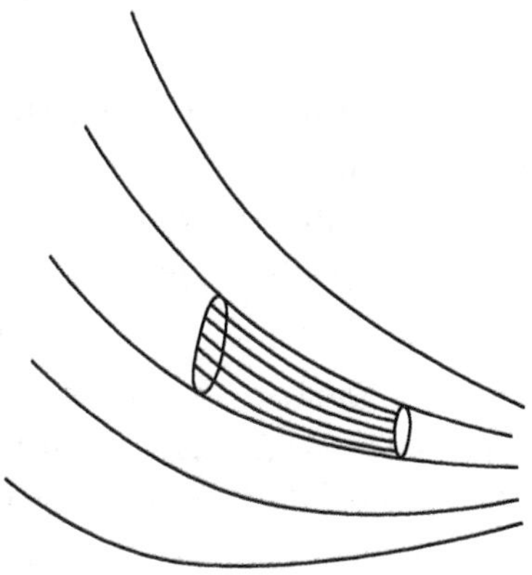

Figure 2-2 The flow tube

When a fluid is performing a steady flow, because the shapes of the streamlines do not change with time, the shape of the flow tube will not change with time. Because the fluid particles at a certain point in the space can only have one velocity at every moment, the streamlines can never be intersectional; meanwhile, the fluid flowing inside the flow tube cannot escape to the outside of the flow tube through the sidewall, and the fluid flowing outside the flow tube cannot flow into the flow tube through the sidewall too. The fluid can only flow into the flow tube from one end and flow out from the other end. If the fluid performs a steady flow in the fixed pipe, the fixed pipe itself can be regarded as a flow tube.

2.1.3 Equation of Continuity for Steady Flow

The equation of continuity is the discussion about the relationship among the rate of flow, the flowing velocity and the area of the section of flow tube on the condition of a fluid performing a steady flow through a flow tube.

As shown in Figure 2-3, assume to select randomly a flow tube with small cross-sectional areas and suppose some incompressible fluid is performing a steady flow inside the flow tube. The velocities at the cross-sectional areas of S_1 and S_2 (both are perpendicular to the flow tube) are respectively v_1 and v_2. After a short time Δt, the volumes flowed through the areas of S_1 and S_2 are respectively

$$V_1 = S_1 v_1 \Delta t$$
$$V_2 = S_2 v_2 \Delta t$$

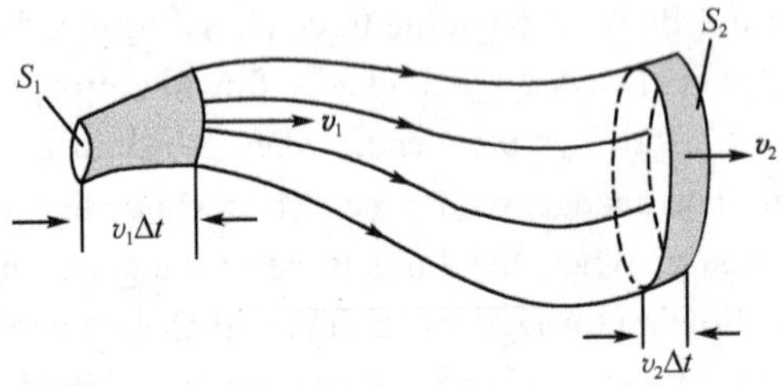

Figure 2-3 The derivation of the equation of continuity

Because the fluid being researched is incompressible and keeps on a continuous flow, according to the principle of mass conservation, during the same time, the volume of the fluid flowing through any cross sections of the flow tube should be equal, i.e.

$$S_1 v_1 \Delta t = S_2 v_2 \Delta t$$

and

$$S_1 v_1 = S_2 v_2 \qquad (2\text{-}1)$$

This relationship is correct for any cross sections of the flow tube S, which are perpendicular to the flow tube. The volume flowed through any cross section in the flow tube during a unit time i.e. Sv is called the **rate of flow**, denoted as Q, and its unit is m^3/s. The equation of continuity for some incompressible fluid performing a steady flow can be expressed as

$$Q = Sv = \text{constant} \qquad (2\text{-}2)$$

This equation shows that: when an incompressible fluid performs a steady flow, the product of the velocity of the fluid and the cross-sectional area at any points is a constant. Where the cross-sectional area is bigger, the flowing velocity is lower; and where the cross-sectional area is smaller, the flowing velocity is higher. At any point the flow rate is a certain constant value. Therefore, the equations of continuity Equation (2-1) and Equation(2-2) reflect the relationship among three quantities: the rate of flow, the flow velocity and the cross-sectional area.

By using the equation of continuity, we can analyze the relationship between the velocity of blood flow and the vascular cross-sectional area in the circulatory system of human body approximately. Under normal physiological conditions, the average flow rate of blood in all kinds of vessels should be equal. It has also been revealed by physiological measurements that, in general, during one heartbeat period the quantity of flowing blood shot from the left ventricle is equal to the average quantity of blood flowed back into the left atrium and they will be both equal to the blood volume ejected out from the heart during one heartbeat period. That is to say, the flow of blood in the blood vessels is generally continuous. According to the equation of continuity, the average velocity of blood flowing inside any kind of blood vessel should be inversely proportional to the total cross-sectional area of this kind of vessel. The total cross-sectional area of human aorta is the minimum, which is only about 3 cm^2. So the average velocity of blood in the aorta is the maximum, which can reach up nearly to 30 cm/s. As the increase of the vascular branches, the radius of each vessel is constantly decreasing, but the number of blood vessels increases quickly, thus the total cross-sectional area of vessels increases rapidly. The total cross-sectional area of capillaries is the maximum, which is about 900 cm^2, so the velocity of blood flowing in the capillaries is the minimum, which is only about 0.1 cm/s. From capillaries to the vena cava the total cross-sectional area of vessels decreases constantly and it is about 18 cm^2 at the vena cava. Here, the velocity of blood flowing in vena cava is about 5 cm/s. Figure 2-4 shows the curves to indicate the relationship between the total cross-sectional area of all kinds of blood vessels in the circulation of human body and the average velocities of blood flowing within them.

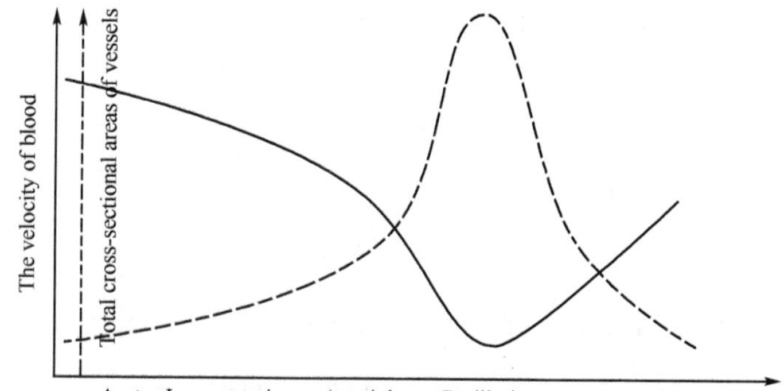

Figure 2-4 The relationship between the total area of vessels and the average flow velocity of blood

2.2 Bernoulli Equation

Bernoulli equation is the fundamental equation in hydromechanics. It reveals the relationship among the pressure, the flowing velocity and the height of an ideal fluid performing steady flow. We can derive this equation with the work-energy theorem.

Figure 2-5 shows a piece of flow tube of an ideal fluid performing steady flow in the gravitational field. The portion of fluid in the section of flow tube *MN* is chosen as the object to research. After a very short time Δt, the position of this portion of flowing fluid flows from *MN* to *M'N'*. Because the flow tube is very narrow and the time interval Δt is very short, the physical quantities inside the fluid segments of *MM'* and *NN'* are thought to be uniform. Their pressures, velocities, heights and cross-sectional areas are respectively P_1, v_1, h_1, S_1 and P_2, v_2, h_2, S_2.

The work-energy theorem points out that the increment of mechanical energy of a system is equal to the work done by the external forces and the non-conservative internal forces.

The increment of mechanical energy of a system includes the increments of its kinetic energy and potential energy. It can be seen from Figure 2-5 that before and after this Δt, the fluid section *M'N* keeps in its original position and the mechanical quantities such as the flowing velocity, the position and the pressure remain unchanged except the fluid particles inside it are replaced, i.e. its mechanical energy remains constant. Therefore, in the process for the fluid flowing from *MN* to *M'N'*, the increment of mechanical energy is equal to the difference of the mechanical energies in the fluid segment of *NN'* and the fluid segment of *MM'*. Because the ideal fluid is incompressible, the volume and mass of the fluid segment *MM'* must be equal to the volume and mass of the fluid segment *NN'*. The volume and the mass are denoted as *V* and *m* respectively. In this way, the mechanical energy of fluid segment *MM'* is

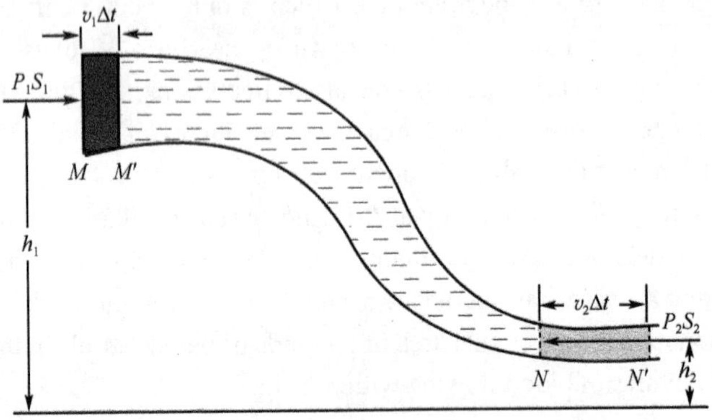

Figure 2-5 The derivation of Bernoulli equation

$$E_1 = \frac{1}{2}mv_1^2 + mgh_1$$

The mechanical energy of fluid segment *NN'* is

$$E_2 = \frac{1}{2}mv_2^2 + mgh_2$$

The total increment of mechanical energy of the fluid section *MN* in this time Δt will be

$$\Delta E = E_2 - E_1 = \frac{1}{2}mv_2^2 + mgh_2 - \frac{1}{2}mv_1^2 - mgh_1$$

When we analyze the work done by the forces to the fluid, we only need to consider the external forces i.e. the surrounding pressures on this portion of fluid, because the object discussed here is the ideal fluid and there isn't any viscosity, namely the non-conservative internal force.

The pressure acting on the sidewall of this section of fluid tube is always perpendicular to the sidewall, so it does not do any work and the only work is done by the pressures acting respectively from the two-end faces of S_1 and S_2. The force acting on S_1 pushes the fluid forward and does a positive work of $A_1 = P_1S_1 \cdot v_1\Delta t$; the force acting on S_2 impedes the fluid to flow forward, and does a negative work of $A_2 = -P_2S_2 \cdot v_2\Delta t$. The total work done by the external forces is

$$A = A_1 + A_2 = P_1S_1v_1\Delta t - P_2S_2v_2\Delta t$$

According to the equation of continuity

$$S_1v_1 = S_2v_2$$

and

$$S_1v_1\Delta t = S_2v_2\Delta t = V$$

so

$$A = P_1V - P_2V$$

By applying the work-energy theorem, we have $\Delta E = A$, i.e.

$$\frac{1}{2}mv_2^2 + mgh_2 - \frac{1}{2}mv_1^2 - mgh_1 = P_1V - P_2V$$

To divide every term with V and then make a transposition, we have

$$P_1+\frac{1}{2}\rho v_1^2+\rho g h_1 = P_2+\frac{1}{2}\rho v_2^2+\rho g h_2 \tag{2-3}$$

In the equation, $\rho = m/V$ is the density of the fluid. Because the section of fluid MN is chosen arbitrarily, Equation (2-3) can also be written as

$$P+\frac{1}{2}\rho v^2+\rho g h = \text{constant} \tag{2-4}$$

Equation (2-3) or Equation (2-4) is called Bernoulli equation, which is one of the fundamental laws in hydromechanics. It shows that when an ideal fluid in a thin flow tube is performing a steady flow, the sum of the gravitational potential energy in per unit volume, the kinetic energy in per unit volume and the pressure at this point is a constant.

If the cross-sectional area of the flow tube is chosen to approach to infinity, the equation will show the relationship among the pressures, the heights and the flowing velocities at any points on a streamline.

Example 2-1 Water is performing a steady flow in a section of horizontal tube. The cross-sectional area at the outlet of the tube is 2 times of the cross-sectional area of the finest point of the tube. If the flowing velocity at the outlet is 2 m/s, determine the pressure of the finest point (it is known that the pressure at the outlet is the pressure of atmosphere).

Solution: Assume that the finest location is at point 1 and the outlet is at point 2. From the hints in the question we know that

$$S_2 = 2S_1,\quad v_2 = 2\ \text{m/s},\quad P_2 = P_0 = 1.013\times10^5\ \text{Pa}$$

According to the equation of continuity we have

$$S_1 v_1 = S_2 v_2$$

And we can get

$$v_1=\frac{S_2}{S_1}v_2 = \frac{2S_1 v_2}{S_1}=2v_2=4\ \text{m/s}$$

Because the water is flowing in a horizontal tube, we know that $h_2 = h_1$. According to Bernoulli equation we can get

$$P_1 = P_0+\frac{1}{2}\rho v_2^2 - \frac{1}{2}\rho v_1^2 = 1.013\times10^5+\frac{1}{2}\times10^3(4-16) = 9.53\times10^4\ \text{Pa}$$

i.e. the pressure at the finest point is 9.53×10^4 Pa.

2.3 Applications of Bernoulli Equation

Bernoulli equation and the equation of continuity are widely applicable in hydromechanics. We can solve many practical problems in hydromechanics by using them. Now, let's illustrate them with some examples.

2.3.1 The Relationship Between Pressure and Flow Velocity in a Horizontal Tube

In many cases the fluid is flowing in horizontal tubes, here $h_1 = h_2$ and Bernoulli equation is simplified as

$$P_1+\frac{1}{2}\rho v_1^2 = P_2+\frac{1}{2}\rho v_2^2 \tag{2-5}$$

By Equation (2-5) we can draw the conclusion that if an ideal fluid is flowing in a horizontal tube, where the flow velocity is lower, the pressure of the fluid is higher; and where the velocity is higher, the pressure is lower.

And by the Equation (2-1) of continuity we can also get a conclusion: When an ideal fluid is performing a steady flow in a horizontal tube with uneven thickness, where the cross-sectional area is bigger, the flowing velocity is lower and the pressure of the fluid is higher; and where the cross-sectional area is smaller, the flowing velocity is higher and the pressure is lower. In this way, when the fluid flows through a tube with a higher velocity, the flowing velocity at the point narrow enough can be so high that the pressure there is lower than the atmosphere pressure. If this narrow part is connected with the outside, this negative pressure can inhale the small particles in the container connected with this part of tube and the inner suction and the particles will be taken to flow away by the fluid flowing quickly. This kind of phenomenon, inhaling the small particles outside the tube by the fluid flowing in the tube, is called the **suction effect**. According to this principle, we can design and manufacture equipment such as sprayers, aspirators, nebulizers, flow-meters and so on.

1. Sprayer

Figure 2-6 is the schematic diagram of the principle of the sprayer. When pushing the piston rod rapidly, the air in the cylinder is forced to rush out through the narrow part with a high speed, so the pressure there could be lower than the pressure of atmosphere. Under the action of atmospheric pressure at point b on the surface of liquid medicine in the bottle, the liquid medicine in the bottle will rise along the vertical fine tube to point a then be blown into the mist and be sprayed from the nozzle by the high-speed flowing air.

2. Aspirator

The schematic diagram of the aspirator used in medicine is shown in Figure 2-7. Water is flowing in from point A and flowing out from point C; the higher the velocity at the narrow cone nozzle D is, the smaller the pressure is. When the pressure at point D is lower than the pressure of the gas in the container B, which is connected with the aspirator, the gas in the container will be mixed with water at point D and flow out from C; in this way, the pumping process is then completed.

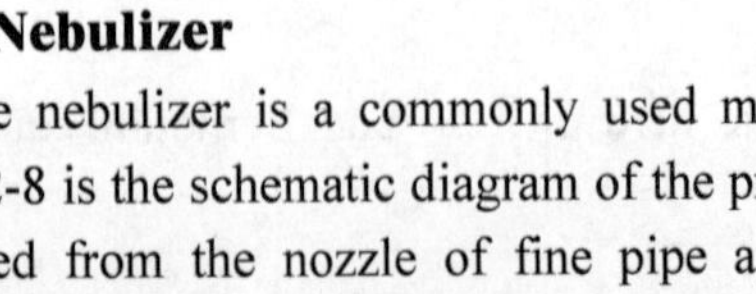

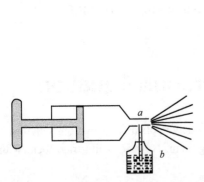

Figure 2-6 The principle of the sprayer

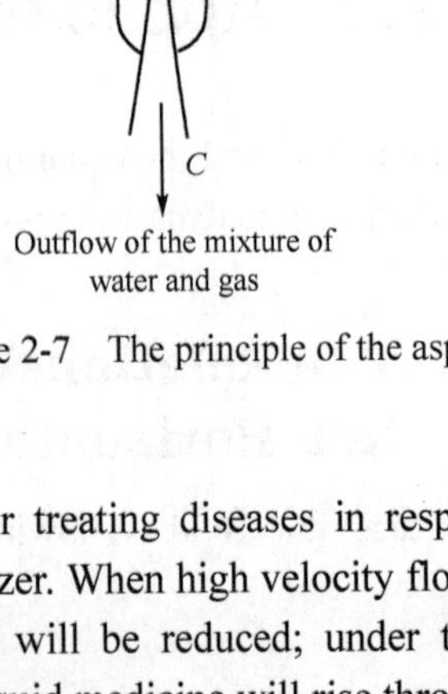

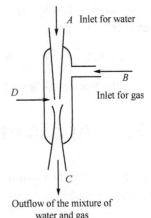

Figure 2-7 The principle of the aspirator

3. Nebulizer

The nebulizer is a commonly used medical instrument for treating diseases in respiratory tract, Figure 2-8 is the schematic diagram of the principle of the nebulizer. When high velocity flowing oxygen is ejected from the nozzle of fine pipe a, the pressure there will be reduced; under the action of atmospheric pressure on the surface of the liquid medicine, the liquid medicine will rise through tube b to the nozzle and be blown into the mist by the highvelocity flowing oxygen. The mist is then led into the patient's trachea, bronchus and lung through an inhaling tube; in this way, the direct regional administration could be completed with the oxygen uptake, to the patient's lungs, bronchi and trachea.

4. Flow Meter

In order to measure the flow rate of liquid flowing in a pipeline, we can join up a venturi flow meter in the pipeline, as shown in Figure 2-9. It is composed of a main tube with the uneven cross-sectional areas and two fine tubes fixed on the main tube respectively at the points with the known cross sectional areas of S_1 and S_2. Each of the fine tubes is kept vertical and connected with the main tube and the atmosphere by its two ends. When the liquid flows through the horizontal main tube, the difference of the heights of liquid levels in the vertical fine tubes Δh can be measured. By using Bernoulli equation and the calculating formula for the flow rate we can measure the flow rate of the liquid flowing in the main tube. Because the liquid in the horizontal main tube has the same height, here Bernoulli equation is expressed as

$$P_1+\frac{1}{2}\rho v_1^2 = P_2+\frac{1}{2}\rho v_2^2$$

It can be seen from Figure 2-9 that $h_1 > h_2$, so we have

$$P_1 > P_2$$

and

$$P_1 - P_2 = \rho g \Delta h$$

By the equation of continuity

$$S_1 v_1 = S_2 v_2$$

and by simplifying the three simultaneous equations we have

$$v_1 = S_2\sqrt{\frac{2g\Delta h}{S_1^2 - S_2^2}}$$

That is, the flow rate in the main tube is

$$Q = S_1 v_1 = S_1 S_2\sqrt{\frac{2g\Delta h}{S_1^2 - S_2^2}} \tag{2-6}$$

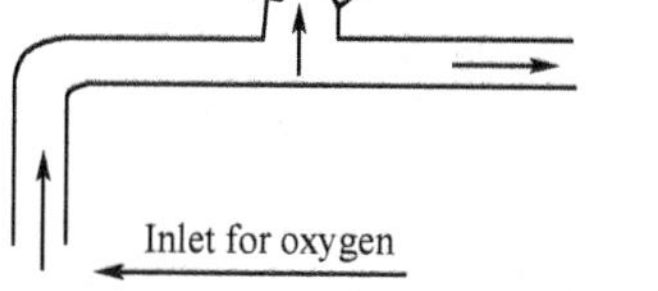

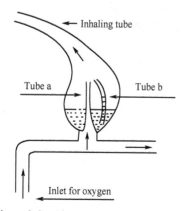

Figure 2-8 The principle of the nebulizer

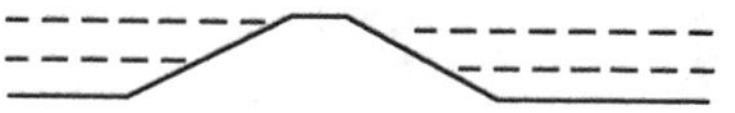

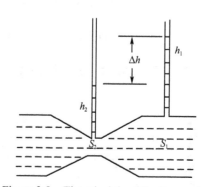

Figure 2-9 The principle of the flow meter

2.3.2 Relationship Between the Pressure and the Height in an Even Tube

If a fluid flows in a pipeline with a uniform degree of thickness, according to the equation of continuity, the velocity will be constant, and Bernoulli equation can be simplified as

$$P_1+\rho gh_1 = P_2+\rho gh_2$$

We can see from the equation above that the fluid flows in the uniform pipeline, where the height is higher the pressure is lower, and where the height is lower the pressure is higher. In this way, we can qualitatively explain the reasons for the change of a person's blood pressure when his position changes. The pressure of blood acting on the vascular lateral wall is the blood pressure, and the value of a blood pressure measured clinically is the number of the exceeded part of this pressure more than the atmospheric pressure; and its unit is kPa. As shown in Figure 2-10, when the human body is in the supine position, the head, feet and the heart have the same height, the arterial pressures of these three locations are almost the same, and the venous pressures are almost the same as well. The only slightly differences are caused by the viscosity of the flowing blood. When the human body is in the upright position, the arterial pressures and venous pressures of these three locations will be significantly different. It is mainly caused by the differences in height. However, no matter the upright position or the supine position is taken the arterial and venous pressures of the heart are not varied. That is to say, the blood pressure of the heart does not vary with the change of the height. This is because the heart is a pump for the flow of blood. So that, when we measure the blood pressure, we often choose the arm at the same height of the heart as the measurement site.

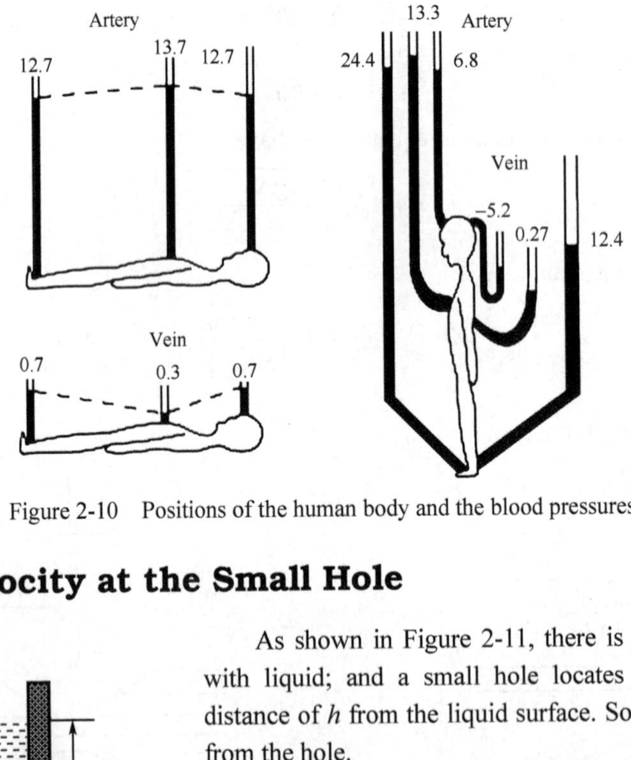

Figure 2-10 Positions of the human body and the blood pressures

2.3.3 Velocity at the Small Hole

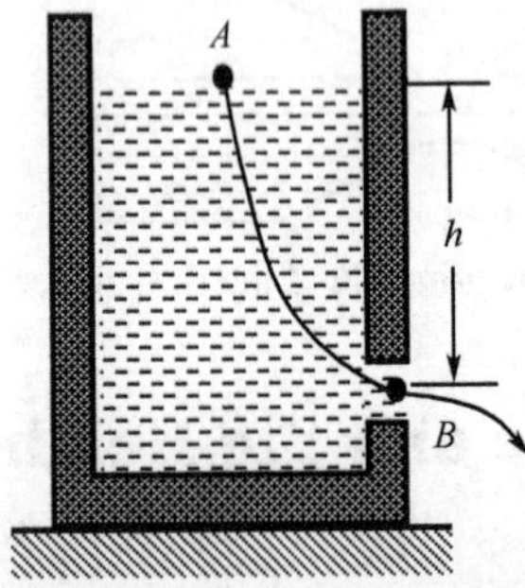

Figure 2-11 Velocity at the small hole

As shown in Figure 2-11, there is a huge container filled with liquid; and a small hole locates at the place with the distance of h from the liquid surface. So the liquid will outflow from the hole.

Assume that A and B represent respectively two points at the liquid surface and at the small hole, and the flow velocities at these two points are respectively v_A and v_B. Because the area of the liquid surface is much higher than the area of the small hole, according to the equation of continuity, the velocity at the small hole is much higher than the velocity at the liquid surface, the velocity at the liquid surface can be regarded as $v_A \approx 0$. Here, both the liquid surface and the small hole contact with the atmosphere, so the pressures at point A and point B are both equal to the atmospheric pressure P_0. Therefore, Bernoulli equation for point A and point B can be rewritten as

$$P_0+\rho gh = P_0+\frac{1}{2}\rho v_B^{2}$$

By this equation we can get the velocity at the small hole

$$v_B = \sqrt{2gh} \tag{2-7}$$

2.4 Flow of the Viscous Fluid

What we have discussed previously is about the laws of motion of the ideal fluid. Because there are internal frictions in actual fluids, the fluids display their viscous properties as they are flowing. This property is called the viscosity. For some fluids, such as glycerol, blood, heavy oil, and so on, they have higher viscosities; and for some others, such as water and ethanol, their viscosities are much lower, but in the long-distance transportation, the loss of energy caused by the viscosity must be considered. When motions of these fluids are studied, their viscosities cannot be ignored. The model of ideal fluid is no longer suitable.

The fluid, which cannot be ignored of its viscous property, is called the viscous fluid. In this section, we are going to discuss the properties and the flow laws of the viscous fluid.

2.4.1 Newton Viscosity Law

1. Internal Friction Phenomenon of Liquid

In the demonstration shown in Figure 2-12, some colorless glycerin is injected in a vertical tube and a section of colored glycerol is injected above it, so there is a distinct boundary between the colored glycerin and the colorless glycerin. If the valve at the lower part of tube is opened, the glycerol will flow out slowly; after a period of time, there will be a tongue-like interface formed at the bottom of the colored glycerol. This indicates that when the glycerol flows out, the flow velocity along the central axis of the tube is the maximum; and as the distance from the axis increases, the corresponding flow velocity becomes lower and lower. It is visible that, the flow of glycerol is stratified.

The glycerol flowing in the tube can be assumed to form many coaxial cylindrical layers, as shown in Figure 2-13. Because there is a relative motion between any two adjacent layers, the faster flow layer will put a forward force on the slower adjacent flow layer and the slower flow layer will put a backward force on the faster adjacent flow layer. This pair forces are parallel to the contact surface and equal in magnitude but opposite in direction. This kind of force is called the **internal friction** or the **viscous force**.

2. New ton Viscosity Law

As shown in Figure 2-14, the fluid flowing in z direction is assumed to be divided into many thin liquid films, which are all perpendicular to the x direction and parallel to each other. So, there will be relative sliding between any layers. Suppose there is a difference of velocity $\mathrm{d}v$ between two liquid layers with $\mathrm{d}x$ apart from each other in x direction, then the quantity of $\mathrm{d}v/\mathrm{d}x$ is the rate of change of the velocity in the direction perpendicular to the flow velocity, it is called the **velocity gradient**.

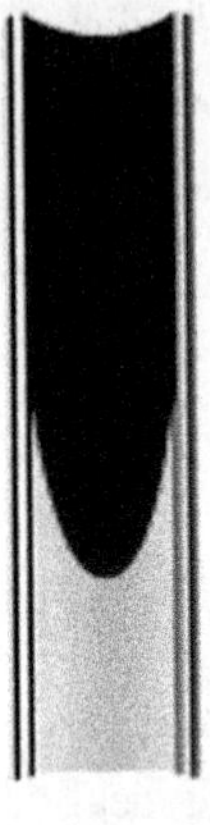

Figure 2-12 The flow of the viscous fluid

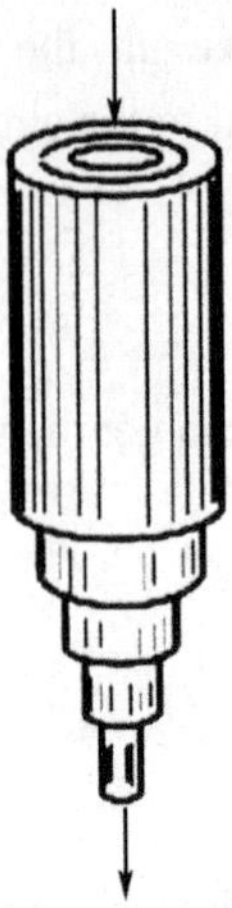

Figure 2-13 Diagram of the stratified flow

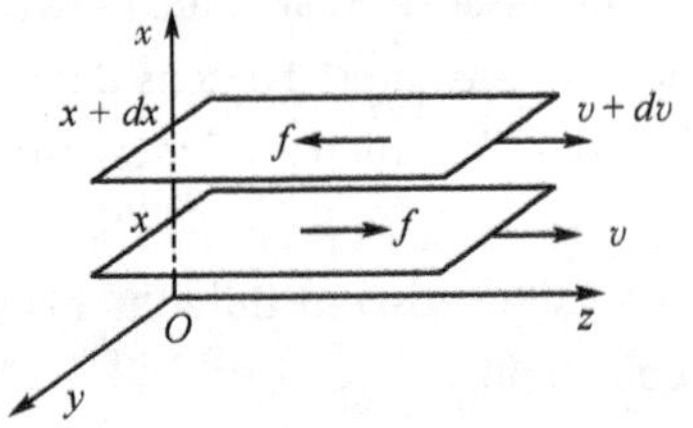

Figure 2-14 Diagram of the distribution of velocity

Experiments show that, the magnitude of the internal friction f at the contact surface of two adjacent layers is proportional to the area of contact surface S and the velocity gradient dv/dx, i.e.,

$$f = \eta S \frac{dv}{dx} \tag{2-8}$$

Equation (2-8) is called the **Newton viscosity law**. In the equation, the proportional coefficient η is called the **coefficient of viscosity** or the **viscosity**. In the international system of units, the unit of the viscosity is Pascal second (Pa·s). Its value depends on the nature of the viscous fluid; the fluid of more viscous has the higher viscosity of η.

Experiments indicate that, the magnitude of the viscosity is also related to temperature. In general, for liquids, the viscosities decrease as temperature increases; and for gases, the viscosities increase as temperature increases. Table 2-1 lists several numerical viscosity coefficients of fluids.

If the viscosity of a fluid is a constant under certain temperature and the fluid follows the Newton viscosity law, this kind of fluid is called the **Newton fluid**. The homogeneous fluids like water, ethanol, plasma, serum, and so on are all Newton fluids. If the viscosity of a fluid is not a constant under a certain temperature and the fluid does not follow Newton viscosity law, this kind of fluid is called the **non-Newton fluid**. Most of the fluids containing suspended or diffused particles are non-Newton fluids. Blood, which contains a large amount of suspended blood cells, is a non-Newton fluid; Newton viscosity law is only applicable for it in some special conditions.

Table 2-1 Several numerical viscosity coefficients of fluids

Liquid	Temperature (℃)	η (Pa·s)	Liquid	Temperature (℃)	η (Pa·s)
Water	0	1.729×10^{-3}	Ethanol	20	1.2×10^{-3}
	20	1.005×10^{-3}	Mercury	20	1.55×10^{-3}
	37	0.69×10^{-3}	Castor oil	17.5	1225×10^{-3}
	100	0.284×10^{-3}	Glycerol	20	0.830
Air	0	1.709×10^{-5}	Blood	37	$(2.5\text{-}4.0)\times10^{-3}$
	20	1.808×10^{-5}	Plasma	37	$(1.0\text{-}1.4)\times10^{-3}$
	100	2.175×10^{-5}	Serum	37	$(0.9\text{-}1.2)\times10^{-3}$

2.4.2 Laminar Flow, Turbulent Flow and Reynolds Number

The flows of fluids have two basic forms, namely laminar flow and turbulent flow; so are the physiological flows of body fluids in human body.

1. Laminar Flow

If the flow velocity of a viscous fluid is not very high, it performs a stratified flow; because of the difference of the flow velocities, the adjacent layers have a relative sliding, but they do not mix to each other and the particles of the flowing fluid have no transversal motion. This flow form is called the laminar flow.

2. Turbulent Flow

As the flow velocity of the viscous fluid increases, the laminar flow is destroyed. There will be transverse components of velocity emerged in the flowing fluid, the former layers will be confused and a disorder flow state emerges; meanwhile, there may even be the emergence of vortexes. This flow form is called the **turbulent flow**. The energy losses and the resistances in turbulent flows are much bigger than that in laminar flows. Turbulent flows can also cause mechanical vibrations, which produce noises, but a laminar flow is a silent form.

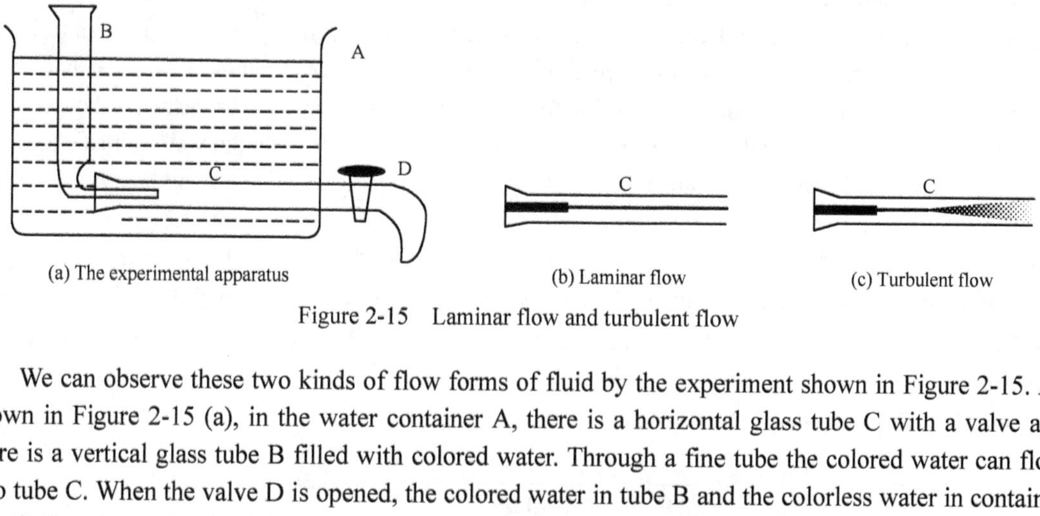

(a) The experimental apparatus (b) Laminar flow (c) Turbulent flow

Figure 2-15 Laminar flow and turbulent flow

We can observe these two kinds of flow forms of fluid by the experiment shown in Figure 2-15. As shown in Figure 2-15 (a), in the water container A, there is a horizontal glass tube C with a valve and there is a vertical glass tube B filled with colored water. Through a fine tube the colored water can flow into tube C. When the valve D is opened, the colored water in tube B and the colorless water in container A will flow into tube C. If the flow velocity is not high, the colored water in tube C flows as a stable linear trickle, as shown in Figure 2-15 (b), the flow in tube C is a laminar flow. When the valve D is opened more widely and the flow velocity increases to a certain extent, the flow is no longer stable and the colored water trickle spreads and mixes with the colorless water, as shown in Figure 2-15 (c), and the flow becomes the turbulent flow.

3. Reynolds Number

Whether a fluid flows as a laminar flow or as a turbulent flow is dependent not only on the flow velocity v, but also on the viscosity η and the density ρ of the fluid and on the shape, the size and the rigidness of the pipeline. In 1883, after many experimental researches the British physicist Reynolds proposed a unit-less pure number as the deciding basis for judging the transition from laminar flow to turbulent flow for the fluid flowing in a rigid long straight cylindrical pipeline, i.e.

$$Re = \frac{\rho v r}{\eta} \tag{2-9}$$

where Re is called **Reynolds number**, and r is the radius of the pipeline. The experimental results show that, if $Re < 1000$, the fluid performs a laminar flow; if $Re > 1500$, the fluid performs a turbulent flow; and if $1000 \leqslant Re \leqslant 1500$, the flow form is unstable, and the fluid may perform a laminar flow or a turbulent flow. It can be seen from Equation (2-9) that, the lower the viscosity of the fluid is, the higher the flow velocity, the radius of the pipeline and the density of the fluid are, the more easily a turbulent flow will take place; on the contrary conditions, a turbulent flow will not take place easily. Whether a turbulent flow appears or not, it is not only related to the radius of the pipeline, the velocity, the density and the viscosity, but also affected by the shape and the smoothness of the inner wall of the pipeline. The sections with sharp bends, branches or sudden changes in the diameter of the pipeline are all the places where turbulent flows appear easily.

The study on the turbulent flow has significant meanings in medicine. The blood vessels, trachea and other pipelines in a healthy human body have good elasticity. Pipe walls can absorb the disturbing energy and play the role of stabilizing, so the blood in the circulatory system and the gas in respiratory system of the normal body are mostly flowing in the form of laminar flow. But at the location where the pipeline has a sharp bend, or branches, or the sudden change of diameter, if the inner wall of the blood vessel or the trachea is rough enough, a turbulent flow may occur even in the situation where Reynolds number is lower. Meanwhile, the high energy of the turbulent flow will cause further damage to the pipe wall and this is so-called "the theory of pathopoiesia by the turbulent flow". The decrease of the blood viscosity caused by the reduce of red blood cells or the decrease of pipeline's elasticity will also make a turbulent flow easier. When a turbulent flow takes place, there will be of a sound accompanied. This also has a very practical value in medicine. At some locations in the human heart, aorta and the bronchus, turbulent flows are easier to take place. According to the sounds from the turbulent flows, with the well-trained ears and a simply structured stethoscope, a clinician can identify whether the blood flow and the breath are normal or not.

Example 2-2 The radius of a artery of somebody is supposed to be 2 mm, the average velocity of the blood flow is 50 cm/s; and it is known that: The coefficient of viscosity of blood is $\eta = 3.0 \times 10^{-3}$ Pa·s and the density of blood is $\rho = 1.05 \times 10^3$ kg/m^3. Find its Reynolds number and decide the flow form of the blood.

Solution: From Equation (2-9) we know that

$$Re = \frac{\rho v r}{\eta} = \frac{1.05 \times 10^3 \times 0.5 \times 2 \times 10^{-3}}{3.0 \times 10^{-3}} = 350$$

This value is far less than 1000, so the flow of the blood here is in the form of a laminar flow.

2.5 Poiseuille's Law and Stokes' Law

2.5.1 Poiseuille's Law

In nineteenth century, the French physiologist Poiseuille researched the case in which the viscous fluid flowed in a thin glass tube and found the following regularity: when the viscous fluid with the coefficient of viscosity of η is performing a steady flow in a horizontal tube with the radius of R and the length of L, the volume flow rate of the fluid is proportional to the difference of the pressure on both ends of the tube ΔP, i.e.

$$Q = \frac{\pi R^4 \Delta P}{8\eta L} \tag{2-10}$$

Equation (2-10) is called **Poiseuille's law**. By using Poiseuille's law, we can analyze problems about the flow of blood qualitatively. For example, the change of a vessel's radius will affect the flow of blood greatly. When the drop of the blood pressure is fixed, the flow rate of blood will change with the 4th power of the radius; and when an organ's demand of the flow rate of blood is certain for keeping functions, if the vessel's radius becomes smaller, the drop of the blood pressure must be increased with corresponding to the 4th power of the vessel's radius to ensure the adequate blood flow for the organ. And it is an effective way to reduce the blood pressure by dilating blood vessels. In addition, it is also an effective action to reduce the drop of the blood pressure by reducing the viscosity of blood on the condition to ensure the blood perfusion of a certain amount.

Let

$$Z = \frac{8\eta L}{\pi R^4} \tag{2-11}$$

Then Equation (2-11) can be rewritten as

$$Q = \frac{\Delta P}{Z} \tag{2-12}$$

where Z is called the **flow resistance**, in medicine, it is usually called the peripheral resistance, which is decided by the viscosity of the liquid η and the geometric shape of the pipeline. Its unit is Pa·s/m^3. It should be particularly noted that the flow resistance is inversely proportional to the 4th power of the radius of the circular tube. The effects on the flow resistance caused by any subtle change of the radius should not be ignored. Because the elasticity of blood vessels is very good, their sectional areas can be changed in certain ranges, which exert a very strong effect on controlling the flow rate of blood. Especially, the small arteries in human body have very sensitive and effective function on controlling the flow rate of blood.

Equation (2-12) is applicable for any fluid flowing in the pipeline of any shape. For a Newton fluid flowing in a circular tube, Z can be calculated by Equation (2-11); for a non-Newton fluid or for the fluid flowing in a non-circular tube, Z is generally determined by experiments.

Similar to the situation of the electric resistance, if the fluid is flowing through several "serial" flow tubes, the total flow resistance equals to the sum of the flow resistances of these flow tubes; if several flow tubes are in "parallel", the reciprocal of the total flow resistance equals to the sum of the reciprocals of the branch flow resistances.

It should be particularly noted that, as the electric resistance, the flow resistance is not the resistant force, and there is no unit of the resistant force, it is only a factor affecting the flow rate. In medical researches on the cardiovascular system, the flow resistance is used to being called the peripheral resistance. By applying Equation (2-12) we can analyze the relationship among the cardiac output of blood, the pressure of blood and the peripheral resistance.

2.5.2 Stokes' Law

When a solid is performing a relative motion in a viscous fluid, it will be affected by the viscous resistance. The reason is that there is a layer of fluid adhering on the surface of the solid and moving together with the solid piece; thus there will be a relative motion between this layer and the surrounding fluid and an internal frictional force is set up. This force will hinder the motion of the solid piece in the fluid.

Experiments show that, if the moving object in the viscous fluid is a small ball and its velocity is very low (Reynolds number $Re < 1$), the resistant viscous force f acting on it is proportional to the radius of the ball r, the velocity of the ball's motion v, and the coefficient of viscosity of the fluid η; the proportional coefficient is only related to the shape of the object. Stokes derived theoretically that, for the sphere, the proportional coefficient is 6π. That is to say, for a sphere with the radius of r moving with velocity of v in the viscous fluid with the coefficient of viscosity of η, the viscous resistance is

$$f = 6\pi\eta v r \tag{2-13}$$

Equation (2-13) is called **Stokes' law.**

Stokes' law can be used to measure the viscosity of a fluid or the radius of a ball. As a small ball is descending in some viscous fluid, the forces acting on the ball are the gravity, the buoyancy and the viscous resistance, and the resultant force is

$$F = \frac{4}{3}\pi r^3 \rho_1 g - \frac{4}{3}\pi r^3 \rho_2 g - 6\pi\eta v r$$

where ρ_1 is the density of the ball, ρ_2 is the density of the liquid. Under the action of this resultant force, the ball will descend with acceleration; but the resistant viscous force will increase as the descending velocity increases. When the velocity increases to a certain value these three forces become balanced, the ball will descend with a uniform velocity. When the ball is performing a motion of a uniform velocity, this corresponding velocity is called the **terminal velocity**, and it follows the relation of

$$\frac{4}{3}\pi r^3 g(\rho_1 - \rho_2) = 6\pi\eta r v_{\text{terminal}}$$

or, to be finished as

$$v_{\text{terminal}} = \frac{2}{9\eta} r^2 (\rho_1 - \rho_2) g \tag{2-14}$$

Equation (2-14) indicates that, when a spherical object is descending in a viscous fluid (such as a particle dust in the air or a blood cell in the plasma), the terminal velocity is proportional to acceleration of gravity, the difference of ball's density and the fluid's density and the square of the radius of the ball, but inversely proportional to the viscosity of the fluid.

Equation (2-14) has been widely used in the field of medicine. For example, when liquid medicines are produced in the pharmaceutical factories, in order to prevent precipitation, the terminal velocities of particles in the solutions should be minimized. From Equation (2-14) we see that, the purpose to reduce the terminal velocity can be achieved by increasing the density of solution and reducing the size of the particle and other measures.

For particles in the suspension liquids, such as blood cells in plasma, biomacromolecules and micelles in viscous liquids, because the sizes of these particles are extremely small, their terminal velocities are very slow. If the sedimentation method is taken to separate particles from the suspension liquid, it has to spend a long time and get a poor effect. In this situation, the suspension liquid is usually put into a high-speed centrifuge, which can increase the effective value of g (acceleration), according to Stokes' law, the centrifugation can shorten the separation time and improve the separation performance.

A Brief Summarization of This Chapter

(1) An ideal fluid: It is a fluid that is absolutely incompressible and has no viscosity completely.

(2) Steady flow: It is a flow form in which at any certain point in the space the flow velocity does not change with time.

(3) Streamlines: Some imaginary curves used to describe vividly the distribution of the velocity of the fluid flowing in the space; the tangential direction at each point on any curve is always agreed with the velocity direction

of the fluid flowing through that point.

(4) The flow tube: In the field where the fluid is performing a steady flow, the tubular region surrounded by many streamlines.

(5) The equation of continuity: Under the condition of a steady flow, the relationship among the flow rate, the flow velocity and the cross-sectional area of the flow tube is

$$Q = Sv = \text{constant}$$

(6) Bernoulli equation: It reflects the relationship among the pressure, the velocity and the height on a streamline for an ideal fluid performing a steady flow.

$$P + \frac{1}{2}\rho v^2 + \rho g h = \text{constant}$$

(7) Laminar flow: When a viscous fluid is flowing with a flow velocity of not too high, the flow will be performed as the stratified flow; because the flow velocities of adjacent layers are different and there will be the relative sliding between the layers, but they will not mix to each other. This flow form of the fluid is called the laminar flow.

(8) Turbulent flow: As the velocity of the flowing viscous fluid increases, the laminar flow is destroyed, the transversal components of velocity will appear in the fluid and the liquid layers will be mixed. A disorder and confused flow state is formed; meanwhile, there may even be the emergence of vortexes. This flow form is called the turbulent flow.

(9) Reynolds number: It is a unit-less pure number used as the basis for deciding the transition from the laminar flow to the turbulent flow.

$$Re = \frac{\rho v r}{\eta}$$

(10) Newton Viscosity Law: In a viscous fluid performing a laminar flow, the magnitude of viscous force f between two adjacent layers is proportional to the area of the contact surface of the liquid layers S and the velocity gradient at the location of the contact surface of the two layers $\mathrm{d}v/\mathrm{d}x$.

$$f = \eta S \frac{\mathrm{d}v}{\mathrm{d}x}$$

(11) Poiseuille's law: When the viscous fluid with the coefficient of viscosity of η is performing a steady flow in the horizontal tube with the radius of R and the length of L, the volume flow rate is proportional to the difference of the pressures at the two ends of tube ΔP.

$$Q = \frac{\pi R^4 \Delta P}{8\eta L}$$

(12) Stokes' law: When a ball with the radius of r is moving with the relative velocity v in the fluid which has the coefficient of viscosity of η, the viscous resistance is

$$f = 6\pi \eta v r$$

Exercises 2

2-1. What is the ideal fluid?

2-2. What is the steady flow?

2-3. Are the streamlines and the flow tube objectively existent?

2-4. When the water column spouts from the fire pump toward the sky, why does its cross-sectional area increase with the increase of the height? When water is poured from a kettle to a bottle, why does the cross-sectional area of the water column decrease with the decrease of the height?

2-5. What are the conditions on which the equation of continuity is applicable? What are the conditions on which Bernoulli equation is applicable?

2-6. When two parallel ships voyage forward, why is it not allowed for them to keep too near?

2-7. Water is performing a steady flow in one flow tube. The flow velocity at the location with the cross-sectional area of 0.5 cm^2 is 12 cm/s. What is the cross-sectional area of the flow tube at the location where the flow velocity is 4 cm/s?

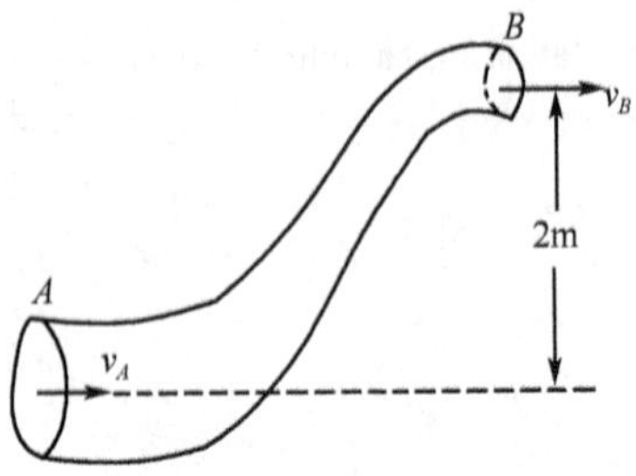

Figure for Exercise 2-8

2-8. With the flow rate of 0.012 m^3/s, water is flowing through a section of pipeline as shown in Figure for Exercise 2-8. At point A the pressure is 2×10^5 Pa, and the cross-sectional area is 100 cm^2, while the cross-sectional area at point B is 60 cm^2, and point B is 2 m higher than point A. Determine the flow velocities at point A and point B; and find the pressure at point B. Here water is regarded as an ideal liquid.

2-9. Water is flowing in a circular pipeline. At some location the cross-sectional area of the pipeline is 5 cm^2, the flow velocity is 2 m/s and the pressure is 1.5×10^4 Pa which is higher than the atmospheric pressure. At another location the cross-sectional area of the pipeline is 10 cm^2 and the pressure is 3.3×10^4 Pa which is higher than the atmospheric pressure. Determine the difference of the heights of these two points.

2-10. A big container is filled with water and the distance from the bottom to the water surface is H. At the bottom of the container, there is a hole with the area of a. Determine the flow rate of the water flowed out from the hole in the beginning.

2-11. In the infusion device shown in Figure for Exercise 2-11, the height difference from the liquid surface inside the hanging infusion bottle to the injection needle is 1.25 m. Determine the flow velocity of the liquid flowed out from the tip of the needle.

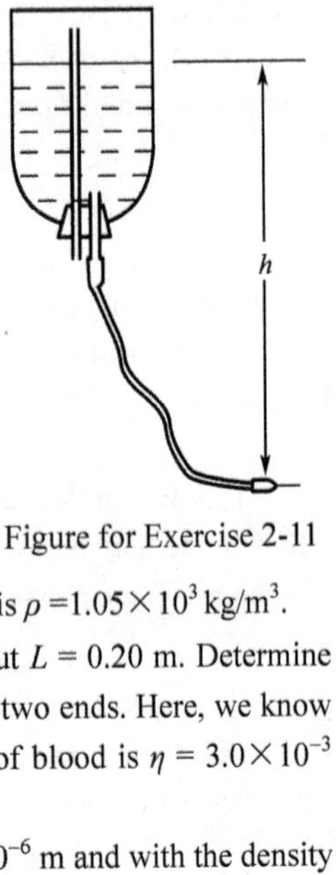

Figure for Exercise 2-11

2-12. A big circular container, whose top is opened, at the center of its bottom there is a hole with the cross-sectional area of 1 cm^2. When water is injected continuously from the top of the circular container with the flow rate of 100 cm^3/s, what will be the maximum height of the water surface that can be reached inside the container?

2-13. A hard plaque exists in a artery which have the normal diameter of 6.0 mm. Therefore, at this location the effective diameter becomes 4.0 mm, and the average flow velocity of blood is 5.0cm/s. Determine:

(1) The average flow velocity at the normal unchanged place in the artery;

(2) Whether a turbulent flow will take place at this stenosed location. Here, we have known the coefficient of viscosity of blood is $\eta = 3.0\times10^{-3}$ Pa·s, and its density is $\rho = 1.05\times10^3$ kg/m^3.

2-14. Generally, the radius of the adult aorta is about $R=1.0\times10^{-2}$m, and its length is about $L = 0.20$ m. Determine the flow resistance of this section of the aorta and the pressure difference between its two ends. Here, we know the flow rate of the cardiac output is $Q=1.0\times10^{-4}m^3/s$, the coefficient of viscosity of blood is $\eta = 3.0\times10^{-3}$ Pa·s.

2-15. A red blood cell can be approximately regarded as asmall ball with the radius of 2×10^{-6} m and with the density of 1.3×10^3 kg/m^3. Determine the time required for the red blood cell to sedimentate a distance of 1.0 cm after becoming the uniform sedimentation under the action of the gravity at 37℃ (Here, we have known the coefficient of viscosity of blood is $\eta = 3.0\times10^{-3}$ Pa·s, and the density of blood is $\rho = 1.05\times10^3$ kg/m^3).

Chapter 3 Molecular Physics

Molecular physics is a branch of thermotics based on microstructures of matters and the kinetic theory of molecules. By using the statistical averaging method, we are able to illuminate thermal phenomena, establish the relations between the macroscopic and microscopic quantities of matters, and interpret the microscopic natures of macroscopic properties of gases.

Any kind of matter in any phase is composed of numerous molecules. And all the molecules are performing the irregular thermal motion ceaselessly. Comparing with the mechanical motion, it is a much more complex motional form. Thermal phenomena are common expressions of the thermal motions of numerous molecules. Every moving molecule has its volume, mass, velocity, energy, and so on, and these physical quantities to express the property and motion state of an individual molecule are called microscopic quantities; the physical quantities which can be observed with the general experiments, such as pressure, temperature, and so on, are the physical quantities to describe the common properties of numerous molecules, i.e., the macroscopic quantities. In addition, there are inevitably intrinsic relations between macroscopic and microscopic quantities.

In this chapter, we'll use the viewpoint of kinetic theory of molecules to explain some macroscopic properties and regularities of gases; meanwhile, we'll give a brief description to the surface phenomena of liquid and corresponding applications.

3.1 Pressure Formula of an Ideal Gas

3.1.1 Microscopic Model of an Ideal Gas

1. Equilibrium State

Suppose there is a closed container, and we can divide it into two parts, A and B, by a separator, as shown in Figure 3-1. Part A is filled with some kind of gas and part B is in vacuum. When we move the separator away, the gas in part A will move to part B. At first, the states of the gas at any points in A or B are not uniform and may vary with time. But they will become uniform and steady everywhere at last. After that, if there is no other surrounding effect, the gas in the container will always maintain this state and will not change macroscopically any more. Another example is, when two objects with different temperatures are contacted with each other, the hot object becomes colder and colder, and the cold object becomes hotter and hotter, until the two objects reach the state that there is the same degree of cold and hot uniformly everywhere at last. Here, if there is no any influence from the surroundings, the two objects will always maintain this state and will not change macroscopically any more. There are many other similar phenomena that can be given. From these phenomena we can conclude that if there is no any influence from the surroundings, a thermal system will reach a certain state and there will not be any macroscopic change. On the condition that there is no any influence from the surroundings, the system will reach the state in which the macroscopic properties of the system do not vary with time, and this state is called the

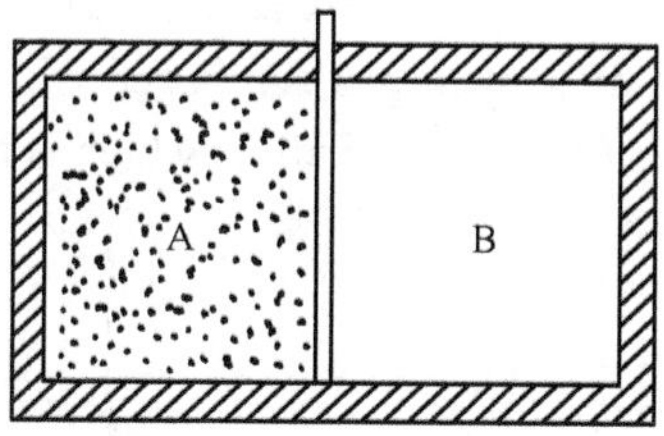

Figure 3-1 initial status

equilibrium state.

We should point out that the equilibrium state refers to the macroscopic properties of a system do not change with time. From the microscopic viewpoint, in an equilibrium state, the molecules which compose the system are keeping moving, but the average effect of the molecular motions remains unchangeable with time, and this average unchanged effect indicates that the system reaches the equilibrium state from the macroscopic viewpoint. Therefore, we often call this equilibrium the **thermal equilibrium**, and call the equilibrium state the **thermal equilibrium state.**

2. Microscopic Model of an Ideal Gas

In order to derive the pressure formula of an ideal gas, let's give the following assumptions to the molecular model of an ideal gas according to the characteristics of an ideal gas and thermal equilibrium.

(1) Comparing with the average distance between any molecules, the dimension of the molecule is negligible, i.e., a molecule can be regarded as a particle without size;

(2) Except at the moments when collisions take place, it is considered that, there is no any interaction between molecules or between a molecule and the wall of the container, meanwhile, the gravitational force acting on the molecule is also ignored;

(3) Collisions between the molecules or between molecules and the container walls can be regarded as perfectly elastic collisions;

(4) Any molecules have the equal opportunity to move along any direction, i.e., at any moment along any directions, there is an equal number of moving molecules; and in any direction the average values of the component speeds of the numerous molecules are equal.

The above assumptions are based on some experiments. And the results derived from them can not only conform to the actual situation of an ideal gas, but also reflect the properties of real gas in a certain range.

3.1.2 Pressure Formula of an Ideal Gas

1. Derivation of the Pressure Formula of an Ideal Gas

According to the assumptions of the model of an ideal gas and the kinetic molecular theory, let's calculate the pressure of the ideal gas, and explain the microscopic essence of the pressure of the gas.

Suppose there is a cubic container with the side length of l, as shown in Figure 3-2, and the container is filled with gas composed with N molecules; the mass of each molecule is m. Now let's calculate the pressure on the wall A_1 which is perpendicular to the x axis.

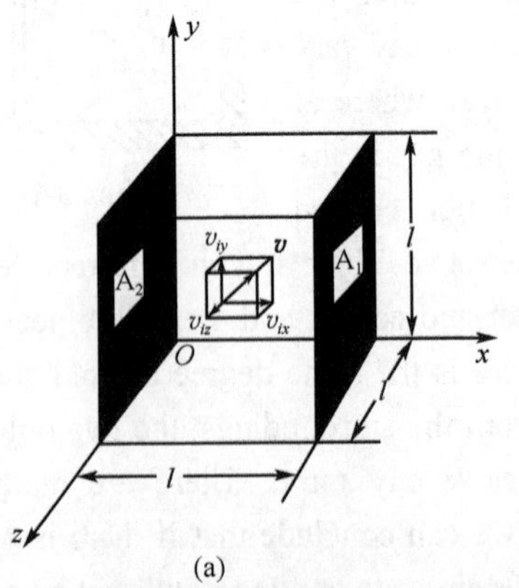

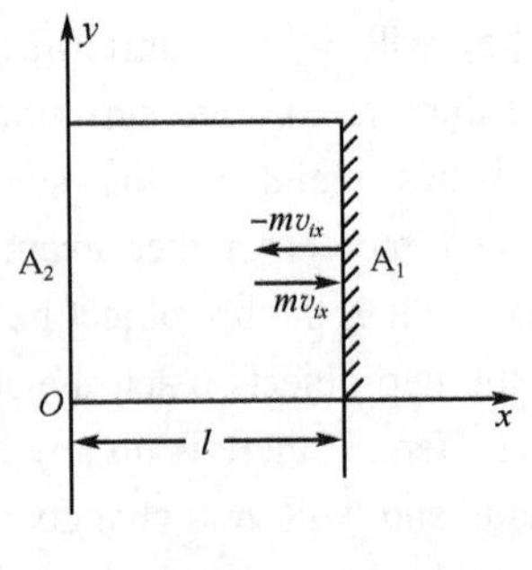

Figure 3-2 Derivation of the pressure formula of an ideal gas

Firstly, let's consider the impulse of one collision acted on the wall A_1 by the molecule i. Assume the velocity of the molecule i is υ_i, and its components along the three coordinate directions x, y, z are respectively υ_{ix}, υ_{iy} and υ_{iz}. Because the collision of the molecule with A_1 is perfectly elastic, the component of the velocity along x direction will change to $-\upsilon_{ix}$ from υ_{ix} after the collision, i.e., the velocity component before the collision and the velocity component after the collision have the same magnitude and opposite directions. So the change of the momentum for the molecule after one collision is

$$-m\upsilon_{ix}-(m\upsilon_{ix})=-2m\upsilon_{ix}$$

According to the theorem of momentum, this quantity is equal to the impulse acted on the molecule i by the wall of A_1. And referring to Newton's third law, the impulse acted on the wall of A_1 by the molecule i is $2m\upsilon_{ix}$.

Secondly, calculate the impulse acted on the wall of A_1 by the molecule i in the time interval dt. Although the path for a molecule proceeding two successive collisions on the wall of A_1 is zigzag, the distance proceeded along the direction of x axis must be $2l$. Therefore, the time interval for the molecule i to undergo two successive collisions on A_1 is $2l/\upsilon_{ix}$, and the number of times of collisions on A_1 in the time interval dt is

$$\frac{\mathrm{d}t}{2l/\upsilon_{ix}}=\frac{\upsilon_{ix}\cdot\mathrm{d}t}{2l}$$

Because the impulse of one collision on the wall of A_1 by the molecule i is $2m\upsilon_{ix}$, the total impulse in the time interval dt on A_1 by it will be

$$2m\upsilon_{ix}\cdot\frac{\upsilon_{ix}\cdot\mathrm{d}t}{2l}=\frac{m\cdot\mathrm{d}t}{l}\upsilon_{ix}^2$$

Thirdly, calculate the impulse on the wall of A_1 by N molecules in the time interval dt

$$I=\overline{F}\cdot\mathrm{d}t=\sum_{i=1}^{N}\frac{m\cdot\mathrm{d}t}{1}\upsilon_{ix}^2=\frac{m\cdot\mathrm{d}t}{1}\sum_{i=1}^{N}\upsilon_{ix}^2$$

So the average impulsive force F is

$$\overline{F}=\frac{m}{1}\sum_{i=1}^{N}\upsilon_{ix}^2 \tag{3-1}$$

Although the impulsive force of a single molecule on a wall is intermittent, but the result of continuous collisions on the wall by numerous of molecules gives a sustaining force in macroscopic scale.

Since the area of the wall A_1 of the container is l^2, the pressure P exerted by the N molecules of the gas on this wall is

$$P=\frac{\overline{F}}{l^2}=\frac{m}{l^3}\sum_{i=1}^{N}\upsilon_{ix}^2=\frac{m}{V}\sum_{i=1}^{N}\upsilon_{ix}^2 \tag{3-2}$$

where V is the volume of the container, i.e., the volume of the gas. And P can also be expressed as

$$P=\frac{mN}{V}\left(\frac{\upsilon_{1x}^2+\upsilon_{2x}^2+\upsilon_{3x}^2+\cdots+\upsilon_{Nx}^2}{N}\right) \tag{3-3}$$

The number of the molecules in a unit volume is $n=\frac{N}{V}$, and it is also called numeral density of molecules. Because $\frac{\upsilon_{1x}^2+\upsilon_{2x}^2+\cdots+\upsilon_{Nx}^2}{N}=\overline{\upsilon_x^2}$, where, $\overline{\upsilon_x^2}$ is the molecular mean square speed component along x axis. Therefore, Equation (3-3) can be rewritten as

$$P=nm\overline{\upsilon_x^2} \tag{3-4}$$

In the equilibrium state, the molecules of the gas have equal opportunity to move towards any directions (the fourth assumption), we acquire that $\overline{v_x^2}=\overline{v_y^2}=\overline{v_z^2}$, and because $\overline{v^2}=\overline{v_x^2}+\overline{v_y^2}+\overline{v_z^2}$, where $\overline{v^2}$ is the molecular mean square speed. From the above two equations we have $\overline{v_x^2}=\frac{1}{3}\overline{v^2}$, and substitute this result into Equation (3-4), we obtain

$$P=\frac{2}{3}n\left(\frac{1}{2}m\overline{v^2}\right) \tag{3-5}$$

Equation (3-5) is called the pressure formula of an ideal gas, where $\frac{1}{2}m\overline{v^2}$ is the average translational kinetic energy of one molecule of the gas. Equation (3-5) indicates that, the pressure P of an ideal gas is proportional to the molecular numeral density of the gas n, and is proportional to the average translational kinetic energy of one molecule.

2. Several Explanations About the Pressure Formula of an Ideal Gas

(1) The essence of the pressure of the ideal gas explained from the viewpoint of the kinetic theory of molecules: The macroscopic pressure, acted on the wall of the container by the gas, is the result of the continuous collisions on the wall by numerous molecules, rather than the reason that the molecules of the gas have the weight. By the derivation process of the pressure formula we see that, the pressure of the gas is equal to the average impulsive force acted on the unit area of the wall by all the molecules in the unit time interval, it depends on the numeral density of molecules n and the average translational kinetic energy of one molecule $\frac{1}{2}m\overline{v^2}$, which quantitatively explains the essence of the pressure of gas. Furthermore, we should deeply understand the significance of the macroscopic quantity of pressure from the microscopic essence. If the molecular numerous density n is bigger, i.e., the number of molecules in a unit volume is more, the number of times of the collisions on a unit area of the wall in a unit time interval by the molecules will be more, so the pressure P will be higher. And on average, if the kinetic energy of every molecule $\frac{1}{2}m\overline{v^2}$ gets bigger, i.e., the intense degree of the random motions of molecules gets higher. On the one hand, the molecules will move back and forth more frequently, the number of times of the collisions on a unit area of the wall by the molecules in a unit time interval will be more; on the other hand, for every collision, the impulse acted on the wall by a molecule will also be bigger. It is these two reasons that lead to the pressure P getting higher.

(2) The pressure formula is a result of statistical regularity. In the derivation process of the pressure formula, we have used not only the principles of mechanics, but also the statistical rules and methods. Because the collisions of molecules on the wall are intermittent, the impulses on the wall by the molecules are fluctuating or not fixed, so the average impulsive force acted by the molecules in a unit time interval on a unit area of the wall, i.e., the pressure P is a statistical average quantity; it is the statistical average quantity for a large number of molecules, certain time and area; so it requires the molecules to be more enough, the time to be long enough, and the area to be large enough. Of course, these three "enough" are relative. In gas, the molecular number in a unit volume is uncertain, so n is also a statistical average quantity. Therefore, the pressure formula is a statistical regularity to characterize the relationships among the three statistical average quantities of P, n and $\frac{1}{2}m\overline{v^2}$, rather than a normal mechanical law.

(3) The pressure formula can not be directly verified by experiments. Although the pressure P can be

measured directly, however, the quantity of $\frac{1}{2}m\overline{v^2}$ can not be measured directly by experiments. But by applying this formula we can explain or deduce some experimental laws that has been demonstrated for ideal gases satisfactorily. It shows that the pressure formula and the assumptions for deriving the pressure formula can reflect the objective reality to some extent.

3.1.3 Relation Between Temperature and the Average Translational Kinetic Energy of a Molecule

Comparing the pressure formula with the equation of state of an ideal gas, we can get the expression of the relationship between the temperature T and the average translational kinetic energy of a molecule $\frac{1}{2}m\overline{v^2}$, thus, we can reveal the microscopic essence of the macroscopic quantity of temperature.

Referring to Equation (3-5), that is the pressure formula of an ideal gas

$$P = \frac{2}{3}n\left(\frac{1}{2}m\overline{v^2}\right)$$

The equation of state of an ideal gas is

$$PV = \frac{M}{\mu}RT$$

where M is the mass of the gas, μ is the molar mass of the gas, R is the universal gas constant, and T is the thermodynamic temperature of the gas.

Comparing the above equations and cancelling the quantity P, we have

$$\frac{1}{2}m\overline{v^2} = \frac{3}{2}\frac{MRT}{n\mu V}$$

Because $n = \frac{N}{V}$, $N = \frac{M}{\mu}N_{\mathrm{A}}$ and $N_{\mathrm{A}} = 6.022\times10^{23}\,\mathrm{mol}^{-1}$, represent the number of the molecules contained in one mole gas, which is called **Avogadro constant**, the above equation can be rewritten as

$$\frac{1}{2}m\overline{v^2} = \frac{3}{2}\frac{R}{N_{\mathrm{A}}}T$$

where R and N_{A} are both constants, so the ratio of them can be expressed by another constant k, k is called **Boltzmann constant**, and it has the value of

$$k = \frac{R}{N_{\mathrm{A}}} = 1.38\times10^{-23}\,J/K$$

Then

$$\frac{1}{2}m\overline{v^2} = \frac{3}{2}kT \tag{3-6}$$

Equation (3-6) shows that, the average translational kinetic energy of a molecule of an ideal gas is only dependent on the temperature and proportional to the absolute temperature. Equation (3-6) illustrates the following three main points:

(1) By the viewpoint of kinetic theory of molecules, this equation explains the essence of the temperature, i.e., the temperature is the mark of the intense degree of the irregular motions of the molecules inside an object; or, the temperature is a measuring scale of the average translational kinetic energy of a gas molecule. It indicates that the higher the temperature of an object is, the more intense the motions of the molecules inside the object will be.

(2) It reveals the relationship between the macroscopic quantity of temperature T and microscopic quantity of the average translational kinetic energy of a molecule $\frac{1}{2}m\overline{v^2}$. Because the temperature is related with the average value of translational kinetic energies of numerous molecules, the temperature is the collective performance of the thermal motions of numerous molecules; it has the statistical significance; for an individual molecule, it is meaningless to say it has the temperature.

(3) It actually provides one of the essential regularities of kinetic theory of molecules, i.e., the application of the theorem of the equipartition of energy (we will discuss it in the next section) in the case of translation of the molecules of an ideal gas.

From Equation (3-5) and Equation (3-6), we have

$$P=\frac{2}{3}n\left(\frac{1}{2}m\overline{v^2}\right)=\frac{2}{3}n\left(\frac{3}{2}kT\right)=nkT$$

that is

$$P=nkT \tag{3-7}$$

Equation (3-7) is called **Avogadro law**.

Example 3-1 A container is filled with oxygen with the pressure of $P=1.0\times10^5\,\text{Pa}$ and the temperature of $0℃$. What is the rms (root-mean-square) speed of a molecule of the oxygen and how many molecules are there in per cubic meter?

Solution: According to Equation (3-6), we know that

$$\frac{1}{2}m\overline{v^2}=\frac{3}{2}kT$$

So

$$\overline{v^2}=\frac{3kT}{m}=\frac{3kT}{\dfrac{\mu}{N_A}}=\frac{3RT}{\mu}$$

That is

$$\sqrt{\overline{v^2}}=\sqrt{\frac{3RT}{\mu}}=\sqrt{\frac{3\times8.31\times273}{32\times10^{-3}}}=461\text{ m/s}$$

From Equation (3-7), we know that

$$P=nkT$$

So

$$n=\frac{P}{kT}=\frac{1.0\times10^5}{1.38\times10^{-23}\times273}=2.65\times10^{25}\,\text{m}^{-3}$$

That is, there are 2.65×10^{25} oxygen molecules in per cubic meter.

3.2 Degrees of Freedom and the Theorem of Equipartition of Energy

3.2.1 Degrees of Freedom

We have only discussed the average translational kinetic energy of a molecule previous. In fact, except the monatomic molecules, other complicatedly structured molecules not only have the translational kinetic energy, but also have the rotational and vibrational energies. In order to determine the statistical regularity of the molecules' energies in various moving forms, we need to introduce and understand the concept of the degrees of freedom. **The number of independent coordinates required to determine the position of an object in the space is called the degrees of freedom of the object**. It is often denoted be the letter i.

1. Number of Degrees of Freedom of a Particle

If a particle is moving freely in the space, 3 independent coordinates are required to determine its position, such as x, y, z, so this particle has 3 degrees of freedom; if a particle is moving in a plane or curved surface, it has only 2 degrees of freedom for its position; similarly, if the particle is restricted to move in a straight line or curve, it has only 1 degrees of freedom. If an airplane, a ship or a train is regarded respectively as a particle, then, the airplane has 3 degrees of freedom, i.e., $i = 3$; the ship has 2 degrees of freedom, i.e., $i = 2$; and the train has only 1 degree of freedom, i.e., $i = 1$.

2. Number of Degrees of Freedom of a Rigid Body

A molecule composed of 2 or more than 2 atoms can be approximately regarded as a rigid body at room temperature, so it is necessary to discuss the degrees of freedom of a rigid body first. The motion of a rigid body can be decomposed into the translation of its center of mass and rotation about an axis through the center of mass, so degrees of freedom of a rigid body should be the sum of the translational and rotational degrees of freedom, specifically, the position of a rigid body is determined as follows:

(1) To determine the position of the center of mass with 3 independent coordinates, such as x, y, z.

(2) To determine the orientation of the rotational axis through the center of mass with 2 independent coordinates, such as α and β (here, only two of the three azimuths are independent, the reason is that, $\cos^2\alpha+\cos^2\beta+\cos^2\gamma=1$).

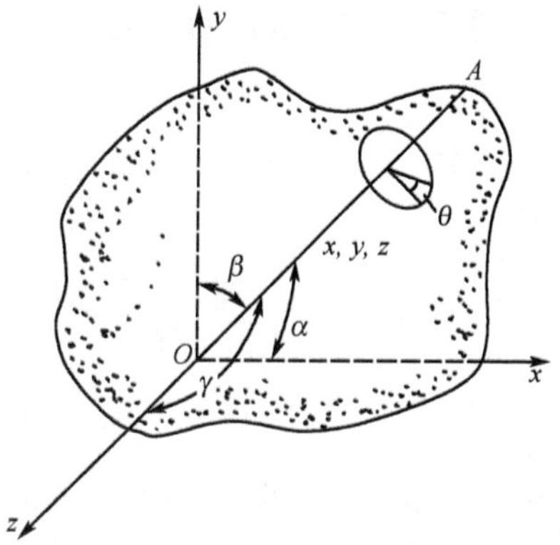

Figure 3-3 Degrees of freedom of a rigid body

(3) For the molecules composed by 3 or more than 3 atoms, determine the angular coordinate of the rigid body, i.e. the turning angle from the original position with 1 extra independent coordinate, such as θ. Therefore, a free rigid body has 6 degrees of freedom (i.e., $i = 6$), among them, there are 3 translational degrees of freedom and 3 rotational degrees of freedom, as shown in Figure 3-3. If the motion of a rigid body is restricted, the number of degrees of freedom will be reduced. A rigid body rotating about a fixed axis has only 1 degree of freedom. However, when a molecule is consisted by 2 atoms, there is no such a degree of freedom of θ, which is a tiny slope.

3. Number of Degrees of Freedom for the Motions of Molecules

For a monatomic molecule such as the molecule of helium, or neon, or argon, it can be looked as a freely moving particle, so it has 3 degrees of freedom ($i = 3$). For a diatomic molecule like the molecule of oxygen, or carbon monoxide, if the relative position between the two atoms is fixed, the molecule of such kind can be regarded as a "dumbbell"-styled rigid molecule composed of two particles, because 3 independent coordinates will be required to determine the position of its center of mass, and 2 independent coordinates will be required to determine the orientation of the line connecting the 2 atoms, the diatomic molecule has 5 degrees of freedom ($i = 5$), i.e., a rigid diatomic molecule has 3 translational degrees of freedom and 2 rotational degrees of freedom. Molecules composed of 3 or more than 3 atoms, if regarded as rigid bodies, should have 6 degrees of freedom ($i = 6$). At room temperature, molecules are generally regarded as rigid molecules. For non-rigid molecules, according to the results of molecular spectroscopy, atoms have the slight vibrations along the directions of the connecting lines, and the non-rigid molecule can be described by the model of "the two particles connected by a spring of negligible mass". Therefore, except the translational and rotational degrees of freedom, the molecule of this kind has also its vibrational degrees of freedom. For example, a non-rigid diatomic molecule has 6 degrees of freedom ($i = 6$): 3 translational degrees of freedom, 2 rotational degrees of freedom and 1 vibrational degree of freedom. Generally speaking, a non-rigid molecule composed of n atoms ($n \geqslant 3$) has $3n$ degrees of freedom at most, among them, there are 3 translational degrees of freedom, 3 rotational degrees of freedom, and the rest of the $3n-6$ are the vibrational degrees of freedom.

It should be pointed out that, the moving status of identical molecules of a gas also depends on the temperature of the gas; if the temperature changes, the degrees of freedom will be different. For example, a molecule of hydrogen can be regarded as two particles connected by a rigid bond at room temperature, and only at high temperature its molecular model becomes two particles connected by a spring of negligible mass.

3.2.2 Theorem of Equipartition of Energy

In the previous section we have determined the relationship between the average translational kinetic energy of a molecule of the ideal gas and the temperature, i.e.,

$$\frac{1}{2}m\overline{v^2} = \frac{3}{2}kT$$

While,

$$\frac{1}{2}m\overline{v^2} = \frac{1}{2}m\overline{v_x^{\,2}} + \frac{1}{2}m\overline{v_y^{\,2}} + \frac{1}{2}m\overline{v_z^{\,2}}$$

It has indicated that, for numerous gas molecules at the equilibrium state, they have the equal opportunity to move along any directions. So we have

$$\overline{v_x^{\,2}} = \overline{v_y^{\,2}} = \overline{v_z^{\,2}} = \frac{1}{3}\overline{v^2}$$

From the above formula an important result can be obtained

$$\frac{1}{2}m\overline{v_x^{\,2}} = \frac{1}{2}m\overline{v_y^{\,2}} = \frac{1}{2}m\overline{v_z^{\,2}} = \frac{1}{2}kT$$

That is, a molecule has the same average kinetic energy in each translational degree of freedom, whose value is $\frac{1}{2}kT$, that is to say, the average translational kinetic energy of the molecule of $\frac{3}{2}kT$ is evenly distributed to each translational degree of freedom.

This conclusion can be extended to the rotational and vibrational degrees of freedom of molecules. According to the essential regularity of classical statistical physics, we can deduce a general theorem—the **theorem of equipartition of energy**: **At the equilibrium state and the temperature of *T*, for any matters (gas, liquid or solid), every degree of freedom of one molecule has the same average kinetic energy, and its value is $\frac{1}{2}kT$**. Therefore, if a molecule of some gas has t translational degrees of freedom, r rotational degrees of freedom and s vibrational degrees of freedom, the average translational kinetic energy, the average rotational kinetic energy and the average vibrational kinetic energy of the molecule will be respectively $\frac{t}{2}kT$, $\frac{r}{2}kT$ and $\frac{s}{2}kT$; then, the average total kinetic energy of the molecule will be

$$\overline{e_k} = \frac{i}{2}kT = \frac{(t+r+s)}{2}kT \tag{3-8}$$

The theorem of equipartition of energy is the statistical regularity about the kinetic energy of thermal motions of molecules; it is a statistical averaging result of numerous molecules. For an individual molecule at any time moment, its energies of various forms and its total energy may extremely differ from the average values derived with the theorem of equipartition of energy, and the energy of every form can not necessarily be uniformly distributed according to the degrees of freedom. For numerous molecules as a whole, the equipartition of the energy is the result of molecular random collisions. In the process of a collision, the energy of one molecule can be transmitted to another molecule, one form of energy can be converted into another form, and the energy can be transferred from one degree of freedom to another degree of freedom. If the energy of one form or of a degree of freedom is more, at the moment of the collision, the probability for the energy to be converted from this form into other forms or to be transferred from this degree of freedom to the other degrees of freedom will be bigger. Therefore, at the equilibrium state, the energy is uniformly distributed according to the degrees of freedom.

Referring to the knowledge of vibration mechanics, we know that the average kinetic energy is the same as the average potential energy in a period of a harmonic motion. Because the slight vibration of the atoms in a molecule can be regarded as harmonic motion, for each vibrational degree of freedom, there is not only the average vibrational kinetic energy of $\frac{1}{2}kT$, but also the average vibrational potential energy of $\frac{1}{2}kT$. Therefore, if the vibrational degrees of freedom of a molecule is s, the average vibrational kinetic energy and the average vibrational potential energy of the molecule will be $\frac{s}{2}kT$ respectively; the average total energy of a molecule will be

$$\overline{e} = \frac{1}{2}(t+r+2s)kT \tag{3-9}$$

Example 3-2 Try to find the average translational kinetic energy, the average total kinetic energy and the average total energy of a monatomic molecule, a diatomic molecule with the rigid bond, and a diatomic molecule with the non-rigid bond.

Solution: (1) For a monatomic molecule, $t = 3$, $r = 0$, $s = 0$,

the average translational kinetic energy is $\frac{3}{2}kT$

the average total kinetic energy is $\frac{3}{2}kT$

and the average total energy is $\frac{3}{2}kT$

(2) For a diatomic molecule with rigid bond, $t = 3$, $r = 2$, $s = 0$,

the average translational kinetic energy is $\frac{3}{2}kT$

the average translational kinetic energy is $\overline{e_k} = \frac{1}{2}(t+r+s)kT = \frac{5}{2}kT$

the average total energy is $\overline{e}=\frac{1}{2}(t+r+2s)kT=\frac{5}{2}kT$

(3) For a diatomic molecule with the non-rigid bond, $t=3$, $r=2$, $s=1$

the average translational kinetic energy is $\frac{3}{2}kT$

the average translational kinetic energy is $\overline{e_k}=\frac{1}{2}(t+r+s)kT=3kT$

the average total energy is $\overline{e}=\frac{1}{2}(t+r+2s)kT=\frac{7}{2}kT$

3.2.3 Internal Energy of an Ideal Gas

In addition to various forms of the kinetic energy and the vibrational potential energy of the atoms inside the molecules, due to the existence of the conservative interacting forces among molecules, the molecules of normal gases also have the potential energy associated with such forces. The sum of various forms of the kinetic energy and the potential energy of all the molecules in a gas is called the **internal energy** of the gas. Because there is no conservative interacting force existed among the molecules of ideal gases, an ideal gas has no potential energy associated with such force. So the internal energy of an ideal gas is the sum of various forms of the kinetic energy of all the molecules and the vibrational potential energy of all the atoms inside all the molecules of the gas. According to Equation (3-9), if the mass of the ideal gas is *M*, its internal energy is

$$E=\frac{M}{\mu}N_A\cdot\frac{1}{2}(t+r+2s)kT$$

That is,

$$E=\frac{1}{2}\frac{M}{\mu}(t+r+2s)RT \qquad (3\text{-}10)$$

From the above result we can infer that, for the ideal gas with a fixed number of moles, the internal energy is dependent only on the degrees of freedom of the molecules and the temperature of the gas, and is independent of its volume and pressure.

Example 3-3 What are the values of the internal energy of 1 mol of O_2 and the internal energy of 1 mol of N_2 at the temperature of 27℃? (O_2 and N_2 can be regarded as the gases with rigid bond).

Solution: The molecules of O_2 and N_2 have the same degrees of freedom, i.e., $t=3$, $r=2$, $s=0$, so the internal energies of them are equal.

$$E_{O_2}=E_{N_2}=\frac{5}{2}RT=\frac{5}{2}\times 8.31\times(273+27)=6.23\times 10^3\ \text{J}$$

3.3 Phenomena on Liquid Surfaces

The distance between the molecules in liquid is much shorter than the one between the molecules of gas. The order of magnitude of the average distance r_0 is about 10^{-10} m. When the distance between two molecules is longer than r_0, or is in $10^{-10}-10^{-9}$ m, the force between the molecules is an attractive force. When the distance between the molecules is longer than 10^{-9} m, the attractive force may tend to be zero rapidly. Therefore, we can consider the range of action of the attractive forces among the molecules as a sphere with the radius less than 10^{-9} m. And only the molecules within the sphere can have the attractive forces to the molecule at the center of the sphere. So we call the radius of this sphere is **radius of action of molecular attraction**. The liquid layer beneath the liquid surface with the thickness of being approximately equal to the radius of action of molecular attraction is called **surface layer** of the liquid.

3.3.1 Surface Tension of a Liquid and Surface Energy

For a molecule C inside a liquid, as shown in Figure 3-4, it will be subject by the forces of the molecules around it. Inside the range of action of the attractive forces, the arrangement of molecules is spherically symmetric, so the vector sum of the attractive forces acting on the molecule C is zero. For the molecule of A or B which is in the surface layer of the liquid, the situation is different. It is subject by the attractive forces of the molecules in the liquid on the one hand, and by the forces from the gas molecules outside the liquid on the other hand. Because the density of the gas is much lower than the density of the liquid, the action from the gas can be generally ignored. Thus, for every molecule in the surface layer of the liquid, the vector sum of the attractive forces acted on it by the surrounding molecules is perpendicular to the surface and point to the inside of the liquid, and the closer the molecule is to the liquid surface, the bigger the magnitude of this vector sum will be. So if a molecule is moved from the inside of a liquid to the surface, a work must be done to overcome this resultant force, thus the potential energy of the molecule is increased. That is to say, comparing with the molecule inside the liquid, a molecule inside the surface layer has more potential energy, and this potential energy is called the **surface energy**. Because every molecule in the liquid surface is acted by a force pointing to the inside of the liquid, all the molecules in the surface layer have the tendency to squeeze into the inside of the liquid, so the liquid surface is at a state of being tightened, as if a tensed elastic film with a shrinking tendency. From the viewpoint of the surface energy, if a system is in a steady equilibrium, the system will have minimal potential energy, so all of the liquid surfaces have the shrinking tendency. In this way, from the macroscopic viewpoint, there exists the **surface tension** in the surface layer of the liquid. For examples, when mercury falls on the desktop, it will reduce into small balls; water on a leave will be in the form of dews; putting a small coin gently on a surface of water, the coin will float on the water surface, etc. An experiment is shown in Figure 3-5 (a): a fine wet cotton thread loop is put on the soap film supported by a metal ring. Here, for any segment of the thread, the tensions on both sides of it are equal in magnitude but opposite in the directions, the cotton thread is in a state of balance, thus, its original shape keeps invariant. As shown in Figure 3-5 (b), if the soap film within the cotton thread loop is pierced by a hot needle, the cotton thread loop will be acted only by the soap film outside it, and cotton thread loop is pulled into a circle. From this experiment we can see that, the surface tension is along the liquid surface and tangent with the liquid surface and its direction is perpendicular to the boundary.

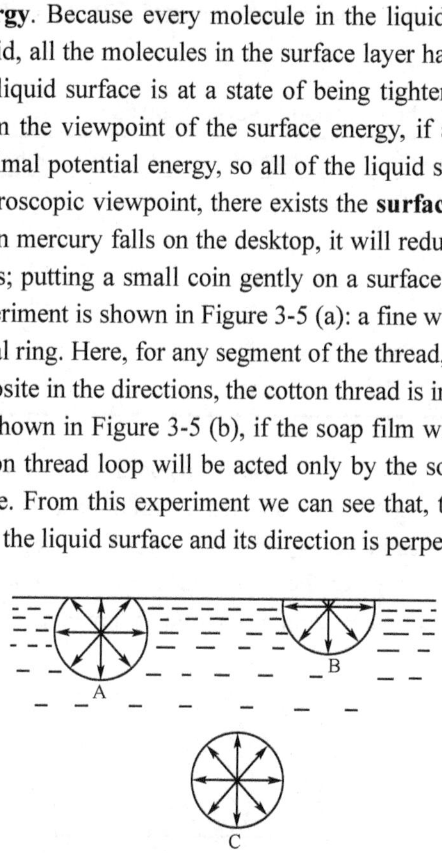

Figure 3-4 The forces acting on the molecules of a liquid

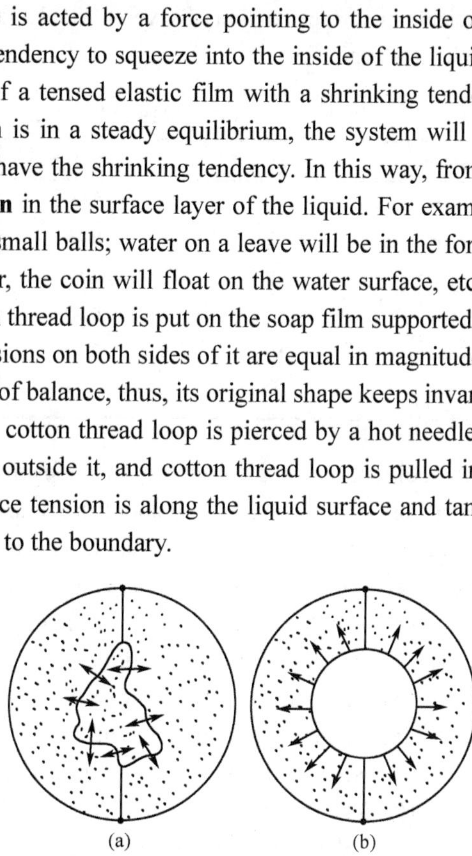

Figure 3-5 The effect of surface tension

Now let's discuss the magnitude of the surface tension. Line segment *MN* represents an assumed boundary on the surface, as shown in Figure 3-6, and it divides the surface into two parts, i.e., Ⅰ and Ⅱ. On each side of the line segment *MN* there is a surface tension along the surface and perpendicular to *MN*. The force f_1 represents the surface tension pulling on surface Ⅱ by surface Ⅰ, and f_2 represents the surface tension pulling on surface Ⅰ by surface Ⅱ. These two forces are equal in magnitude but opposite in direction. The magnitude of the surface tension is the proportional to *l*, i.e., the length of the assumed boundary *MN*, and this can be written as

$$f = \alpha l \tag{3-11}$$

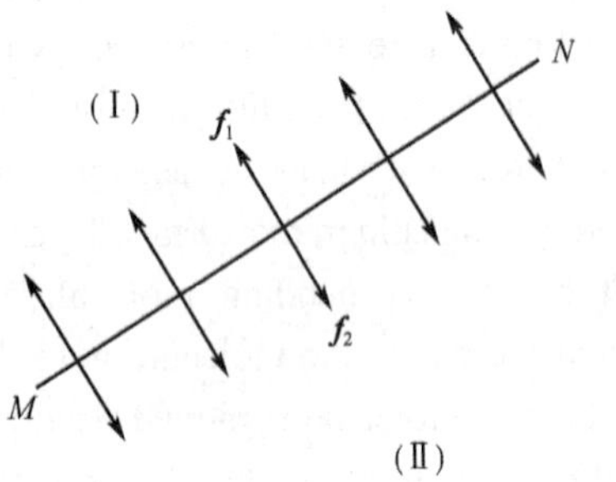

Figure 3-6 Coefficient of surface tension

where the proportional coefficient α is called the **coefficient of surface tension**; its unit is N/m.

In magnitude, the coefficient of surface tension is equal to the surface tension along the liquid surface acted on a unit length of the boundary. The coefficients of surface tension are related with the properties of liquids, for different liquids, the coefficients of surface tension are different. In addition, the coefficient of surface tension is related with the property of the matter, which contacts the liquid and is outside liquid surface, and the temperature of the liquid. In general, the higher the temperature is, the smaller the coefficient of surface tension will be. Table 3-1 gives the quantities of the coefficients of surface tension of several liquids. In this table, the outer matter contacted with the surfaces of the liquids is air.

Table 3-1 The values of the coefficients of surface tension of several liguids

Liquid	Temperature (℃)	α (10^{-3} N/m)	Liquid	Temperature (℃)	α (10^{-3} N/m)
Water	0	75.64	Soap-bubble	20	40
Water	20	72.75	Alcohol	20	22
Water	40	69.56	Mercury	20	470
Water	60	66.18	Plasma	20	60
Water	80	62.62	Normal urine	20	66
Water	100	58.85	Urine of the icteric patient	20	55

In addition, let's explain the physical meaning of the coefficient of surface tension from the relation between work and energy. As mentioned previously, comparing with the same amount of molecules inside the liquid, the molecules in the surface layer have more potential energy, and this potential is called the **surface energy** of the liquid. It is clear that the bigger the area of the liquid surface is, the more the surface energy will be, and vice versa. When a system is in a steady equilibrium state, its potential energy is always a minimum value. So the liquid surface will shrink as far as possible, till the area of the surface becomes the smallest. Now, let's analyze the value of the surface energy. Assume that there is a liquid film supported by a metal frame of *ABCD* as shown in Figure 3-7, and the side *CD* can slide freely. Let the length of the side *CD* is *L*. The film has a tendency of shrinking, so *CD* will move to the left to prevent the motion of the side *CD*, an external force ***F*** to the

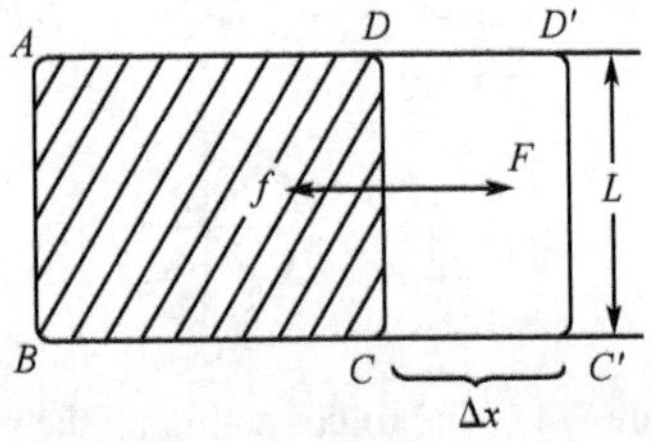

Figure 3-7 The magnitude of surface energy

right must be acted on the side *CD*, and the magnitude of ***F*** should be equal to the magnitude of the surface tension acted on the side *CD*. Because the film has two surfaces, the magnitude of the surface tension acted on the side *CD* will be

$$f = F = 2\alpha L$$

If the sliding side *CD* moves a distance of Δx the right with a constant speed under the action of external force, the work done by the external force is

$$\Delta W = F\Delta x = 2\alpha L\Delta x = \alpha \cdot \Delta S$$

where ΔS is the increment of the surface area of the liquid film, it can be derived from this equation:

$$\alpha = \frac{\Delta W}{\Delta S}$$

Thus, **the numerical value of the coefficient of surface tension is equal to the work done by external force when liquid surface is increased a unit area.**

From the above experiment we can see that the effect of the work done by the external force is to increase the surface area of the liquid film, or to move more molecules from the inside of the liquid to the surface layer, thereby, to increase the surface energy of the liquid. So we say that the work done by the external force is for increasing the surface energy of the liquid. If the increment of surface energy is denoted as ΔE, then

$$\Delta E = \Delta W = \alpha \cdot \Delta S$$

Or

$$\alpha = \frac{\Delta E}{\Delta S} \tag{3-12}$$

Thus, **the coefficient of surface tension** can also be defined as the **increment of the surface energy of the liquid when the liquid surface increases a unit area.** Its unit can also be written as J/m^2.

Example 3-4 Divide a big drop of water with the radius of 1 mm into eight equal small water droplets, what is the increment of the surface energy (suppose the coefficient of surface tension of water is 73×10^{-3} N/m)?

Solution: Suppose the radius of the big drip of water is *R*, and the radius of the small water droplet is *r*, then the increment of the surface energy is

$$\Delta E = \alpha(8 \times 4\pi r^2 - 4\pi R^2)$$

Because the mass of the big drip of water is equal to the masses of the eight small water droplets, so we have

$$\rho\frac{4}{3}\pi R^3 = \rho\frac{4}{3}\pi r^3 \cdot 8$$

$$8r^3 = R^3, \quad r^3 = \frac{R^3}{2^3}$$

$$r = 0.5 \text{ mm}$$

That is

$$\Delta E = 0.9 \times 10^{-6} \text{ J}$$

3.3.2 Additional Pressure of a Curved Surface of Liquid and Air Embolism

In daily life, we can see that the stationary liquid surface is commonly a plane; but there are also curved surfaces, such as the surfaces of soap bubbles, small water droplets, and the surface of liquid which is contacted to a solid, etc.

As shown in Figure 3-8, the three diagrams represent respectively the three cases of the liquid surfaces: the plane, the convex surface and the concave surface.

Let's assume a small area of ΔS on the liquid surface. The surface tension acted on ΔS is along the perimeter and perpendicular to the perimeter line and also tangent with the surface. If the liquid surface is a plane, everywhere on the surface, the direction of surface tension is parallel to the surface. Therefore, there is not any additional pressure whose direction perpendicular to the surface and produced by the surface tension. The pressure at a point beneath the surface will be equal to the external pressure of the atmosphere P_0, i.e., $P = P_0$, as shown in Figure 3-8 (a). If the surface is a convex surface, the direction of the integrated force of the surface tension will point to the inside and this integrated force will exert an additional pressure of P_S to the liquid below the convex surface, now, the pressure P at the point beneath the surface should be equal to the sum of the external pressure P_0 and the pressure P_S which is produced by the surface tension, i.e., $P = P_0 + P_S$, as shown in Figure 3-8 (b). If the surface is a concave surface, the direction of the integrated force of the surface tension will point to the outside and this integrated force will exert a pulling effect to the liquid below the concave surface, so the pressure P_S which is produced by the surface tension should point to the outside of the liquid, so the pressure P at the point beneath the surface should be $P = P_0 - P_S$, as shown in Figure 3-8 (c). **The pressure P_S produced by the surface tension on the curved surface of the liquid is called the additional pressure.**

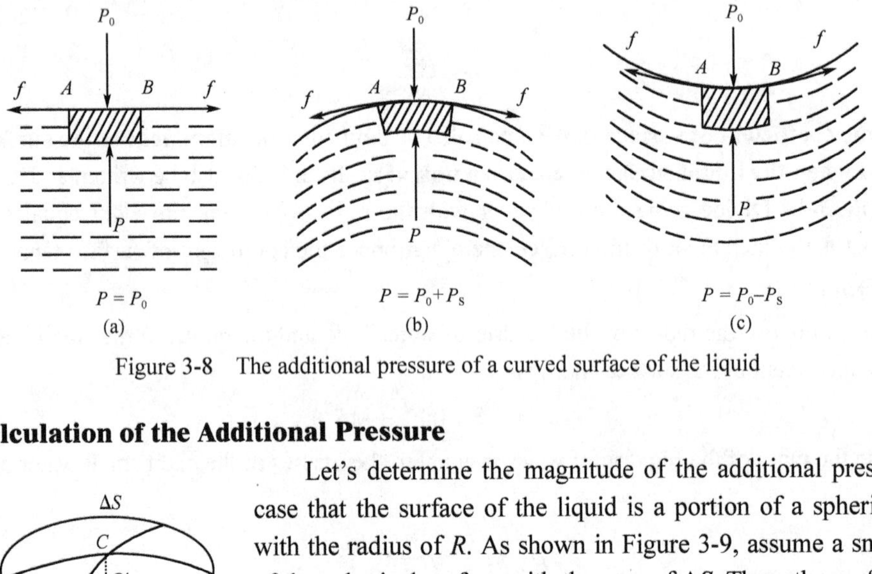

Figure 3-8 The additional pressure of a curved surface of the liquid

1. Calculation of the Additional Pressure

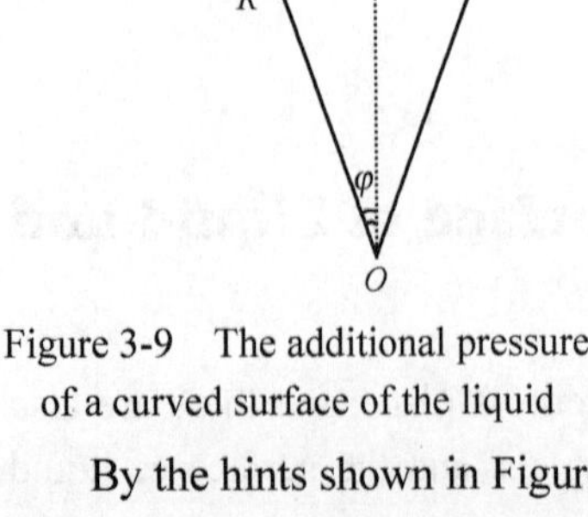

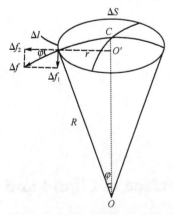

Figure 3-9 The additional pressure of a curved surface of the liquid

Let's determine the magnitude of the additional pressure in the case that the surface of the liquid is a portion of a spherical surface with the radius of R. As shown in Figure 3-9, assume a small portion of the spherical surface with the area of ΔS. Then, the surface tension acting on the perimeter line is tangent to the surface and perpendicular to the perimeter line. We can determine the magnitude of the surface tension acting on a line segment of Δl on the perimeter line by Equation (3-11), i.e. $\Delta f = \alpha \cdot \Delta l$.

Here, Δf can be decomposed into two components. One is Δf_1, which has the direction pointing toward the inside of the liquid. The other one is Δf_2, which has the direction perpendicular to the radius of curvature of OC. The integrated force of these components of Δf_2 along the perimeter line is zero, so every Δf_2 has no effect to the additional pressure, which needn't to be considered.

By the hints shown in Figure 3-9 we can see that

$$\Delta f_1 = \Delta f \sin\varphi = \alpha \cdot \Delta l \sin\varphi$$

The integrated force of the components which is along the perimeter line of ΔS and pointing toward the inside of the liquid is

$$f_1 = \sum \Delta f_1 = \alpha \sin\varphi \sum \Delta l = 2\pi r \cdot \alpha \cdot \sin\varphi$$

By substituting the quantity of $\sin\varphi = \frac{r}{R}$ into the above equation, we have

$$f_1 = \frac{2\pi\alpha r^2}{R}$$

Owing to the effect of f_1, the small surface element ΔS will be compressed toward the inside of the liquid. If ΔS is small enough, it can be considered as a small circular area with the radius of r and the area of $\Delta S = \pi r^2$. We can calculate the magnitude of the additional pressure of liquid surface ΔS exerting to the inside of the liquid with f_1 divided by ΔS, i.e.,

$$P_S = \frac{2\pi\alpha \cdot r^2}{\pi r^2 R} = \frac{2\alpha}{R} \tag{3-13}$$

Thus it can be seen that the magnitude of the additional pressure is proportional to the coefficient of surface tension α, and inversely proportional to the radius of curvature of R. The smaller the radius of curvature is, the bigger the additional pressure will be.

Example 3-5 Try to determine the pressure of the air inside a bubble, which is beneath the surface of water. Suppose that the radius of the bubble is 4×10^{-6} m, the coefficient of surface tension of the water is 73×10^{-3} N/m.

Solution: According to Equation (3-13), we have

$$P_S = \frac{2\alpha}{R} = \frac{2 \times 73 \times 10^{-3}}{4 \times 10^{-6}} = 3.65 \times 10^4 \text{ Pa}$$

Then we can determine the pressure of the air inside the bubble: $P = P_0 + P_S = 1.38 \times 10^5$ Pa.

Example 3-6 Try to determine the pressure difference between the outside and inside of a soap bubble. Assume that the radius of curvature of the bubble is R, and the coefficient of surface tension of it is α.

Solution: From Figure 3-10, we see that the soap bubble has two surfaces, i.e., the inside surface and the outside surface. Since the liquid film is very thin, the radiuses of the inside surface and the outside surface of the bubble can be looked as the same. They are both equal to R. We may choose three points respectively at the places outside of the soap bubble in the liquid of the bubble film and inside the soap bubble , which are denoted by A, B and C.

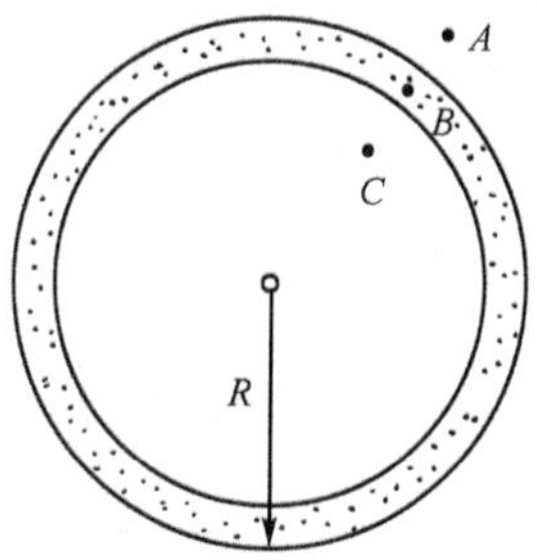

Figure 3-10 Pressure difference between two sides of the bubble

According to Equation (3-13), we know

$$P_B = P_A + \frac{2\alpha}{R}$$

$$P_C = P_B + \frac{2\alpha}{R}$$

From the equations above, we can get $P_C - P_A = \frac{4\alpha}{R}$, that is the pressure difference between the outside and the inside of the soap bubble.

2. Air Embolism

When some liquid flows through a narrow tube, a gas bubble in the tube will hamper the flow of the liquid; if the tube contains a large number of gas bubbles and is blocked, the flow of the liquid in the narrow tube may be completely stopped. This phenomenon is called the **air embolism**.

The reason to produce the air embolism is the existence of the additional pressure on the curved interface between the gas and liquid. As shown in Figure 3-11, let's consider the case that a narrow tube contains a gas bubble. If the liquid pressures on both sides of the bubble are equal (that is, $P_A = P_B$), the two interfaces between the gas and the liquid will be two curved surfaces with the same radius of curvature, as shown in Figure 3-11 (a). According to Equation (3-13), the additional pressures produced by the curved liquid surfaces on both sides of the bubble are equal in magnitude $P_{SA} = P_{SB}$ but opposite in direction. This system is in equilibrium, and the liquid keeps steady. To make the liquid flow toward right from left, the liquid pressure on the left side A should be increased, i.e., $P_A > P_B$. The result is that the shapes of the two interfaces will change, the radius of curvature of the surface on the left side will increase, and the radius of curvature of the surface on the right side will decrease, as shown in Figure 3-11 (b). Because the additional pressure is inversely proportional to the radius of curvature, the additional pressures on the two sides will follow $P_{SA} < P_{SB}$ and have the resultant effect of hampering the flow of the liquid toward right. When the pressure difference of the liquid toward right $\Delta P = P_A - P_B$ is just equal to the difference of the additional pressures produced by the two curved surfaces $\Delta P_S = P_{SB} - P_{SA}$, which is toward left, the system is still in equilibrium and the liquid doesn't flow. In the case that the liquid in the narrow tube separated by n gas bubbles, there will be a resistant additional pressure difference of $n\Delta P_S$, as shown in Figure 3-11 (c). So the more the bubbles are, the bigger the total resistant additional pressure to overcome for moving the liquid column would be. When the total pressure difference of the liquid between the two ends of the tube ΔP is equal to $n\Delta P_S$, it is still impossible for the liquid to flow in the tube, which will cause the phenomenon of air embolism.

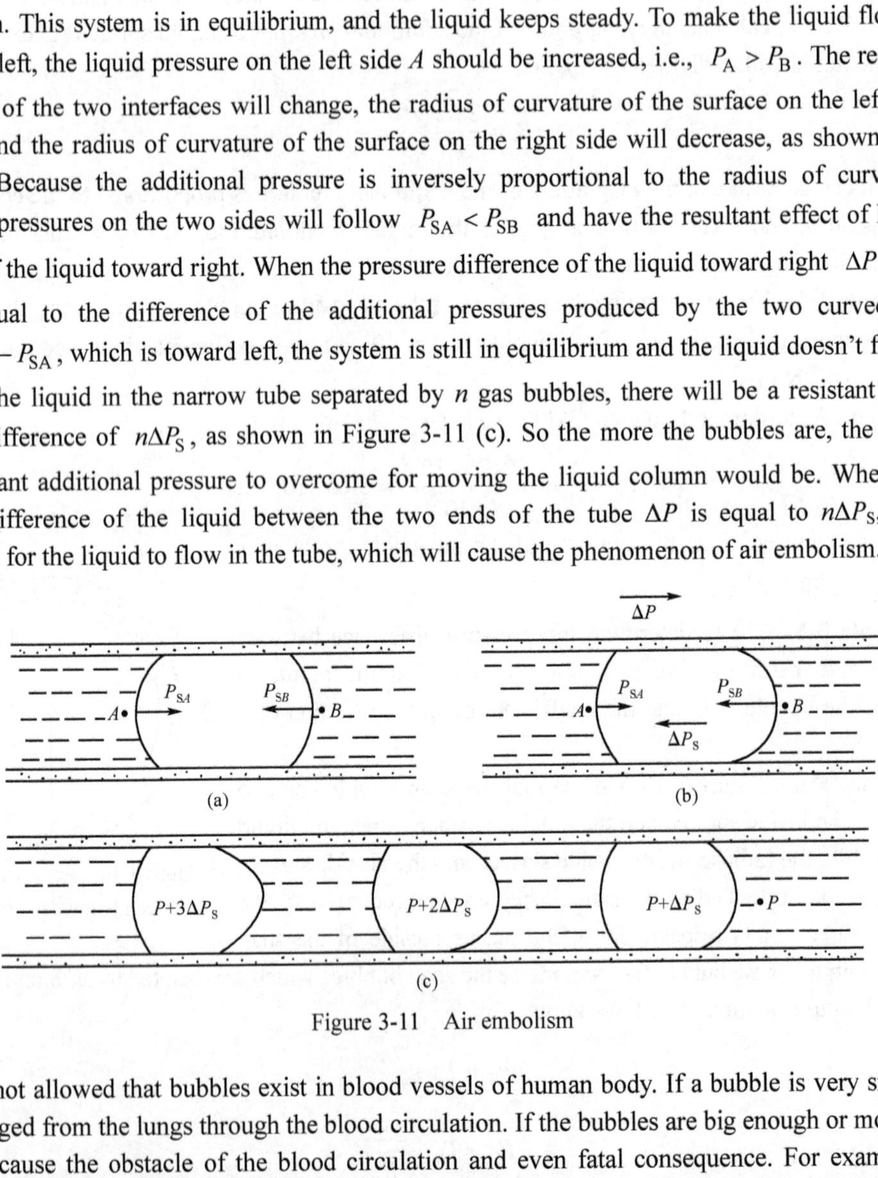

Figure 3-11 Air embolism

It is not allowed that bubbles exist in blood vessels of human body. If a bubble is very small, it can be discharged from the lungs through the blood circulation. If the bubbles are big enough or more enough, they will cause the obstacle of the blood circulation and even fatal consequence. For example, in the process of intravenous injection or transfusion we should pay special attention to prevent the air from being brought into the blood vessels.

In addition, the gas can dissolve in the liquid and the higher the pressure is, the greater the solubility is. For example, when a diver works in deep water, under a high pressure, there will be more gas dissolved in his blood. If he rises to the water surface rapidly, the pressure will suddenly become lower. Then, a large amount of gas dissolved originally in the blood will be freed immediately from the state of dissolution and generate numerous tiny bubbles in the blood; and these tiny bubbles can gather into large bubbles to cause the extensive air embolisms in all organs. This is a life-threatening result known as decompression sickness in medicine. Therefore, when a diver rises from deep water or someone working in a hyperbaric oxygen chamber comes out, there should be an appropriate buffering time to avoid the phenomenon of air embolism.

3.3.3 Surface Adsorption and Surfactant and the Pressure in the Pulmonary Alveoli

1. Surface Adsorption and Surfactant

A small liquid droplet I with the lower density is floating on the surface of another liquid II with the higher density. The upper surface of liquid I is contacted with the air, and its coefficient of surface tension is α_1. The lower surface of liquid I is contacted with the liquid II, as shown in Figure 3-12. There is also the surface tension where the two liquids are in contact with each other, and the coefficient of surface tension of the contacting surface between the two liquids is denoted by α_{12}. For the surface where the liquid II contacts with the air, its coefficient of surface tension is denoted by α_2. At the junction of droplet I, liquid II and the air, three interfaces connect and form a circle. There are three surface tensions acting on the circle, and they are represented respectively by f_1, f_2 and f_{12}, and each of them is tangential to the corresponding surface. There is a tendency for the droplet to be contracted under the actions of the forces f_1 and f_{12}; and there is a tendency for the droplet to be stretched under the force f_2. When the droplet is in equilibrium, the vector sum of f_1, f_2 and f_{12} should be zero. Obviously, only when $f_2 < f_1 + f_{12}$, this situation can exist. So we see that, if it is on the condition of droplet I can remain its shape on the surface of liquid II.

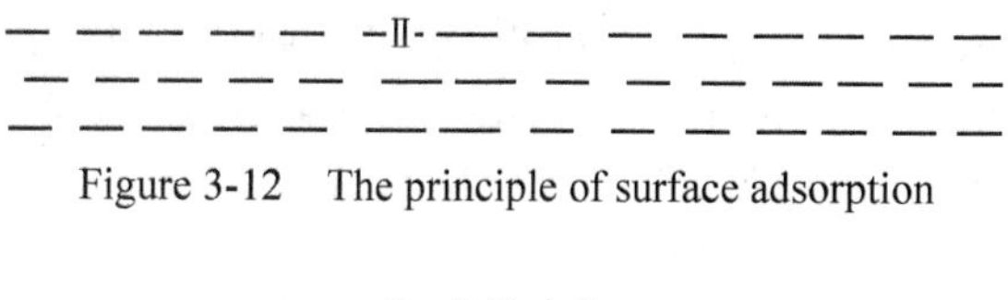

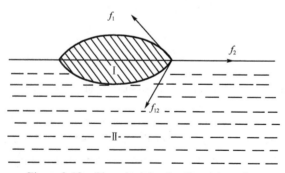

Figure 3-12 The principle of surface adsorption

$$\alpha_2 < \alpha_1 + \alpha_{12}$$

If α_2 is much greater than the other two α_1 or α_{12}, so that

$$\alpha_2 > \alpha_1 + \alpha_{12}$$

In such case, no matter what the shape of the droplet is, the vector sum of f_1 and f_{12} could not be in equilibrium with f_2. Then the droplet I will be stretched into a thin film on the surface of liquid II. The phenomenon that droplet I is stretched into a thin film on the surface of liquid II is called the

surface adsorption. Meanwhile, liquid I is called the **surfactant** of liquid II; liquid II is the **adsorbent** of liquid I. The mass of the surfactant on a unit area of the surface of the adsorbent is called **surface concentration** of the surfactant.

It is relative for a liquid to be a surfactant or an adsorbent. Comparing with its adsorbent, the coefficient of surface tension of the surfactant is smaller. According to Equation (3-12), we know that if put the surfactant into the adsorbent, it will reduce the surface energy and the coefficient of surface tension of the adsorbent. This is the chief character of a surfactant. The coefficient of surface tension of the adsorbent will decrease when the surface concentration of the surfactant increases.

2. Pressure in the Pulmonary Alveoli

Now look at an experiment. Supposing two soap bubbles with different sizes are blown on the two ends of a connecting tube and separated by a closed valve, as shown in Figure 3-13 (a). Bubble A is the larger one with the radius R; and bubble B is the smaller one with the radius r. The pressure outside the bubble is P_0. Here, the pressure in bubble A is

$$P_A = P_0 + \frac{4\alpha}{R}$$

The pressure in bubble B is

$$P_B = P_0 + \frac{4\alpha}{r}$$

Because $R > r$, $P_A < P_B$. When the valve is opened to connect with each other, the air from the smaller bubble will pass into the larger bubble. The smaller one will gradually become atrophic, and the larger one will be expanded gradually, until the bigger bubble's radius of curvature and the radius of curvature of the remaining portion of the smaller one turn into the same, as shown in Figure 3-13 (b).

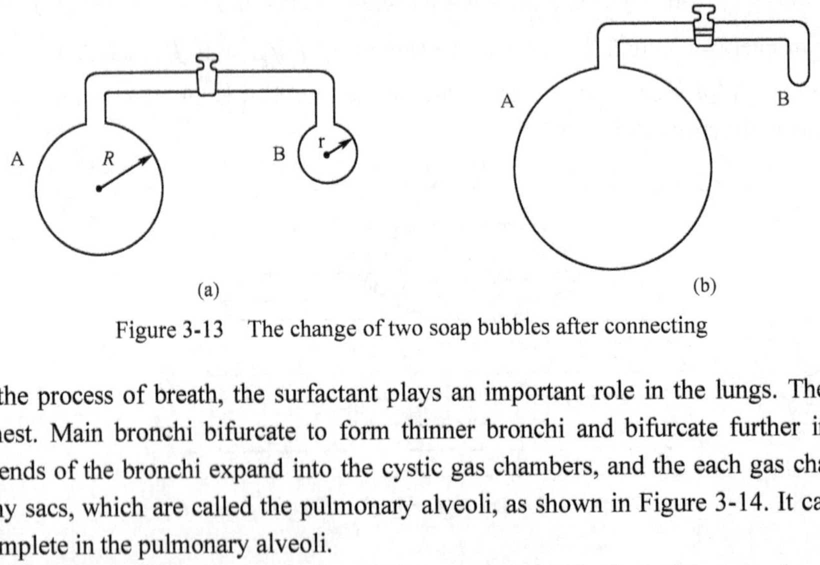

Figure 3-13 The change of two soap bubbles after connecting

During the process of breath, the surfactant plays an important role in the lungs. The lungs locate inside the chest. Main bronchi bifurcate to form thinner bronchi and bifurcate further into more and thinner. The ends of the bronchi expand into the cystic gas chambers, and the each gas chamber divides into many tiny sacs, which are called the pulmonary alveoli, as shown in Figure 3-14. It can be said that the breath complete in the pulmonary alveoli.

For inhaling air into the pulmonary alveoli, the pressure inside the pulmonary alveoli P_i must be lower than the pressure of atmosphere about a quantity about 3 mmHg (i.e., $P_i = -3$ mmHg). Generally, the pressure outside the pulmonary alveoli, i.e., the intrapleural pressure is averagely −4 mmHg, which is 1 mmHg lower than that in the pulmonary alveoli. So the lungs cling to the thoracic wall. During the inspiration, because the diaphragm goes down and the chest expands, a negative pressure of −9 mmHg~10 mmHg forms. It seems capable to enlarge the pulmonary alveoli and accomplish the inspiration. But it is covered by a layer of viscous interstitial fluid with the coefficient of surface tension about 0.05 N/m on the surface of each pulmonary alveolus, the explanation will not be so simple and convenient. If a pulmonary alveolus is looked as a small ball with an average radius of 0.5×10^{-4} m, the additional pressure produced by the surface of the pulmonary alveolus can be determined with Equation (3-13).

$$P_S=\frac{2\alpha}{R}=\frac{2\times0.050\ \text{N/m}}{0.50\times10^{-4}\ \text{m}}=2\times10^{3}\ \text{N/m}^2\approx15\ \text{mmHg}$$

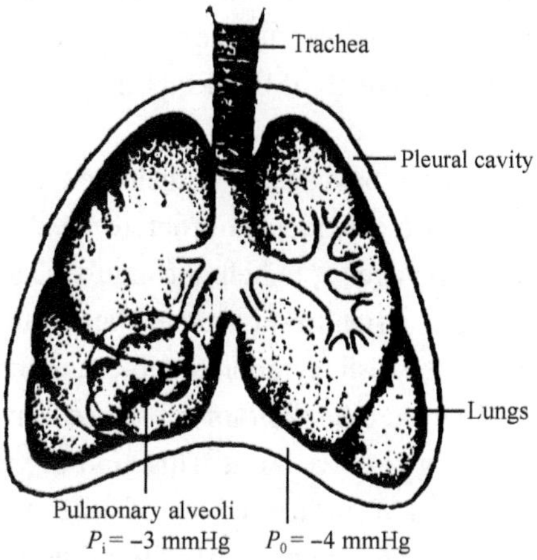

Figure 3-14 Diagram of lungs and pulmonary alveoli

Obviously, the negative pressure produced by the diaphragm's going down and the chest's expanding, is not big enough to overcome this additional pressure and ensure the regular inspiration. This matter is just disposed by the surfactant (something phospholipid) secreted by the walls of the pulmonary alveoli, which could reduce the coefficient of surface tension of the pulmonary alveoli. With the forming of monomolecular layer, this kind of surfactant covers the surface of the viscous liquid on each pulmonary alveolus, and makes the surface tension decrease to 1/15～1/7 of the original value. So that under the negative pressure of the expanded chest, the process of inspiration in the pulmonary alveoli can carry out. On the other hand, because the quantity of surfactant on each pulmonary alveolus is fixed, when the pulmonary alveolus is expanding, the concentration of the surfactant (i.e. the surfactant on a unit area of the surface) will become decreased relatively, results in the relative increase of the surface tension and the additional pressure, so that the expansion of the pulmonary alveolus restricts in a range; when the lungs is shrinking, the concentration of the surfactant on every pulmonary alveolus will become increased relatively, results in the relative decrease of the surface tension and the additional pressure, so that the pulmonary alveolus is kept not atrophying. In this way, for the existence of the surfactant, the surface tension of each pulmonary alveolus could be adjusted and the stabilization of functions of the pulmonary alveoli with different sizes is maintained.

In human lungs there are about 300 million of the pulmonary alveoli with different sizes, and some are connected with each other in the same cystic gas chamber. As the experiment shown in Figure 3-13, if the coefficients of surface tension of the two bubbles are the same, the pressure in the smaller one is higher than the pressure in the bigger one, the gas in the smaller bubble will keep flowing into the bigger one until the smaller one tends to atrophy. But that doesn't take place in the lungs. The reason is also the action of the surfactant as explained above. During the breath, the surfactant can adjust the surface tensions of the pulmonary alveoli of different sizes and stabilize the pressures inside the pulmonary alveoli of different sizes. Thus, the smaller pulmonary alveoli will not become atrophy and the bigger pulmonary alveoli will not be over expanded. During the inspiration, the pulmonary alveoli expands and the concentrations of the surfactant on the pulmonary alveoli decrease, thereby, the coefficients of surface tension and the surface tensions of the pulmonary alveoli are increased, which is beneficial to the expiration; during the expiration, the pulmonary alveoli become smaller and the concentrations of the surfactant on the pulmonary alveoli are increased, thereby, the coefficients of surface tension and the surface tensions of the pulmonary alveoli are decreased, which is beneficial to the inspiration. In the case of the shortage of the surfactant, many pulmonary alveoli can not be stable for the different sizes; and as the surface tensions of the pulmonary alveoli increase, the functions of the pulmonary alveoli are disturbed. That can lead to respiratory distress syndrome, and severe cases can lead to death.

Inside the uterus, fetal pulmonary alveoli are covered by mucus and closed completely under the additional pressures. When the birth is given, although the surfaces of the pulmonary alveoli secrete the surfactant to reduce surface tensions of the mucus, the forceful action of crying loudly is also necessary for the first breath of the newborn baby to overcome the surface tension of the pulmonary alveoli and to survive.

Besides being used in disinfection, sterilization and antisepsis directly, the surfactants are mainly applied in medication to promote the filtration of medicine, to separate the suspension, to be used as suspending agents, to help the emulsification of the oil and the extraction of the effective components, to increase the stabilization of medicine, to improve the absorption of the medicine through the skin, to improve the disintegration of tablets, to intensify the functions of medicines, and so on.

There is other kind of substance which can increase the coefficient of surface tension of the solvent after being dissolved in it. This kind of substance is called the depressant of surface activity. Some of the depressants of surface activity of water are salt, saccharide, starch and so on.

Solid has also the capability of the surface adsorption to the molecules of liquid and gas for reducing its surface energy. Just as the surface of liquid, after being stained with other substances on the surface, the surface energy of the solid will be decreased. The surface of solid has very strong attraction to the molecules adsorbed. In order to removing the adsorbed molecules of the vapor from the surface of a piece of glass thoroughly, the piece of glass will be heated to 400 ℃ in vacuum. The more the area of the surface of the solid is, the stronger the ability of the surface adsorption will be. The amount of the gas adsorbed on the surface of the solid is proportional to the area of the surface of the solid. The amount of the adsorbed gas on a unit area of the surface of the solid is called the **adsorptivity**. When the temperature increases, the adsorptivity will decrease. The adsorptivity is also related with the pressure of the gas and the properties of the solid and the gas. The material of porosity has the larger surface area, so it has the stronger ability of adsorption. For example, the adsorptivity of activated carbon is very high, its ability of adsorption is outstanding especially at low temperature. The volume of the gas adsorbed on a piece activated carbon can be several hundred times of the volume of the activated carbon itself. In medical treatment the kaolin (a kind of white clay powder) the activated carbon are often given to the patients as oral medicine to adsorb bacteria, pigments, toxins decomposed from food, and other organic matters in the gastrointestinal tract. In the production process of medication, the activated carbon and other adsorbents are often used to refine glucose, insulin and other medicines.

Solid can not only adsorb gas but also adsorb the matters dissolved in liquid. In the common used water purifiers, water is lead to flow through the different layers of porous materials in the filter; after being filtered, the harmful substances in the water are adsorbed by the porous materials, so as to achieve the purpose of water purification.

3.4 Phenomenon of Adhesive Layer of Liquid

3.4.1 Soakage and Non-soakage

If some water droplets are put on the surface of clean glass, these droplets will spread the wet the glass; if a drop of mercury is put on the glass, the mercury will automatically reduce into a ball. Thus it can be seen, when the liquid and solid contact, there will be two different phenomena happened at the contacting place. One is that the contacting surface of liquid and solid has the tendency of expanding, so that the liquid can adhere to the solid easily; this phenomenon is called the **soakage**. The other is that the contacting surface of liquid and solid has the tendency of shrinking; this phenomenon is the **non-soakage**.

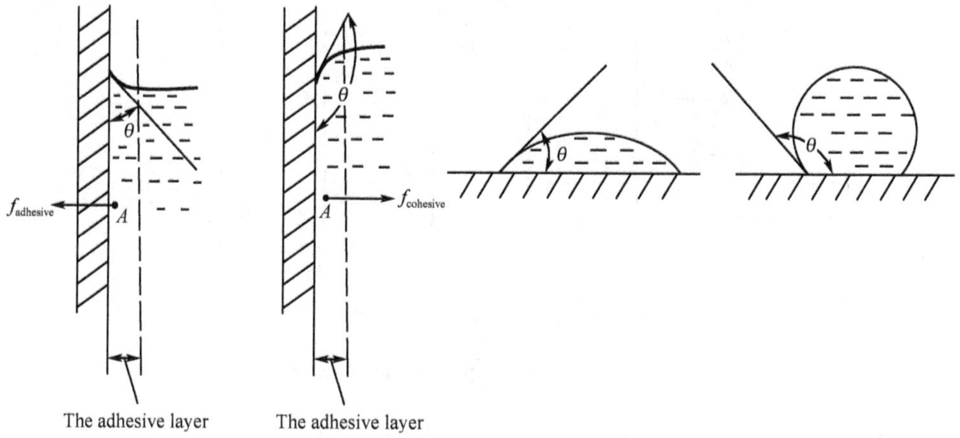

Figure 3-15 Soakage and non-soakage

The phenomena of soakage and non-soakage are usually described by the **contact angle** θ. At the point where the liquid surface and the solid surface are contacted, draw a tangent line of the liquid surface, and the angle between the tangent line and solid-liquid interface is defined as the **contact angle**. As shown in Figure 3-15, when θ is an acute angle, **the liquid soaks the solid**; when θ is zero, **the liquid soaks the solid completely**; when θ is an obtuse angle, **the liquid does not soak the solid**; when θ is 180°, **the liquid can never soak the solid at all.**

The phenomena of soakage and non-soakage depend on the attractions of the molecules of the liquid itself and the molecules of the solid and the liquid. The attractive force between the molecules of the liquid itself is called the **cohesion**. And the attractive force between the molecules of the solid and the liquid is called **adhesion**. Assume that the effective acting distance of the cohesion is l, and the effective acting distance of adhesion is r, there is a layer of liquid at the contacting surface of the liquid and the solid, which has the thickness of the bigger one of l and r, called the **adhesive layer** (as shown in Figure 3-15). For any liquid molecule A within the adhesive layer, it is acted by adhesion on one hand and is acted by the cohesion on the other hand. When the cohesion is bigger than the adhesion, the contacting surface of the liquid and the solid has the tendency of shrinking, i.e., the phenomenon of non-soakage happens. When the adhesion is bigger than the cohesion, the contacting surface of liquid and solid has the tendency of expanding, i.e., the phenomenon of soakage happens.

3.4.2 Capillary Phenomenon

If we put a fine glass tube into a water container with one end, we can see that the level of water inside the tube is higher than the water surface in the container. The smaller the inner diameter of the tube is, the higher the level of the water inside the tube will be, as shown in Figure 3-16 (a). If the glass tube is put into the container filled with mercury, then we can see that the level of the mercury inside the tube is lower than the surface of the mercury in the container, and the finer the tube is, the lower the level of the mercury inside the tube will be, as shown in Figure 3-16 (b). Either the phenomenon that the liquid of soakage rises in the thin tube or the phenomenon that the liquid of non-soakage falls in the thin tube is called the **capillary phenomenon**. The tube which is fine enough for the occurrence of the capillary phenomenon is called **capillary tube**.

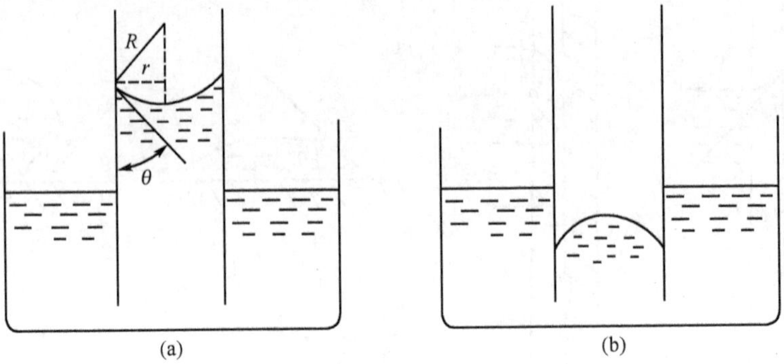

Figure 3-16 The capillary phenomenon

The height to which the liquid rises or falls along the capillary tube can be determined by the additional pressure. As shown in Figure 3-16 (a), the contact angle is assumed to be θ; because water can soak glass, the angle θ is an acute angle and the liquid level inside the tube is a concave surface, so the pressure at the point beneath the surface is less than atmospheric pressure outside the surface; as a result, the liquid inside the tube will rise along the tube wall until the pressure produced by the liquid column is equal to the additional pressure of the curved surface of liquid, i.e.,

$$P_S = \frac{2\alpha}{R} = \frac{2\alpha}{r}\cos\theta = \rho g h$$

Hence

$$h = \frac{2\alpha\cos\theta}{\rho g r} \tag{3-14}$$

where ρ is the density of the liquid, R is the radius of curvature of the curved surface of liquid, r is the inner radius of the capillary tube, α is the coefficient of surface tension of the liquid, and h is the maximum height to which the liquid can rise along the tube.

Similarly, we can determine the height to which the liquid of non-soakage can fall inside the capillary tube.

Example 3-7 When we put a capillary tube vertically into water, the height to which the water rises in the tube is 4 cm. And if we put it into alcohol, the height to which the alcohol rises in the tube is 2 cm. The coefficient of surface tension of water is 73×10^{-3} N/m and the density of alcohol is 0.8×10^{3} kg/m^3. What is the coefficient of surface tension of alcohol?

Solution: According to Equation (3-14), and substituting $\theta = 0$, we have

$$h_1 = \frac{2\alpha_1}{\rho_1 g r}$$

$$h_2 = \frac{2\alpha_2}{\rho_2 g r}$$

To compare the two equations above, we get

$$\alpha_2 = \frac{\alpha_1\rho_2 h_2}{\rho_1 h_1} = \frac{73\times10^{-3}\times0.8\times10^{3}\times2}{1\times10^{3}\times4} = 29.2\times10^{-3}\ \text{N/m}$$

The coefficient of surface tension of alcohol is 29.2×10^{-3}N/m.

The conceptions of the surface tension of liquid, the surface energy, the surfactant, the surface adsorption, the soakage, the capillary phenomenon, and so on are vitally significant in daily life and the production technology, especially in the production, the storage, the usage, and other aspects of medicines.

In the production and the stability's maintenance of some liquid medicines, injections, ointments, pills and other products, the knowledge about the phenomena on liquid surfaces is requisite.

The capillary phenomenon is commonly involved in daily life and the production technology. There exist a lot of tiny ducts in the tissues of animals and plants. The capillary phenomenon plays an important role in the transportation and the absorption of the nutrient and water in the plants' tiny ducts, and in the flow of blood in animals' blood capillaries.

Most porosity materials, such as wood, paper, cloth, cotton yarn, etc., can absorb liquid. The reason for the absorption of liquid is that the liquid of soakage can go deep into the numerous tiny ducts in the solid materials. The tiny ducts in soil play a significant role in absorbing and preserving moisture.

During the preparations of medicines some materials which could reduce the connect angles of the medicinal liquids are mixed appropriately in the medicines to increase the soakage capacity of the medicines and promote the absorption of the medicines, so as to improve curative effects of the medicines.

A Brief Summarization of This Chapter

(1) The pressure formula of an ideal gas: $P=\frac{2}{3}n\left(\frac{1}{2}m\overline{v^2}\right)$ $\overline{e}_k$ or $P=\frac{2}{3}n\overline{e}_k$, where $\overline{e}_k$ is the average transla- tional kinetic energy of a molecule

(2) Avogadro law: $P = nkT$

(3) The relationship between the temperature and the average translational kinetic energy of a molecule of an ideal gas: $\overline{e}_k=\frac{3}{2}kT$

(4) The theorem of equipartition of energy: At the equilibrium state at the temperature of T, for every degree of freedom of one gas molecule has the same average kinetic energy of $\frac{1}{2}kT$

(5) The internal energy of an ideal gas with the mass of M: $E=\frac{M}{\mu}\frac{i}{2}RT=\frac{M}{\mu}\frac{t+r+2s}{2}RT$

(6) The surface tension and the surface energy: $f=\alpha l$; $\Delta E=\alpha\cdot\Delta S$

(7) The additional pressure of a curved surface of liquid: $P_S=\frac{2\alpha}{R}$

Exercises 3

3-1. The gas of hydrogen and the gas of helium are at the same temperature and have the same mole number. Try to answer the following questions about these two kinds of gases:

(1) If they have the same average kinetic energy of a molecule?

(2) If they have the same average translational kinetic energy of a molecule?

(3) If they have the same internal energy?

3-2. When an ideal gas is compressed, its pressure has an increment of 1.01×10^4 Pa and its temperature is kept as 27℃. Determine the number of molecules increased in a unit volume.

3-3. Some ideal gas with the pressure of 1.33 Pa and the temperature of 27℃ is stored in a container. Try to determine the following quantities:

(1) The average translational kinetic energy of a molecule of this gas;

(2) The total average kinetic energy of the molecules in the volume of 1 cm^3.

3-4. When the temperature is increased with 1℃, what is the increment of the internal energy of 1 mole of helium gas?

3-5. Explain the physical meanings of the following expressions:

(1) $\frac{1}{2}kT$ (2) $\frac{3}{2}kT$ (3) $\frac{1}{2}(t+r+s)\ kT$

(4) $\frac{1}{2}(t+r+2s)\ kT$ (5) $\frac{M}{\mu}\frac{1}{2}(t+r+2s)RT$ (6) $\frac{M}{\mu}\frac{3}{2}RT$

3-6. The pressure difference between the inside and the outside of a soap bubble with the radius of 10 cm is 16×10^{-3} Pa. What is the coefficient of surface tension of the liquid soap?

3-7. It is observed that in a capillary the alcohol with the density of 790 kg/m^3 (and with the coefficient of surface tension of 22.7×10^{-3} N/m) rises to the height of 2.5 cm. If the contact angle is assumed to be 30°, what is the radius of the capillary?

3-8. It is know that the coefficient of surface tension of the interface of oil and water is 1.8×10^{-2} N/m. If 1 g of the oil is broken up into small oil drops with the radius of 1.0×10^{-6} m in water. Determine the work done for this process (the density of the oil is supposed to be 900 kg/m^3).

3-9. A U-form tube is positioned vertically and some water is poured into it. The inner radiuses of the two sides of the tube are respectively r_1 and r_2; the contact angle of the water surface is zero; and the coefficient of surface tension of water is α. Determine the height difference between the water levels on the two sides of the U-form tube.

Chapter 4 Thermodynamics

Thermodynamics is a subject for studying the forms and conversional regularities of substances' thermal motions; the theoretical foundations of thermodynamics are the first law of thermodynamics and the second law of thermodynamics. The first law of thermodynamics is the law to study the conservation of energy including heat phenomena; while the second law of thermodynamics specifies the directions and the conditions of processes.

The field for applying these basic thermodynamic laws is very extensive. For example, in animal metabolism processes: a human or animal body, regardless of rest or work, always transforms the chemical energy stored in food into other necessary forms continuously, for maintaining the functions of various organs, systems, tissues and cells of the body. In the metabolic process, the internal energy in an animal body reduces constantly; in order to compensate the reduction of energy, the animal must eat food. The catabolism of part of the food provides the function for the body to do work to the outside system, another part of the food is transformed into the body's heat conducted to the surroundings. This metabolic activity of the animal follows the first law of thermodynamics. The other example is the processes of the traditional Chinese medicine composition and dosage forms, or the extraction and separation of traditional Chinese medicine preparation, in which some problems of chemical reactions and phase changes are often encountered. For solving these problems, we need thermodynamic theories combining with the measured data in practice and the corresponding calculations.

So it is very important for us to learn the content of this chapter well. This chapter focuses on the basic discussion about the first and the second laws of thermodynamics.

4.1 Several Fundamental Concepts of Thermodynamics

In order to discuss the basic theory of thermodynamics more clearly and deeply, we must understand some basic concepts used in thermodynamics first.

4.1.1 Thermodynamic Systems

In thermodynamics, the object (or a group of objects) researched is usually called a **thermodynamic system** (or a **system** for short). And the outside substances are often called the **external surroundings** (or the **surroundings** for short).

4.1.2 Equilibrium State

For a system at some moment, there are a series of characters corresponding to its state, and for a state, we often use one or several physical quantities to describe its characters. In order to describe the state and the change of the state of the system, we can choose some physical quantities from them. These physical quantities for describing the change of the state are called the **state parameters**. The state in which the system exists in the beginning is called the **initial state**, and after a series of changes, the state in which the system exists is called the **final state**.

For a system, when all the state parameters do not change with time, i.e., in each part of the system any one of the physical quantity has the same and unchanged value, we say that this system is in a certain **equilibrium state**. Conversely, in different parts of this system, any one of the state parameters has different values or any one of the state parameters in the system changes with time, and the system is called in a **non-equilibrium state**. In fact, it is impossible to have a system in which all the characters remain unchanged forever in the world. A so-called equilibrium state of a system is only an ideal concept; it is an idealized abstraction for the state of a system under the certain conditions. In this chapter, unless there is a special indication, all the states are considered as the equilibrium states. It should be noted that: an equilibrium state refers to the state in which the macroscopic properties of the system does not change with time. On the microscopic viewpoint, the molecules consisting the system in the equilibrium state are still moving constantly, but only the average effect of molecular motion does not change with time. and in the macroscopic viewpoint, the invariance of this average effect indicates that the system reaches the equilibrium state.

4.1.3 Quasi-static Equilibrium Process

When the state of a system changes with time, or in other words, the system changes from one equilibrium state to another, we say that the system undergoes a **thermodynamic process**. Generally, at any tiny step in the process the state of the system will change and the change of the state must cause the destruction of equilibrium, and before reaching a new equilibrium state, the system will continuously undergo the following tiny step of the process. So in this process the system must experience a series of non-equilibrium states, and this process is called the **non-static equilibrium process** (or the **non-stationary process**).

In thermodynamics, a significant concept is the **quasi-static equilibrium process** (or the **quasi stationary process**). The so-called quasi stationary process is: at every moment in the process, the state of the system is always infinitely close to an equilibrium state, or in other words, the process underwent by the system is composed of a series of equilibrium states.

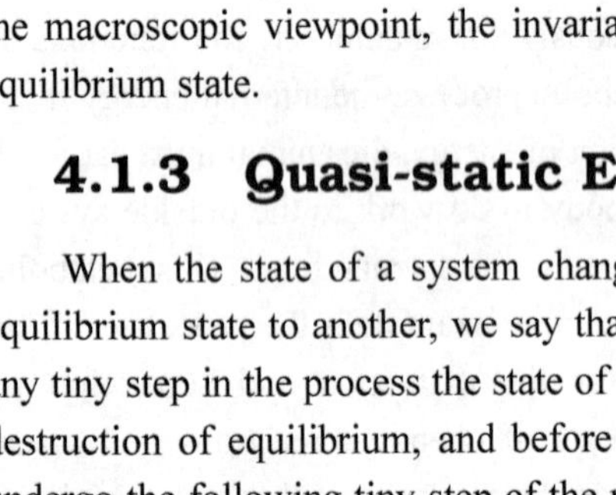

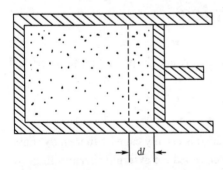

Figure 4-1 The surroundings push the piston to compress the gas

Here, taking the quasi stationary process for an example. A container with a piston contains some gas, as shown in Figure 4-1. The gas inside the container is in thermal equilibrium with the outside (the temperature outside T_0 remains unchanged). The state parameters of the gas are represented by P_0 and T_0. When the gas expands, we assume that the piston is frictionless with its outside in the expansion process. If we make the pressure outside of the gas be less than the pressure inside by a little amount, the gas inside will be allowed to expand slowly. During the expansion process, a process can be regarded as a quasi stationary process if the time for every small expansion step of the gas is longer than the time for the system to reach the next new equilibrium state, and the system is nearly in an equilibrium state at any moment.

Here please think about what process the system will undergo if the piston is compressed rapidly by a strong force.

For a gas system with a certain mass, the state parameters are the pressure *P*, the volume *V* and the temperature *T*. If any two of these parameters are given, the corresponding state of the system will be at an equilibrium state. So in the P–V diagram (or in V–T diagram or P–T diagram) any point corresponds to an equilibrium state, and any curve or straight line corresponds to a quasi-static equilibrium process.

The quasi stationary process is an infinitely slow and idealized process, the actual processes are all carried out in the finite time, i.e., they can not be infinitely slow, but in many cases, the practical processes can be approximated to the quasi stationary processes. In the following discussions, the processes are mainly regarded as the quasi stationary processes.

4.2 First Law of Thermodynamics

4.2.1 Heat and Work

Many facts show that the change of a thermodynamic system's state is always completed by the system through doing work to the surroundings or by the surroundings through transferring heat to the system or by both of them.

Now let's study the work done by a system in a quasi stationary process. As shown in Figure 4-1, a sealed cylindrical container with a movable piston contains a certain amount of gas, and the piston can move around without any friction. Suppose the pressure inside the container is P when the piston moves a little distance of $\mathrm{d}l$, the work done by the expansion of the gas to push the piston is $\mathrm{d}A$

$$\mathrm{d}A = P \cdot S \cdot \mathrm{d}l$$

where S is the area of the piston. Because the volume of the gas increases a quantity of $S \cdot \mathrm{d}l$, or $\mathrm{d}V = S \cdot \mathrm{d}l$, the above equation can be rewritten as

$$\mathrm{d}A = P \cdot \mathrm{d}V \tag{4-1}$$

We can see from the above, if the gas expands, $\mathrm{d}V > 0$, and $\mathrm{d}A > 0$, it suggests that the system does work to the surroundings; if the gas is compressed, $\mathrm{d}V < 0$, and $\mathrm{d}A < 0$, it suggests that the surroundings do work on the system.

Generally speaking, when changing the state of a system through different processes, the works done by the system to the surroundings will be different.

In a quasi stationary process, the work done by the system can be expressed in the P-V diagram, as shown in Figure 4-2, where A and B represent respectively the initial state and the final state of the system, the curve AB represents a quasi stationary compression process. Assume that the volume of the gas in the initial state is V_1, and the volume of the gas in the final state is V_2, by Equation (4-1) we can get the total work done by the system to the surroundings.

$$A = \int_{V_1}^{V_2} P \cdot \mathrm{d}V \tag{4-2}$$

So we know that the area under the curve AB represents the work done by the system to the surroundings. Therefore, the different areas under different curves represent different works done by the system to the surroundings. So we say that the work done by the system to the surroundings is dependent not only on the system's initial and final states but also on the process itself, i.e., the work done by the system to the surroundings is dependent on the path underwent.

As mentioned above, doing work is one of the manners of interactions between the thermodynamic system and surroundings. The surroundings can change the state of a system by doing work on it. Another method to change the state of a thermodynamic system is to transfer heat between the thermodynamic system and the surroundings. Experiments show that, when the system changes from the initial state A to the final state B, which is undergoing different processes, the quantities of heat transferred from the surroundings to the system are different. That is, the quantity of heat absorbed by the system from the surroundings is also dependent on the process path which the system undergoes. Now, we define that, **when a system absorbs heat from the surroundings, the quantity of heat itself is positive; when the system transfers heat to the surroundings, the quantity of heat itself is negative.**

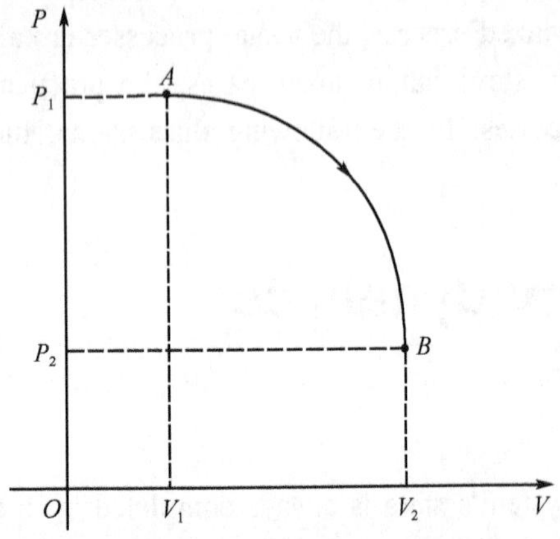

Figure 4-2 The work done by the system to the surroundings is equal to the area under the curve

The fact that the work done by the system to the surroundings and the quantity of heat transferred from the surroundings to the system are both dependent on the process path indicates that the work and the quantity of heat are not the characteristics of the system itself. That is to say, the work and the heat are not dependent on the state of the system, and both of them are not the state parameters of the system. So it is meaningless to say the system's work or the system's heat. The work and the transfer of heat are always accompanied by a specific process which a system undergoes. And it is only meaningful to say the work or the quantity of heat in a process. Well, in thermodynamics what quantity is the state parameter?

In thermodynamics, the internal energy of a system is a quantity, which is dependent only on the system's state and independent of the process, underwent by the system, i.e., the internal energy is the monotropic **function of the state** of the system.

4.2.2 First Law of Thermodynamics

A large number of facts show that, after undergoing a process, for the quantity of heat absorbed by a system Q, one part of it serves as increasing the system's internal energy ΔE, and the other part turns into the work done by the system to the surroundings A. The mathematical expression for this conclusion is

$$Q = \Delta E + A \tag{4-3}$$

This is the **first law of thermodynamics**. When using Equation (4-3), we'd better pay attention to the stipulation for the signs: if the internal energy of a system is increased, ΔE is positive, on the contrary, ΔE is negative; if the system does work to the surroundings, A is positive, on the contrary, if the surroundings do work to the system, A is negative; if the system absorbs heat from the surroundings, Q is positive, on the contrary, if the system releases heat to the surroundings, Q is negative. The first law of thermodynamics is the universal form of the law of conservation and transformation of energy including heat.

4.3 Applications of the First Law of Thermodynamics

As simple applications of the first law of thermodynamics, let's study the transformation of the energy of the ideal gas in some processes.

4.3.1 Isochoric Process

The so-called isochoric process refers to the changing process of the system in which the volume of the gas remains constant. In an isochoric process, because the change of the gas' volume $dV = 0$, we know from Equation (4-2), $A = 0$, and according to the first law of thermodynamics, we have

$$Q = \Delta E$$

It shows that the whole quantity of heat absorbed from the surroundings by the system is served as the increment of the internal energy of the system. Every isochoric process corresponds to a straight line segment parallel to the P-axis in the P-V diagram, as shown in Figure 4-3. If temperatures of the system in the initial and final states are respectively T_1 and T_2, from the knowledge of Chapter 3 we know that the internal energy of the ideal gas is a monotropic function of the temperature, i.e.

$$\Delta E = \frac{M}{\mu}\frac{1}{2}(t + r + 2s)R(T_2 - T_1)$$

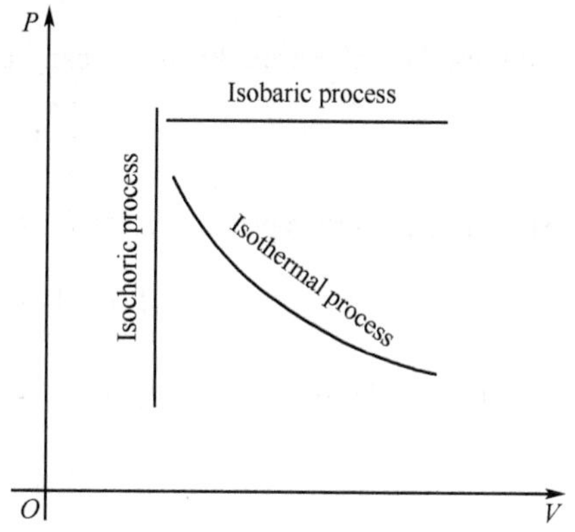

Figure 4-3 Isochoric, isobaric and isothermal processes of the ideal gas

If it is defined that $i=t+r+2s$, we have

$$\Delta E = \frac{M}{\mu}\frac{i}{2}R(T_2 - T_1)$$

where R is the universal gas constant.

For calculating the quantity of heat absorbed by the system from the surroundings, we use the following calculating formula.

$$Q = \frac{M}{\mu}C_V(T_2 - T_1)$$

where C_V is called the **isochoric molar heat capacity**. C_V expresses the quantity of heat absorbed or released by 1 mol of certain gas through an isochoric process, when the temperature increases or decreases 1 degree. The unit of C_V is J/(mol · K).

In an isochoric process, because $Q = \Delta E$, we have

$$\frac{M}{\mu}C_V(T_2 - T_1) = \frac{M}{\mu}\frac{i}{2}R(T_2 - T_1)$$

and

$$C_V = \frac{i}{2}R \tag{4-4}$$

4.3.2 Isobaric Process

An isobaric process refers to the process in which the pressure of system remains constant; every isobaric process corresponds to a straight line parallel to the V axis in the P-V diagram, as shown in Figure 4-3.

In an isobaric process, because the pressure of the gas P is a constant, the work done by the system to the surroundings is

$$A = \int_{V_1}^{V_2} P\mathrm{d}V = P(V_2 - V_1)$$

where V_1 and V_2 represent the volumes in the initial and final states respectively. Then, according to the first law of thermodynamics, we can get

$$Q = \Delta E + P(V_2 - V_1)$$

If C_P represents the quantity of heat absorbed or released by one mole of certain gas in an isobaric process when temperature increases or decreases 1 degree, i.e., what is called the **isobaric mole heat capacity**, the quantity of heat absorbed by the system can be expressed as

$$Q=\frac{M}{\mu}C_P(T_2-T_1)$$

So, the first law of thermodynamics can be rewritten as

$$\frac{M}{\mu}C_P(T_2-T_1)=\Delta E+P(V_2-V_1) \tag{4-5}$$

Because in an isobaric process, $P_1 = P_2$ comes into existence, so we have

$$A=P(V_2-V_1)=P_2V_2-P_1V_1=\frac{M}{\mu}R(T_2-T_1)$$

For the increment of the internal energy, ΔE is

$$\Delta E=\frac{M}{\mu}\frac{i}{2}R(T_2-T_1)$$

So, Equation (4-5) can be rewritten as

$$\frac{M}{\mu}C_P(T_2-T_1)=\frac{M}{\mu}\frac{i}{2}R(T_2-T_1)+\frac{M}{\mu}R(T_2-T_1)$$

In this way, we have

$$C_P=\frac{i}{2}R+R=C_V+R \tag{4-6}$$

Equation (4-6) is called **Mayer's formula**.

4.3.3 Isothermal Process

For a system in an entire process, if the temperature of the system remains constant, this process is called the isothermal process. And an ideal gas should follow the equation of state

$$PV=\frac{M}{\mu}RT$$

In an isothermal process, the temperature of T is fixed, so from the above equation we see that

$$PV=\text{constant}$$

Thus, every isothermal process in the P-V diagram corresponds to a hyperbolic curve called **isotherm**, as shown in Figure 4-3.

Because the internal energy of an ideal gas depends only on the temperature, in an isothermal process, the internal energy of an ideal gas will also be invariant, i.e. $\Delta E = 0$, so from the first law of thermodynamics we know

$$Q=A=\int P\cdot dV=\frac{M}{\mu}RT\int_{V_1}^{V_2}\frac{\mathrm{d}V}{V}=\frac{M}{\mu}RT\ln\frac{V_2}{V_1}=\frac{M}{\mu}RT\ln\frac{P_1}{P_2} \tag{4-7}$$

where T is the thermodynamic temperature of the system, P_1, V_1 and P_2, V_2 represent the pressures and volumes of the system at the initial and final states respectively.

4.3.4 Adiabatic Process

For a system in an entire process, if there is no heat exchange with the surroundings, the process is called **adiabatic process**. In an adiabatic process, because there is no heat exchange, we see that $Q = 0$, and from the first law of thermodynamics we can get

$$A=-\Delta E=-(E_2-E_1)$$

That is, the work done by the system to the surroundings relies completely on the internal energy of the system itself.

Now let's derive the adiabatic equation. We write down the first law of thermodynamics in differential form.

$$dQ = dA + dE \tag{4-8}$$

Because it's an adiabatic process, $dQ = 0$, we have

$$dA = -dE$$

That is

$$PdV = -\frac{M}{\mu}C_V dT \tag{4-9}$$

We make differentials to both sides of the state equation of an ideal gas $PV = \frac{M}{\mu}RT$, then we get

$$PdV + VdP = \frac{M}{\mu}RdT \tag{4-10}$$

With simultaneous Equation (4-9) and Equation (4-10) to eliminate dT, then referring to $C_P = C_V + R$, and after simplifying, we have

$$C_V VdP + C_P PdV = 0$$

To divide the above equation with $C_V P$ and to assume $\gamma = \frac{C_P}{C_V}$, we have

$$\frac{dP}{P} + \gamma\frac{dV}{V} = 0$$

After the integral to the above equation, we have

$$\ln P + \ln V^{\gamma} = \text{constant}$$

That is

$$PV^{\gamma} = \text{constant} \tag{4-11}$$

To combine Equation (4-11) with the state equation of ideal gas simultaneously and to eliminate P or V, we have

$$V^{\gamma-1}T = \text{constant} \tag{4-12}$$

and

$$P^{\gamma-1}T^{\gamma} = \text{constant} \tag{4-13}$$

Equation (4-11), Equation (4-12) and Equation (4-13) are all **equations of an adiabatic process**. Moreover, Equation (4-11) is also called **Poisson formula**, where γ is called the **ratio of the specific heat** of the gas. According to Poisson formula, we can draw a curve in P-V diagram, which is called the **adiabat**. Since $\gamma = \frac{C_P}{C_V} > 1$ for any ideal gas, the adiabat on the P-V diagram is steeper than the isotherm on the P-V diagram, as shown in Figure 4-4.

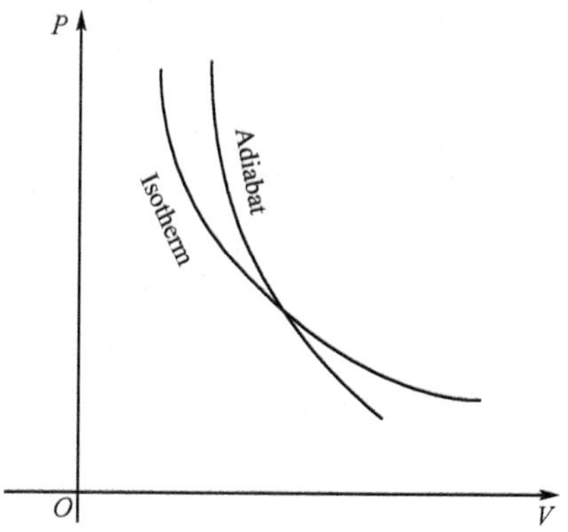

Figure 4-4 An adiabat and an isotherm

Example 4-1 Try to prove that when an ideal gas is in an adiabatic process, the work done by the system to its surroundings follows the formula below.

$$A=\frac{1}{\gamma-1}(P_1V_1-P_2V_2)$$

where γ is the ratio of the specific heat.

Prove: Because the system is in an adiabatic process, then it must follow Equation (4-11), i.e.

$$P_1V_1^\gamma=PV^\gamma=P_2V_2^\gamma$$

The work done by the gas during an adiabatic process is

$$A=\int P\mathrm{d}V=\int_{V_1}^{V_2}P_1V_1^\gamma\frac{\mathrm{d}V}{V^\gamma}=P_1V_1^\gamma\int_{V_1}^{V_2}\frac{\mathrm{d}V}{V^\gamma}$$

$$=\frac{P_1V_1^\gamma}{1-\gamma}(V_2^{1-\gamma}-V_1^{1-\gamma}) \tag{4-14}$$

$$=\frac{1}{\gamma-1}(P_1V_1-P_2V_2)$$

4.4 Carnot Cycle and Efficiency of a Heat Engine

4.4.1 Cyclic Process

If a thermodynamic system changes its state from an initial state by undergoing a series of processes and coming back to the original state or the initial state, and this situation goes round and round, these series of changing processes compose a **cyclic process** (or a **cycle** for short). Each process contained in a cyclic process, or in other words, each process that participates in the composition of the cyclic process is called a **component process**. In the discussion of a cyclic process, the substance underwent the cycle is often called the **working substance**.

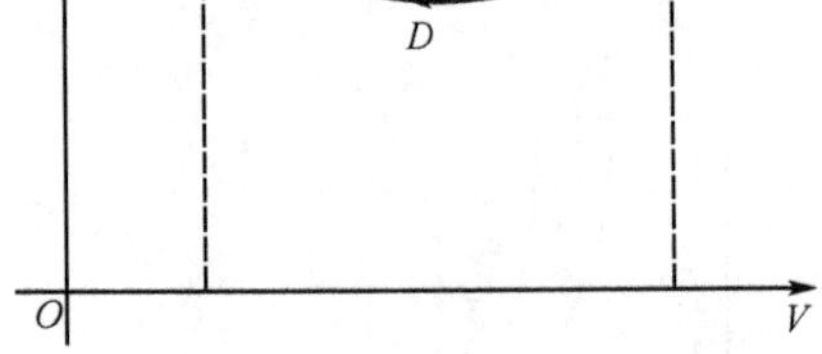

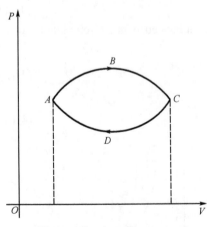

Figure 4-5 A cyclic process

In the P-V diagram, a cyclic process can be represented by a closed curve. As shown in Figure 4-5. Because the internal energy is the monotropic function of the state when the working substance is undergoing a cycle, its internal energy can not change, i.e. after a cycle $\Delta E=0$, which is the main property of the cycle process. If a cyclic process is in the clockwise direction in the P-V diagram, we call this cycle a **direct cycle**; if the cycle is in the counterclockwise direction it is called a **reverse cycle**. For a direct cycle, as shown in Figure 4-5, in the process of *ABC*, the system keeps expanding continuously and doing work to the surroundings, the work is numerically equal to the area under the curve of *ABC*. In the process of *CDA*, the system compresses continuously, the surroundings do work on the system, and the magnitude of the work is equal to the area under the curve of *CDA*. We know that the value of work is positive when the system does work to the surroundings, while it is negative when the surroundings do work on the system. So, we conclude that after undergoing a positive cycle, the system does positive work to the surroundings, the numerical value of the work is the area surrounded by the closed curve of *ABCDA*, and this work is usually called the **useful work** in a cyclic process. For the working substance, after undergoing a cycle and coming back to the initial state, its internal energy keeps unchanged.

According to the first law of thermodynamics, we know that, after an entire cycle, the sum of the quantity of heat absorbed by the system from the surroundings Q_1 must be more than the sum of the quantity of heat released to the surroundings by the system $|Q_2|$. The difference of the total heat absorbed and the total heat released is equal to the useful work of this cycle, denoted by A_{useful}, i.e.

$$A_{useful} = Q_1 - |Q_2| \tag{4-15}$$

We can obtain that, after undergoing a positive cycle, the working substance dispends a part of the heat absorbed from the surroundings for doing work to the surroundings and releases the other part of the heat back to the surroundings then makes the system come back to its initial state.

In the production practice, the devices that utilize the working substances for transforming continuously the quantity of heat absorbed into the work to the surroundings are called **heat engines**.

4.4.2 Efficiency of a Heat Engine

One of the efficacy symbols for a heat engine doing work to the surroundings is its efficiency; that is to say, the efficiency of a heat engine represents that the percentage of heat is transformed into the useful work by the working substance in all the heat it absorbed. The bigger the ratio of the useful work done by the heat engine to the total heat absorbed by the system is, the higher the efficiency of the heat engine will get. The efficiency of a heat engine is denoted by η and defined as

$$\eta = \frac{A_{useful}}{Q_1}\% = \frac{Q_1 - |Q_2|}{Q_1}\% \tag{4-16}$$

The efficiency of a heat engine is expressed in percentage.

Besides heat engines, the devices which can help to obtain the low-temperature is called the **coolers** (or **refrigerators**). A refrigerator operates on the reverse cycle of the working substance.

4.4.3 Carnot Cycle and Its Efficiency

In the practical production, people always search for the heat engine with the maximum efficiency. In 1824 a French engineer Carnot presented a kind of ideal heat engine and proved that the efficiency of this kind of heat engine was the maximum. A heat engine of this kind takes an ideal gas as the working substance and undergoes a quasi stationary cyclic process; in the cycle, all the component processes will go on between two heat reservoirs with constant temperatures. The heat engine of this kind is called the **Carnot heat engine**, the cycle that it undergoes is called the **Carnot cycle**.

A quasi stationary Carnot cycle consists of two isothermal processes and two adiabatic processes. The working substance we discuss is the ideal gas, and the Carnot cycle can be represented by the diagram in Figure 4-6. The curve AB in the diagram is the isotherm with the temperature T_1, the curve CD is the isotherm with the temperature T_2, and curves BC and AD are two adiabats.

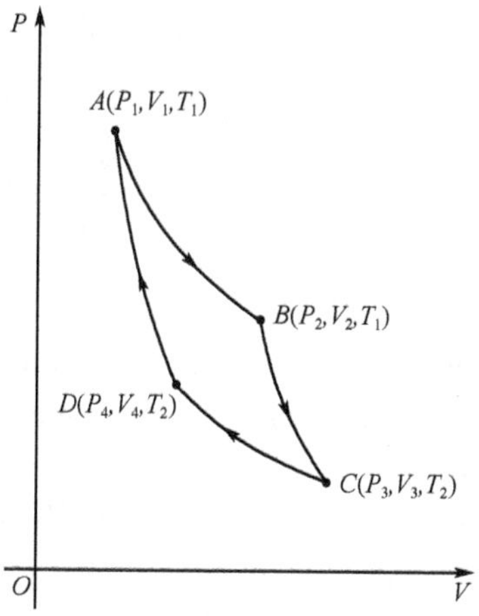

Figure 4-6 Carnot Cycle

Now let's discuss the situations of energy conversion in four component processes and the efficiency of the Carnot cycle.

(1) The process from state A to state B is an isothermal expansion process. In this process, the ideal gas absorbs heat from the surroundings, and the quantity of heat can be derived from Equation (4-7).

$$Q_1 = \frac{M}{\mu} RT_1 \ln \frac{V_2}{V_1}$$

(2) The process from state B to state C is an adiabatic expansion process. The temperature of the ideal gas decreases from T_1 to T_2; it does not have the exchange of heat with the surroundings; due to the expansion, the working substance continues to do work to the surroundings.

(3) The process from state C to state D is an isothermal compression process. In this process, the surroundings do work to the gas and the ideal gas releases heat to the surroundings, the quantity of heat is

$$|Q_2| = \frac{M}{\mu} RT_2 \ln \frac{V_3}{V_4}$$

(4) The process from state D to the initial state A is an adiabatic process, there is no heat exchange between the system and the surroundings, but the surroundings continue to work to the gas, so the temperature of the gas gets back to T_1 from T_2.

From the analysis above we see that, after undergoing an entire Carnot cycle, the total quantity of heat absorbed by the gas is Q_1, the quantity of heat released by the gas is Q_2; because the system gets back to the initial state, the internal energy of the ideal gas is constant. According to the first law of thermodynamics, the useful work done by the working substance (i.e. the ideal gas) to the surroundings is

$$A_{\text{useful}} = Q_1 - |Q_2| = \frac{M}{\mu} RT_1 \ln \frac{V_2}{V_1} - \frac{M}{\mu} RT_2 \ln \frac{V_3}{V_4}$$

In this way, we can get the efficiency of the Carnot cycle.

$$\eta_{\text{Carnot}} = \frac{A_{\text{useful}}}{Q_1} = \frac{Q_1 - |Q_2|}{Q_1} = 1 - \frac{|Q_2|}{Q_1} = 1 - \frac{T_2 \ln \frac{V_3}{V_4}}{T_1 \ln \frac{V_2}{V_1}}$$

The above equation can be simplified; the reason is that states A, D and states B, C are respectively in two adiabats, and the working substance is the ideal gas, so it should meet the adiabatic Equation (4-12), i.e.,

$$T_1 V_2^{\gamma-1} = T_2 V_3^{\gamma-1}, \quad T_1 V_1^{\gamma-1} = T_2 V_4^{\gamma-1}$$

By doing the division of the above two equations and rearranging the result, we have

$$\frac{V_2}{V_1} = \frac{V_3}{V_4}$$

So the efficiency of the Carnot cycle is

$$\eta_{\text{Carnot}} = 1 - \frac{T_2}{T_1} \tag{4-17}$$

This is the efficiency of the Carnot cycle. The above equation shows that the efficiency of a Carnot engine is dependent only on the temperatures of the two heat reservoirs. The higher the temperature of the reservoir with the high temperature is, and the lower the temperature of the heat reservoir with the low temperature is, the higher the efficiency of the Carnot cycle will be. The above equation also shows that the temperature of the heat reservoir with a high temperature can not be infinite, and the temperature of the heat reservoir with a low temperature can not be zero, so the efficiency of a Carnot cycle can never be 100%. That is to say, it is impossible to transform the quantity of heat absorbed from the heat reservoir with the high temperature into the useful work completely; a part of this heat must be transferred to the heat reservoir with low temperature.

Example 4-2 For 1 mole of some monatomic ideal gas, it undergoes a cyclic process as shown in Figure 4-7, where AB is an isotherm, AC is an isochore, and BC is an isobar. $V_A = 3\ \text{m}^3$ and $V_B = 6\ \text{m}^3$

are known. What is the efficiency of this cyclic process?

Solution:

(1) $A \to B$ is a process of isothermal expansion, so the system absorbs heat from its surroundings, and the numerical value of the heat is

$$Q_{AB} = RT_A \ln \frac{V_B}{V_A} = RT_A \ln 2$$

(2) $B \to C$ is a process of isobaric compression, so the system releases heat to its surroundings, and the numerical value of the heat is

$$|Q_{BC}| = C_P (T_B - T_C)$$

(3) $C \to A$ is an isochoric process and its temperature rises in this process; then the system absorbs heat, and the numerical value of the heat is

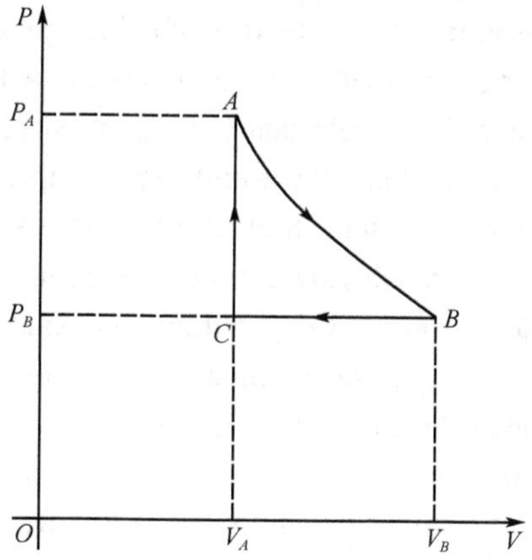

Figure 4-7 Diagram for Example 4-2

$$Q_{CA} = C_V (T_A - T_C)$$

Because $A \to B$ is an isothermal process, then $T_A = T_B$; because $B \to C$ is an isobaric process, then $\frac{V_C}{T_C} = \frac{V_B}{T_B}$, that is $T_C = \frac{1}{2} T_B = \frac{1}{2} T_A$. The efficiency is

$$\eta = \frac{Q_{AB} + Q_{CA} - |Q_{BC}|}{Q_{AB} + Q_{CA}} = \frac{RT_A \ln 2 + C_V (T_A - T_C) - C_P (T_B - T_C)}{RT_A \ln 2 + C_V (T_A - T_C)}$$

The working substance is a monatomic ideal gas, so $C_V = \frac{3}{2} R$. Substitute $T_A = T_B$ and $T_C = \frac{1}{2} T_A$ to the above formula, we have

$$\eta = \frac{RT_A \ln 2 + \frac{3}{4} RT_A - \frac{5}{2} R \cdot \frac{1}{2} T_A}{RT_A \ln 2 + \frac{3}{2} R \cdot \frac{1}{2} T_A} = \frac{\ln 2 + \frac{3}{4} - \frac{5}{4}}{\ln 2 + \frac{3}{4}} = 13.4\%$$

4.5 Second Law Thermodynamics

The first law of the thermodynamics confirms that the energy in any changing process must be conservational in nature. However, some of the changing processes of energy conservation can not necessarily realize, that is to say, the first law of thermodynamics does not indicate the directions of the processes, it was the second law of thermodynamics that can determine the problem of processing directions. The second law of thermodynamics is found gradually in researches on the cases of how to improve the efficiencies of heat engines; it is another basic law independent of the first law of thermodynamics. The first and the second laws of thermodynamics constitute together the main theory foundations of thermodynamics.

4.5.1 Second Law of Thermodynamics

There are many statements of the second law of thermodynamics in texts. The most common two are Kelvin statement and Clausius statement of the second law of thermodynamics.

Kelvin statement: It is impossible to devise such a cycle, the sole effect of which is to absorb energy in the form of heat from a single thermal reservoir and to deliver an equivalent amount of useful work without producing any other effects. It should be pointed out that in Kelvin statement, "a single thermal" reservoir refers to the thermal reservoir with a uniform and constant temperature. On the other hand, this statement emphasizes that it is impossible for all the quantity of heat absorbed to be converted into the useful work completely without other effects. If there are other effects, it is possible to transform all the heat absorbed from a single thermal reservoir into the useful work completely.

Clausius statement: It is impossible to transfer heat from a lower temperature body to a higher temperature body without causing other changes. Or we can simply say: **Heat can never flow spontaneously from a low-temperature object to a high-temperature object.** Clausius statement indicates that when any two objects with different temperatures are contacted, the heat always passes from the high-temperature object automatically to the lower-temperature object, and finally they reach a common temperature. In daily life, we can never observe the phenomenon that heat passes to the high-temperature object automatically from the low-temperature object, so that the temperature difference between the two objects becomes bigger and bigger. Obviously, this phenomenon, if it would exist, does not violate the first law of thermodynamics, but the changing process corresponding to this phenomenon is impossible, that is to say, any spontaneous changing process of substance has its certain direction.

Although the above two statements of the second law of thermodynamics are in different expressions, they are in fact equivalent. If the first law of thermodynamics shows that the energy conservation is indisputable for any object in any process of change, then the second law of thermodynamics indicates further that not all the changing processes, in which the energy conservation is indeed in existence, can be realized automatically. This law points out that a spontaneous changing process of substance is directional; for some changing processes if the directions are changed, the processes can automatically proceed; while for others if the directions are opposite, the processes can not proceed automatically.

4.5.2 Reversible and Irreversible Processes

To discuss the problems about the directions of thermodynamic processes further, it is necessary to introduce the two basic concepts of reversible and irreversible processes. A system starts from an initial state and reaches another state via a process which consists of a series of component changing processes. If the system can come back from the final state to the initial state along the original path in the reverse direction, meanwhile, the system and the surroundings are fully recovered, then the original process is a **reversible process**; otherwise, the process is an **irreversible process**.

For a simple pendulum, if there is no resistance from the air and other friction, after leaving some position in a period, it will return to the original position, the surroundings and the system itself does not have any change, so this kind swing of the pendulum can be considered as a reversible process. The heat can flow from a high-temperature object to a low-temperature object; although its inverse process, i.e., in which heat transferred from a cooler body to a hotter one can also be realized, it can only be achieved by the help of the work done by the surroundings (such as a refrigerator). It must cause a change of the surroundings. Therefore, the heat transferring process is an irreversible process.

Kelvin statement of the second law of thermodynamics points out that the process of converting work into heat is an irreversible process. Moreover, Clausius statement indicates that the heat transferring process is another irreversible process. So, every expression about an irreversible process can be considered as a statement of the second law of thermodynamics.

4.5.3 Statistical Significance of the Second Law of Thermodynamics

For an isolated thermodynamic system, any process, which happens inside the system, always goes on from the state of small probability towards the one of big probability; or to say that according to the microscopic viewpoint, for an isolated thermodynamic system, any process, which happens inside the system, always goes on from the macroscopic state which includes less microscopic states towards the macroscopic state which includes more microscopic states. This is the statistical significance of the second law of thermodynamics. Now let's interpret the statistical significance of the second law of thermodynamics with the example of the free expansion of gas.

Suppose there is a container with a partition in the middle, as shown in Figure 4-8. A and B are the two parts of the container divided by the partition. A is filled with some gas and B is kept the vacuum. First, assume that there is only one molecule a in part A. After removing the partition, we can guess molecule a will move in A for a while and in B for another while. Molecule a has equal opportunity to be moving in A or B. That is, the probabilities for molecule a to be moving in A and in B are both 1/2.

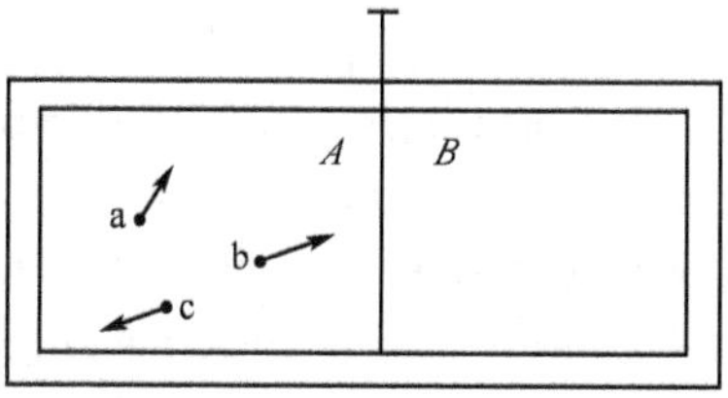

Figure 4-8 Free expansion of a gas

Then, assume there are three molecules a, b and c in part A at first; after removing the partition, we know that the three molecules will be moving in the whole container. Moreover, there can be eight probable distributions of the three molecules in parts A and B, which is listed in Table 4-1.

Table 4-1 Probable distributions of three molecules

	1	2	3	4	5	6	7	8
A	abc	ab	ac	bc	a	b	c	0
B	0	c	b	a	bc	ac	ba	abc

From Table 4-1 we see that, there is only a probability of 1/8 for the three molecules to return back into part A at the same time. It can be proved mathematically that if there are N molecules in the container, then the probable distributions of these N molecules will be $1/2^N$. We all know that any macroscopic system contains numerous molecules or atoms. For 1 mole of gas, the number of its molecules is about 6.02×10^{23}. So after the free expansion the probability for all the molecules to be collected to the original region is only $\dfrac{1}{2^{6.02\times10^{23}}}$. It is so tiny a result that the opportunity of the phenomenon to happen in the real situation for the system of gas is considered impossible. In fact, this essentially reflects that any process occurring inside the system always goes on from the macroscopic state with the smaller probability towards the macroscopic state with the larger probability; and any reverse process can never occur on the condition without any change in the surroundings. This is the statistical significance of the second law of thermodynamics.

4.5.4 Carnot's Theorem

Before the first and the second laws of thermodynamics were found, based on the analysis of various factors deciding the conversions of the heat and the work in steam engines and general heat engines, French engineer Carnot brought forward Carnot's theorem. Its contents are as follows.

(1) All the reversible heat engines working between the same high-temperature heat reservoir and the

same low-temperature heat reservoir have the same efficiency, and this efficiency is independent of the working substances.

(2) The efficiencies of all the irreversible heat engines working between the same high-temperature heat reservoir and the same low-temperature heat reservoir must be less than the efficiency of the reversible heat engine working in the same condition.

All the heat reservoirs mentioned above are the heat reservoirs with the uniform and constant temperatures, and the reversible heat engines are the Carnot's heat engines. Carnot's theorem can be proved with the first and the second laws of thermodynamics.

4.6 Entropy and Principle of Entropy Increase

We have many statement forms to express the second law of thermodynamics, although these statement manners are equivalent, obviously, it is very inconvenient for us to judge whether an arbitrary process can go on automatically by these statements. The reason is that, for the spontaneous processes, each process has its corresponding standard for judging on the possibility. One example is the heat transferring process. In this case, heat always flows automatically from the high-temperature object to the low-temperature object until the two objects get the same temperature; here, the standard for judging on the direction and the limit of heat transferring process is temperature. Another example is the free diffusion process of the gas. The gas molecules are always diffused from the region of higher density to the region of lower density until the two regions have the same uniform density; here, the standard for judging the direction and the limit of the diffusion process is the molecular numerical density. There are many phenomena in nature similar to these, and each process has its own standard for judging, so it was thought that whether a common standard can be found in the thermodynamic systems for judging the directions of the processes. The answer is yes, and this standard is a function of the state **entropy**.

4.6.1 Entropy

According to the Carnot cycle and its efficiency, we know that

$$\eta_{\text{Carnot}} = \frac{Q_1 - |Q_2|}{Q_1} = \frac{T_1 - T_2}{T_1}$$

Rearrange the above equation, we have

$$\frac{Q_1}{T_1} + \frac{Q_2}{T_2} = 0$$

This formula indicates that for the Carnot cycle, the algebraic sum of the ratio $\frac{Q}{T}$ is zero, where Q is the heat that the system absorbed from its surroundings and T was the very temperature that it absorbed the heat.

This conclusion is also suitable for any reversible cycles. The reason is that we can divide this reversible cycle into many infinitesimal Carnot cycles, as shown in Figure 4-9. For each tiny Carnot cycle, the above conclusion is applicable. By summing these infinitesimal Carnot cycles, we have

$$\sum_i \frac{\Delta Q_i}{T_i} = 0$$

In case of the limit, i.e., when the number the tiny Carnot cycles tends to infinity, the sum to the quantity of $\Delta Q_i/T_i$ for all these tiny Carnot cycles will become the integral to the quantity of $\mathrm{d}Q/T$ along the path of this arbitrary cyclic process, so there is

$$\oint \frac{\mathrm{d}Q}{T} = 0 \qquad (4\text{-}18)$$

Equation (4-18) is called **Clausius equality**.

Now let's assume that an arbitrary reversible cycle is divided into two component processes, as shown in Figure 4-10. One process is AL_1B, and the other is BL_2A. So Clausius equality can be rewritten as

$$\oint \frac{\mathrm{d}Q}{T} = \int_{A(L_1)}^{B} \frac{\mathrm{d}Q}{T} + \int_{B(L_2)}^{A} \frac{\mathrm{d}Q}{T} = 0$$

By the equation above we have

$$\int_{A(L_1)}^{B} \frac{\mathrm{d}Q}{T} = \int_{A(L_2)}^{B} \frac{\mathrm{d}Q}{T}$$

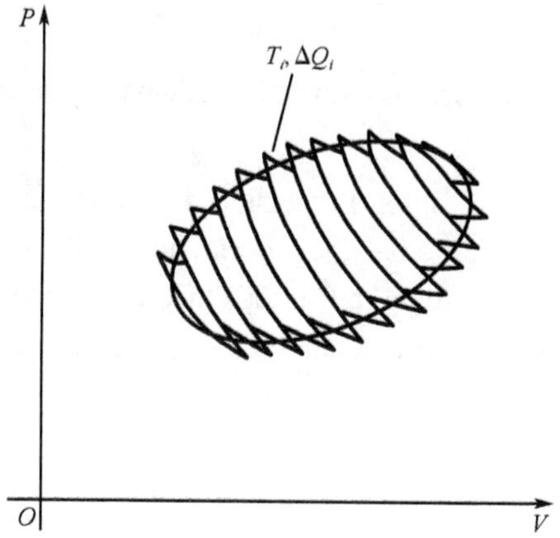

Figure 4-9 A reversible cycle is divided into numerous mini Carnot cycles

It indicates that the integral value of $\int_A^B \frac{\mathrm{d}Q}{T}$ is independent of the path from equilibrium state A to another equilibrium state B, but depends only on the initial and final states.

We know that the work done by a conservative force is independent of the path, but depends only on the initial and final positions, and then we have introduced the difference between the potential energies of a particle at the initial and the final states. Similarly, according to the above conclusion, i.e., the characteristic of $\int_{A(L_1)}^{B} \frac{\mathrm{d}Q}{T} = \int_{A(L_2)}^{B} \frac{\mathrm{d}Q}{T}$, we can now introduce a function, which is only related to the state of the system in thermodynamics. This function is the **entropy**, it is denoted as S, and written as the following formula.

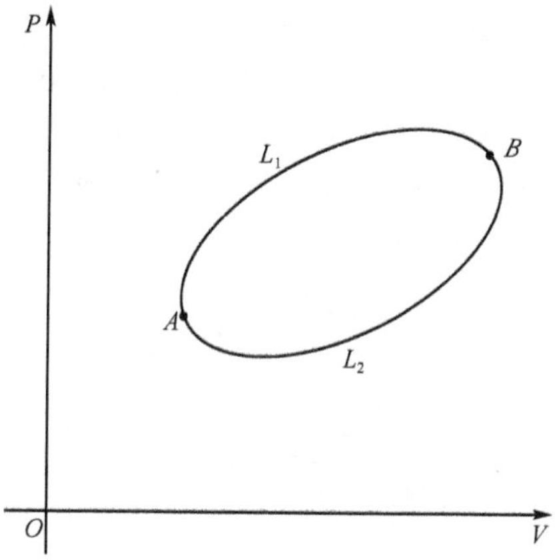

Figure 4-10 A reversible cycle

$$S_B - S_A = \int_A^B \frac{\mathrm{d}Q}{T}$$

where A and B represent the two equilibrium states given arbitrarily, S_A is the entropy of the system in the initial state, and S_B represents the entropy of the system at the final state. We should notice that, the value of the entropy at the final state S_B contains the value of the entropy at the initial state S_A, in general, for a thermodynamic system, the quantity which has the real practical significance is the amount of the change of the entropy from the initial state to the final state, i.e., the **entropy change** or the **difference of entropy** denoted by ΔS

$$\Delta S = S_B - S_A = \int_A^B \frac{\mathrm{d}Q}{T} \qquad (4\text{-}19)$$

The unit of entropy is J/K.

4.6.2 Principle of Entropy Increase

The above discussion shows that, for a reversible process, its entropy difference between the final state and the initial state can be obtained by Equation (4-19), i.e.

$$\Delta S = S_B - S_A = \int_A^B \frac{dQ}{T}$$

If the process is a reversible adiabatic process, then $dQ = 0$, so

$$\Delta S = S_B - S_A = 0$$

That is, for a reversible adiabatic process, the entropy of the system will remain fixed. While for an irreversible adiabatic process, how will the entropy of the system change? Let's discuss it as follows.

According to Carnot's theorem, we know that the efficiency of any irreversible heat engine working between two temperatures is less than the efficiency of the reversible heat engine working in the same conditions, that is

$$\frac{Q_1 - |Q_2|}{Q_1} < 1 - \frac{T_2}{T_1}$$

Then the above formula can be rewritten as

$$\frac{Q_1}{T_1} + \frac{Q_2}{T_2} < 0$$

According to the above analysis to the principle we can infer that for any irreversible cycle, the following formula is suitable.

$$\oint \frac{dQ_{\text{irreversible}}}{T} < 0 \tag{4-20}$$

Equation (4-20) is called Clausius inequality. For further discussion, we assume that there was such a cycle passed through an irreversible process the system proceeds from A to B, expressed as the dotted line in Figure 4-11. Then through a reversible process from B to A, expressed as the solid line in Figure 4-11, the system returns and this constitutes a cycle. Since the former process from A to B is an irreversible process, the whole cycle is still an irreversible cycle. According to Equation (4-20) we have

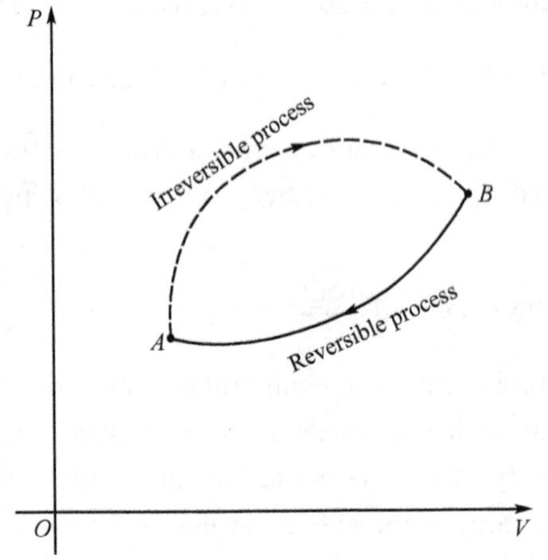

Figure 4-11 An irreversible cyclic process

$$\int_A^B \frac{dQ_{\text{irreversible}}}{T} + \int_B^A \frac{dQ_{\text{reversible}}}{T} < 0$$

That is

$$\int_A^B \frac{dQ_{\text{irreversible}}}{T} - \int_A^B \frac{dQ_{\text{reversible}}}{T} < 0$$

Because

$$\int_A^B \frac{dQ_{\text{reversible}}}{T} = S_B - S_A$$

The above formula can be written as

$$\Delta S = S_B - S_A > \int_A^B \frac{dQ_{\text{irreversible}}}{T} \tag{4-21}$$

Equation (4-21) is a universal inequality for any irreversible processes to obey; it is the mathematical expression of the second law of thermodynamics for any irreversible processes. If the irreversible process is adiabatic, while, $dQ_{\text{irreversible}} = 0$, according to Equation (4-21) we have

$$\Delta S = S_B - S_A > 0$$

To sum up, when the system undergoes a reversible adiabatic process, its entropy is numerically invariant; when the system undergoes an irreversible adiabatic process, its entropy will numerically increase. That is to say, for an isolated thermodynamic system, when it proceeds from an equilibrium state to another equilibrium state, its entropy would never be reduced. This conclusion is called the **principle of entropy increase**.

All the spontaneous processes in nature are irreversible processes. So, for any spontaneous process occurs in an isolated system, its entropy always increases. After getting the equilibrium state, the entropy of the system reaches the maximum. Therefore, the entropy is the standard for judging the direction and the extent of the process proceeding in an isolated system.

4.6.3 Calculation of the Entropy Change

Entropy is a function only of the state of a system regarding the definition of entropy. The entropy is confirmed when a certain equilibrium state of a system is achieved. And the entropy is independent of the path to obtaining the state. We have two very useful methods to calculate the entropy.

(1) For a thermodynamic system, the entropy change between any two given equilibrium states is equal to the integral of $\mathrm{d}Q/T$ along any reversible process, which connects these two equilibrium states.

(2) For a system undergoes an irreversible process from initial equilibrium state to another final equilibrium state, the methods to calculate the entropy change between the initial and final states in the irreversible process are as follows: ①We can assume a reversible process, which connects the same two initial and final states, and then use Equation (4-19) to work out the entropy change. ②We can take the entropy as a state parameter and calculate its function of expression with the state, and then substitute the values of the parameter of the initial and final states into the function to calculate the entropy change. ③For a certain thermodynamic system, we can draw a diagram of the value of entropy with another parameter corresponding to a series of equilibrium states, for example, *T-S* diagram in physical chemistry, then using this diagram we can calculate the entropy change between the initial and final states.

Example 4-3 What is the entropy change in melting 1 kg of ice at 0℃ into water at 0℃ (The heat of fusion of ice is $\lambda = 3.35\times10^5\,\mathrm{J/kg}$)?

Solution: When the process takes place, the temperature is constant, T = 273 K. Therefore, the entropy change is

$$\Delta S = \int\frac{\mathrm{d}Q}{T} = \frac{Q}{T} = \frac{m\cdot\lambda}{T} = \frac{1\times3.35\times10^5}{273} = 1.23\times10^3\,\mathrm{J/K}$$

Example 4-4 What is the entropy change in warming 1 kg of water from 0℃to 10℃ [The isobaric specific heat of water is $C_P = 4.18\times10^3\,\mathrm{J/(kg{\cdot}K)}$]?

Solution:

$$\Delta S = \int\frac{\mathrm{d}Q}{T} = \int\frac{mC_P\mathrm{d}T}{T} = mC_P\int_{273}^{283}\frac{\mathrm{d}T}{T} = 1\times4.18\times10^3\times\ln\frac{283}{273} = 1.5\times10^2\,\mathrm{J/K}$$

A Brief Summarization of This Chapter

(1) The state equation of an ideal gas: $PV = \frac{M}{\mu}RT$

(2) The first law of thermodynamics: $Q = \Delta E + A$

(3) Quantity of heat: $Q = \frac{M}{\mu}C(T_2 - T_1)$

(4) Internal energy: $\Delta E = \frac{M}{\mu}\frac{i}{2}R(T_2 - T_1)$

(5) Work: $A = \int_{V_1}^{V_2} P\mathrm{d}V$

(6) The isochoric molar heat capacity: $C_V = \frac{i}{2}R$

(7) The isobaric molar heat capacity: $C_P = C_V + R$ (Mayer's formula)

(8) The adiabatic process: $PV^{\gamma} = \text{constant}$

(9) The efficiency of a heat engine: $\eta = \frac{A_{\text{useful}}}{Q_1}\% = \frac{Q_1 - |Q_2|}{Q_1}\%$

(10) The efficiency of a Carnot heat engine: $\eta_{\text{Carnot}} = 1 - \frac{T_2}{T_1}$

(11) The calculation of the entropy change: $\Delta S = S_B - S_A = \int_A^B \frac{\mathrm{d}Q}{T}$

Exercises 4

4-1. What are the physical meanings of the signs of the physical quantities Q, A and ΔE in the equation of the first law of thermodynamics $Q = A + \Delta E$? Is it possible to express the first law of thermodynamics with the equation of $Q+A=\Delta E$? If it is possible, how will we define the signs for the quantities of Q, A and ΔE?

4-2. How will the quantities of the pressure P, the volume V and the temperature T change, if an ideal gas is undergoing an adiabatic expansion process or an adiabatic compression process?

4-3. For a certain amount of some gas, it absorbs the quantity of heat of 800 J and does the work of 500 J to the surroundings simultaneously when it changes from one state to another. What is the quantity of the increment of its internal energy?

4-4. Under the fixed pressure of 1.5×10^5 Pa, the volume of gas changes from 0.1 m^3 to 0.5 m^3, and the heat absorbed by the system is 9×10^4 J. Determine the quantity of the increment of the system's internal energy.

4-5. If a system changes from the initial state to the final state through the path of l_1, it absorbs the quantity of heat of 400 J. When the surroundings does the work of 200 J to the system, the system will come back to the final state from the initial state through another path of l_2, and releases a quantity of heat of 500 J. Determine the work done by the system to the surroundings through the path l_1.

4-6. Try to prove the Mayer's formula.

4-7. When a gas is expanded from the volume of V_1 to the volume of V_2, the relationship between the pressure and volume of the gas is $(P + \frac{a}{V^2})(V - b) = K$, where a, b and K are constants. Try to calculate the work done by the gas to the surroundings.

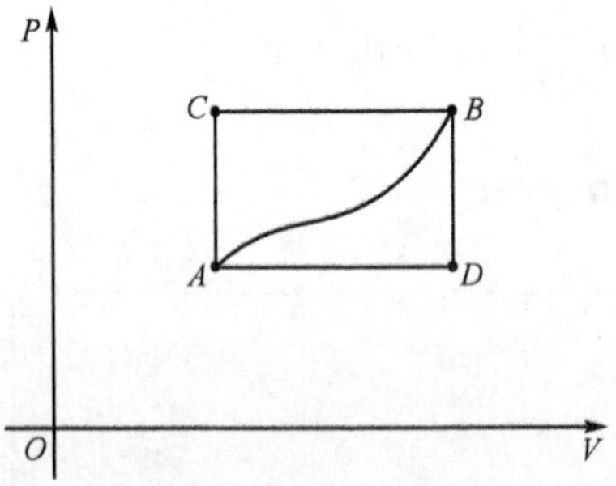

Figure for Exercise 4-8

4-8. As shown in Figure for Exercise 4-8, when a system proceeds from the initial state A to the final state B along the path of ACB, a quantity of heat of 500 J is transferred into the system. Meanwhile, the system does the work of 100 J to the surroundings.

(1) If the system proceeds along the path of ADB, the work done by the system to the surroundings will be 50 J, now, what is the quantity of heat transferred into the system?

(2) if $E_D - E_A = 150$ J, determine respectively the quantities of heat absorbed by the system along the path AD and the path DB.

(3) If the system returns to the state A from the state B along the curve

of *BA*, the work done by the surroundings to the system is 70 J, try to decide: will the system absorb or release heat? And what is the quantity of heat transferred?

4-9. In Figure for Exercise 4-9, a certain changing process of an ideal gas composed of some monatomic molecules is shown. If the system proceeds from state Ⅰ to state Ⅱ along with a straight line, determine the molar heat capacity of the system in this process.

4-10. One mole of some monatomic ideal gas has a quasi stationary cycle along the route ABCDA as shown in Figure for Exercise 4-10. If the isochoric molar heat capacity of the gas is known as $C_V = \frac{3}{2}R$, determine the efficiency of the cycle.

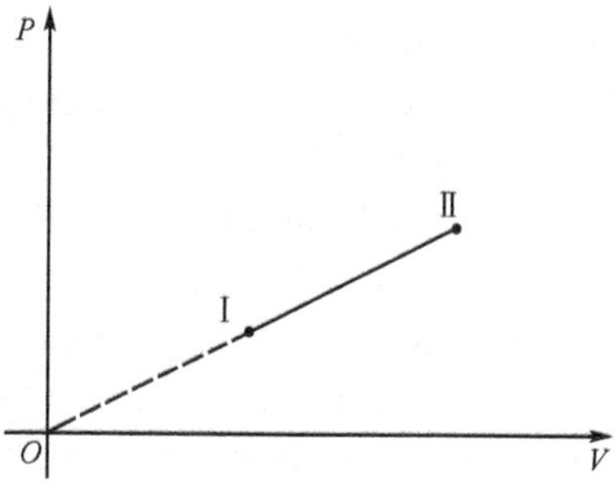

Figure for Exercise 4-9

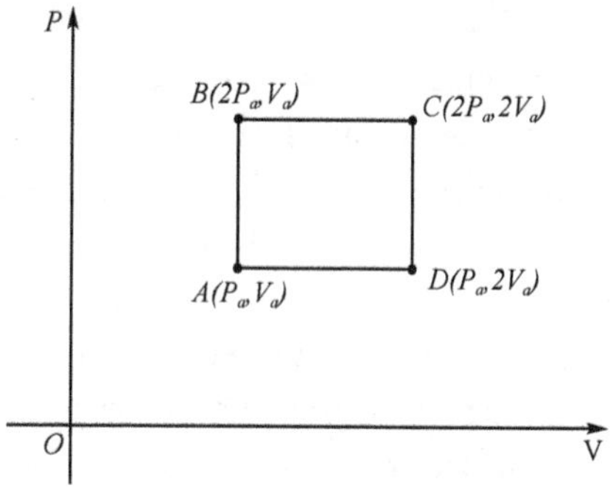

Figure for Exercise 4-10

4-11. A Carnot heat engine is working between the temperatures of 1000 K and 3000 K, depended on the efficiency of this heat engine. If the temperature of the heat reservoir with the high temperature is increased to 1100 K or if the temperature of the heat reservoir with the low temperature is decreased to 200 K, determine how much the efficiency of the heat engine will increase to.

4-12. For a Carnot heat engine, the temperature of the low-temperature heat reservoir is 300 K, and the efficiency of the heat engine is 40%. Now, the efficiency of the heat engine is improved to 50%.

(1) If the temperature of the low-temperature heat reservoir is kept constant, how much should the temperature of the high-temperature reservoir be increased?

(2) If the temperature of the high-temperature heat reservoir is kept constant, how much should the temperature of the low-temperature reservoir be decreased?

4-13. A Carnot heat engine is working between the high-temperature heat reservoir with a temperature of 373 K and the low-temperature reservoir with the temperature of 273 K. After a cycle, the system does a useful work of 800 J to the surroundings. Now, the temperature of the low-temperature heat reservoir remains unchanged, the temperature of the high-temperature heat reservoir is increased, so that the useful work is increased to 1600 J. Determine:

(1) How much the temperature of high-temperature heat reservoir will be increased to.

(2) How much the efficiency of the heat engine will be increased to (It is assumed that the two cycles are both working between the same two adiabats).

4-14. When 1 kg of water is cooled from the temperature of 20℃ to 0℃, what is the entropy change? It is known that the isobaric specific heat of water is a constant of $C_P = 4.18\times10^3$ J/(kg·K).

4-15. 0.5 kg of ice with the temperature of 0℃ is contacted to a heat reservoir, and the ice is melted completely.

(1) What is the entropy change of the ice?

(2) If the heat reservoir is a huge object with the temperature of 20℃, what is the entropy change of this object?

(3) What is the total entropy change of the ice and heat reservoir? What does the result reflect (It is known that the heat of fusion of water is $\lambda = 3.35\times10^5$ J/kg) ?

4-16. Some ideal gas of (M/μ) moles changes from the initial state of (P_1, V_1, T_1) to the final state of (P_2, V_2, T_2). Try to

(1) express the entropy change with the quantities of V and T;

(2) express the entropy change with the quantities of P and T.

Chapter 5 Electrostatic Field and Bioelectric Phenomena

In this chapter, we will study the physical properties of the electric field set up by the charges kept static to the observer relatively, i.e., the **electrostatic field** and the interactions between the electrostatic field and the objects in it; and the electric phenomena accompanying with the living processes of organisms, or the so-called bioelectric phenomena, will also be studied briefly. Bioelectricity exists widely in the phenomena of lives and relates to almost all the functions and activities of human bodies. The content of this chapter is the important theoretical basis of other related knowledge that we'll study in the future. This chapter mainly introduces the basic principles of electrostatics. Starting from the theory of describing the interaction between two point charges i.e. Coulomb's law, it introduces a basic physical quantity to describe the properties of electrostatic field—electric field intensity. On the basis of these, we will discuss the superposition principle of electric field and Gauss' law, which both can reflect the basic properties of the electrostatic field. To discuss the work done by the electrostatic field force acting on the electric charges in the field, we'll introduce the potential of electrostatic field and the principle that the work of electric force is independent of the path. We'll also discuss the properties of dielectrics in electrostatic field and the phenomenon of polarization in electrostatic field. Finally, we are going to introduce the mechanism of bioelectric phenomena, the physical fundamental of ECG and the basic principles of the formation of ECG waves briefly.

5.1 Electric Field Intensity

5.1.1 Coulomb's Law

In 1785, based on previous experiments and theories, a French physicist Coulomb summarized a very important conclusion about the interaction between electric charges: **In the vacuum, there must be interaction force between two point charges with the electric quantities of q_1 and q_2 respectively. The direction of the force is along the direction of the straight line connecting the two point charges, if the two charges are of the same sign, the charges repel each other; if the two charges are of opposite sign, they will attract each other. The magnitude of the force is proportional to the product of the electric quantities of q_1 and q_2, and is inversely proportional to the square of the distance r between the two point charges. This is called Coulomb's law**. Coulomb's law is expressed in mathematical expression as

$$F = \frac{1}{4\pi\varepsilon_0}\frac{q_1 q_2}{r^2} \tag{5-1a}$$

where ε_0 is called the **permittivity of vacuum**, whose value is 8.85×10^{-12} $C^2/(N{\cdot}m^2)$. If taking the vector character of the force into account, the acting force of q_1 on q_2 is written as

$$\boldsymbol{F} = \frac{1}{4\pi\varepsilon_0}\frac{q_1 q_2}{r^2}\hat{\boldsymbol{r}} \tag{5-1b}$$

where $\hat{\boldsymbol{r}}$ expresses the unit vector from q_1 to q_2.

The discussion of Coulomb's law is only about the electrostatic force between two point charges. In a case of more than two point charges in vacuum, another principle—superposition principle should be presented. Its content is the integrated electrostatic force acting on each charge equals to the vector sum of the electrostatic forces acting on it by other point charges when each of them is respectively alone at its location, which is the **superposition principle**.

5.1.2 Electric Field Intensity

In order to research the properties of each point in an electrostatic field, we can imagine to perform an experiment with a point charge q_0. Here, this charge is called the **test charge**. The test charge shall satisfy the following conditions.

(1) q_0 is a positive charge; its dimension must be small enough, so that it can be regarded as a point charge.

(2) The electric quantity of q_0 is small enough, so that the distribution of electrostatic field set up by the original charges can not be disturbed by its appearance.

As we know, even without contacting, there are interactions between any two charged bodies. The reason is that around any charged body there is a special kind substance—the **electrostatic field**. Now, let's discuss the electrostatic field set up by a point charge q in its surrounding space first. We call the point to be studied in the electric field the **field point**. Imagine to place a stationary test charge q_0 at the field point, according to Coulomb's law, we can get the electrostatic field force acting on q_0.

$$\boldsymbol{F} = \frac{1}{4\pi\varepsilon_0}\frac{q\,q_0}{r^2}\hat{\boldsymbol{r}} \tag{5-2}$$

where r is the distance between the point charge q and the field point. It can be seen from the above equation that $\boldsymbol{F}$ associates with both the field point and the test charge q_0. However, the ratio $\boldsymbol{F}/q_0$ is a quantity just associated with the field point but not with q_0. It is dependent only on the ability of exerting force by the electric field itself.

In order to describe the property of exerting force at the field point, we call the ratio of $\boldsymbol{F}/q_0$ at every point in the field the **electric field intensity** (or field intensity) of that point, denoted by E, i.e.

$$\boldsymbol{E} = \frac{\boldsymbol{F}}{q_0} \tag{5-3}$$

Electric field intensity $\boldsymbol{E}$ is a physical quantity representing the nature of the electric field itself at some point in it. **The field intensity is a vector; its magnitude is equal to the electric field force acting on a unit test charge by the field, and its direction is the same as the direction of the force acting on the test charge by the electric field**, i.e., the direction of the electric field force on a positive charge. The unit of electric field intensity is N/C. If the electric field is established by a system of many point charges $q_1, q_2, \cdots, q_n$, in the light of the superposition principle, **the electric field intensity at a field point in space $\boldsymbol{E}$ must be equal to the vector sum of the electric field intensities $\boldsymbol{E}_1, \boldsymbol{E}_2, \cdots, \boldsymbol{E}_n$, which are established respectively by the point charges when each of them is alone at its location**, i.e.

$$\boldsymbol{E} = \boldsymbol{E}_1 + \boldsymbol{E}_2 + \cdots + \boldsymbol{E}_n = \sum \boldsymbol{E}_i \tag{5-4}$$

This regularity is called the **superposition principle of electric field intensity**. By applying it, we can calculate the electric field intensities set up by arbitrary systems of charged bodies.

5.1.3 Calculation of Electric Field Intensity

1. Electric Field Intensity of a Field Set up by a Point Charge *q*

By the definition of the electric field intensity of Equation (5-3) and Coulomb's law, we know that the electric field intensity at a certain point in the field set up by the point charge q should be

$$\boldsymbol{E}=\frac{1}{4\pi\varepsilon_0}\frac{q}{r^2}\hat{\boldsymbol{r}} \tag{5-5}$$

where $\hat{\boldsymbol{r}}$ is the unit vector from point q directing to the field point; r is the distance from q to the field point. When q is positive, the direction of $\boldsymbol{E}$ is the same as $\hat{\boldsymbol{r}}$'s, i.e., the field intensity emits from the point of q; when q is negative, the direction of $\boldsymbol{E}$ is in the opposite direction of $\hat{\boldsymbol{r}}$, i.e., the field intensity points towards the point of q.

2. Electric Field Intensity of a Field Set up by a System of Point Charges

Supposing the field is set up by n point charges $q_1, q_2, \cdots, q_n$, the electric field intensity at a certain point in the field is equal to the vector sum of the electric field intensities which are produced respectively by each point charge. Considering the formula of field intensity for a point charge, we can get the formula for calculating the electric field intensity of the field set up by a system of point charges.

$$\boldsymbol{E}=\sum_{i=1}^{n}\boldsymbol{E}_i=\frac{1}{4\pi\varepsilon_0}\sum_{i=1}^{n}\frac{q_i}{r_i^2}\hat{\boldsymbol{r}}_i \tag{5-6}$$

3. Electric Field Intensity of a Field Set up by a Linear Charge

Suppose the electric charge is distributed continuously in a thin rod. If the distance between the field point and the thin rod is much bigger than its thickness, the thickness can be neglected, and the charge can be looked as distributed on a curve L as shown in Figure 5-1. Assume that the electric quantity on a unit length or the **linear charge density** is λ, it can be expressed as a mathematical formula.

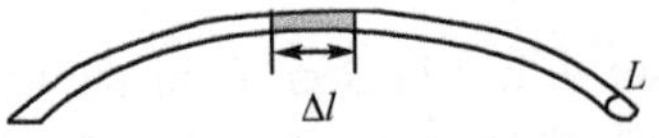

Figure 5-1 A thin rod with electric charge

$$\lambda=\lim_{\Delta l\to 0}\frac{\Delta q}{\Delta l}=\frac{\mathrm{d}q}{\mathrm{d}l}$$

where dq is the electric quantity in a linear element on the thin rod with the length of dl, and $\mathrm{d}q=\lambda\cdot\mathrm{d}l$. Then the field intensity will be calculated as

$$\boldsymbol{E}=\frac{1}{4\pi\varepsilon_0}\int_L\frac{\lambda\,\mathrm{d}l}{r^2}\hat{\boldsymbol{r}} \tag{5-7}$$

where r is the distance from the linear element dl to the field point; $\hat{\boldsymbol{r}}$ is the unit vector from dl pointing to the field point; the integral is throughout the whole curve L.

4. Electric Field Intensity of a Field Set up by a Surface Charge

Suppose the electric charge is distributed continuously on a surface of S. A certain point on a surface element with the area of ΔS is assumed to carry with the electric quantity of Δq, so the electric quantity on a unit area or the surface charge density σ at some point on the surface is

$$\sigma=\lim_{\Delta S\to 0}\frac{\Delta q}{\Delta S}=\frac{\mathrm{d}q}{\mathrm{d}S}$$

When we calculate the field intensity set up by the whole charged surface S, we can regard every surface element dS as a point charge with the electric quantity of $\mathrm{d}q=\sigma\cdot\mathrm{d}S$. So the calculation of the field intensity can be expressed as the following.

$$\boldsymbol{E}=\frac{1}{4\pi\varepsilon_0}\iint_S \frac{\sigma \mathrm{d}S}{r^2}\hat{\boldsymbol{r}} \tag{5-8}$$

where r is the distance from the surface element dS to the field point; $\hat{\boldsymbol{r}}$ is the unit vector from dS pointing to the field point; the integral is throughout the whole charged surface S.

5. Electric Field Intensity of a Field Set up by a Volume Charge

If the electric charge is distributed continuously in a volume of V, a small volume element ΔV is chosen about some point in the volume, and if the electric quantity in ΔV is assumed to be Δq, the electric quantity in the unit volume i.e. the **volume charge density** ρ will be

$$\rho=\lim_{\Delta V\to 0}\frac{\Delta q}{\Delta V}=\frac{\mathrm{d}q}{\mathrm{d}V}$$

When we calculate the field intensity at some point in a field set up by a charged body with the volume of V, we could divide it into numerous volume elements dV, look each dV as a point charge with the electric quantity of d$q=\rho\cdot$dV, and we then get the calculation of field intensity as

$$\boldsymbol{E}=\frac{1}{4\pi\varepsilon_0}\iiint_V \frac{\rho \mathrm{d}V}{r^2}\hat{\boldsymbol{r}} \tag{5-9}$$

where r is the distance from the volume element dV to the field point; $\hat{\boldsymbol{r}}$ is the unit vector from dV pointing to the field point; the integral is throughout the whole charged volume region V.

Example 5-1 A uniformly charged ring with the radius of a get the linear charge density λ. Determine the electric field intensity at point P that is on the central axis of the ring and has a distance of x from the ring's center (here, $\lambda>0$ is known).

Solution: Assuming to choose a segment of linear element with the length of dl on the ring as shown in Figure 5-2. The electric quantity on the element will be d$q=\lambda$dl; and the field intensity dE at point P produced by the charge element dq will have the magnitude of

$$\mathrm{d}E=\frac{1}{4\pi\varepsilon_0}\cdot\frac{\lambda \mathrm{d}l}{r^2}$$

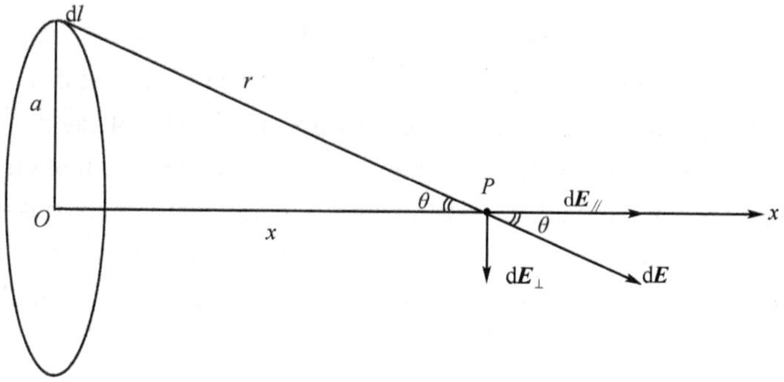

Figure 5-2 The electric quantity on the central axis of a uniformly charged ring

The direction of it is as shown in the figure, where r is the distance between dl and point P. For the electric field intensity d$\boldsymbol{E}$ can be divided into two components: One is d$\boldsymbol{E}_{//}$ which is parallel to the direction of the axis, and the other is d$\boldsymbol{E}_{\perp}$ perpendicular to the axis direction. And because point P is located on the central axis of the ring, in the light of the symmetry, the perpendicular components of field intensities d$\boldsymbol{E}$ produced respectively by the charge elements and the opposite charge elements on the ring are offset each other, so at point P, only the parallel components remain to compose the field intensity there. Then the integrated electric field intensity at point P is the sum of the parallel components of field intensities produced respectively by all the charge elements. So we can get

$$\mathrm{d}E_{//} = \mathrm{d}E \cdot \cos\theta$$

where θ is the angle made by d$\boldsymbol{E}$ and the direction of central axis. The integrated electric field intensity at point P is

$$E = \int \mathrm{d}E_{//} = \int \mathrm{d}E \cos\theta = \int \frac{1}{4\pi\varepsilon_0} \frac{\lambda \mathrm{d}l}{r^2} \cos\theta$$

By the geometric relation of $r^2 = x^2 + a^2$, we know that the electric field intensity at P is

$$E = \frac{\lambda x}{4\pi\varepsilon_0 (x^2 + a^2)^{3/2}} \int_0^{2\pi a} \mathrm{d}l = \frac{2\pi a \lambda x}{4\pi\varepsilon_0 (x^2 + a^2)^{3/2}} = \frac{a\lambda x}{2\varepsilon_0 (x^2 + a^2)^{3/2}}$$

Because the total electric quantity the charged ring carried is $q = 2\pi a\lambda$, the integrated electric field intensity at point P can also be written as

$$E = \frac{1}{4\pi\varepsilon_0} \frac{qx}{(x^2 + a^2)^{3/2}} \tag{5-10}$$

It can be seen from the above equation that, when $x = 0$, $E = 0$, and it indicates the field intensity at the center of the ring is zero; when $x \gg a$, it can be considered $(x^2 + a^2)^{3/2} \approx x^3$, then the electric field at point P is

$$E = \frac{q}{4\pi\varepsilon_0 x^2}$$

It shows that, in a place far away from the ring's center, the electric charge on the ring can be looked as concentrated at the central point as a point charge; this result is exactly the same as the formula for calculating the field intensity of a point charge.

5.2 Gauss' Law in the Electrostatic Field

When the distribution of electric charges of a charged body is known, in principle, the electric field intensity at any point in the field set by the body can be determined by means of Coulomb's law and the superposition principle, but the calculation is often comparatively complicated. If the distribution of charges has certain symmetry, in order to make the calculation of the distribution of the electric field easier, we shall introduce a new method for calculating the field intensities in this section, i.e., to solve problems about the electric field intensity by applying Gauss' law. Before introducing Gauss' law, let's make an expatiation on two basic concepts: the electric field lines (or the lines of electric force) and the electric flux.

5.2.1 Electric Field Lines

In order to describe the distributions and properties of an electric field visually, we can draw a series of curves in the field, and define some restrictions on these curves: ① **The tangential direction at any point on any one of the curves is consistently the direction of the electric field intensity at the point.** ② where the curves are denser, the electric field intensity is bigger; and where the curves are sparse, the electric field intensity is smaller. These curves are what we called the **electric field lines** (or **lines of electric force**). Because the density of field lines can reflect the situation of electric field intensity, around a point in the field, a plan element with the area of $\Delta S_{\perp}$ which is perpendicular to the electric field intensity at the point is taken into consideration. If the number of field lines passing across the surface element is assumed to be $\Delta\Phi$, then the magnitude of the field intensity at that point is defined as

$$E = \frac{\Delta\Phi}{\Delta S_{\perp}} \tag{5-11}$$

5.2.2 Electric Flux

We call **the total number of the field lines that penetrate through an area in the electric field the electric flux of passing through this area** and express it with Φ.

In a uniform electric field, the electric flux through a plane with area of S that is perpendicular to the field is $\Phi = E{\cdot}S$, and if the normal direction $\boldsymbol{n}$ of the plane makes an angle of θ with $\boldsymbol{E}$, the electric flux passing through S should be

$$\Phi = E\,S\cos\theta = \boldsymbol{E}{\cdot}\boldsymbol{S} \tag{5-12}$$

where $\boldsymbol{S}$ is defined as a vector, its magnitude is S, and its direction is the normal direction $\boldsymbol{n}$ of the plane, as shown in Figure 5-3 (a).

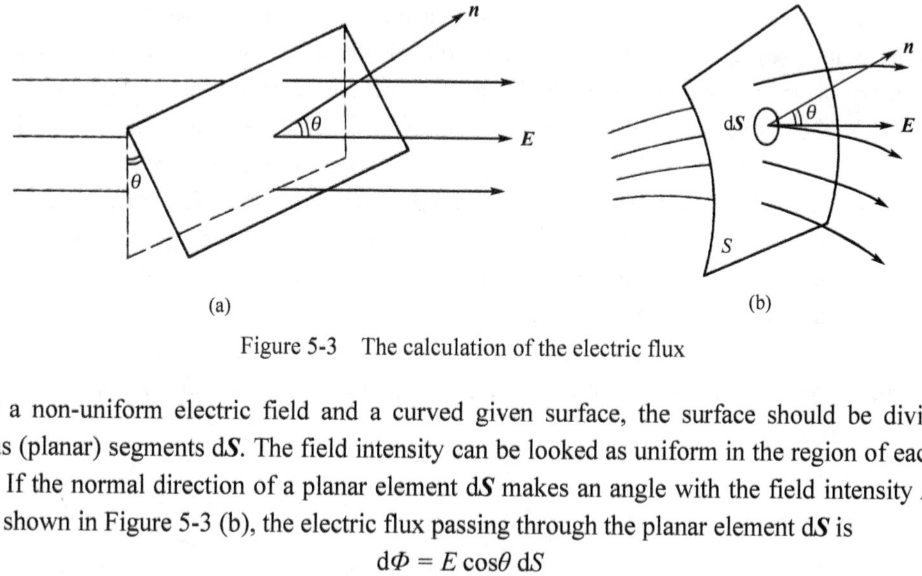

Figure 5-3 The calculation of the electric flux

For a non-uniform electric field and a curved given surface, the surface should be divided into numerous (planar) segments d$\boldsymbol{S}$. The field intensity can be looked as uniform in the region of each planar element. If the normal direction of a planar element d$\boldsymbol{S}$ makes an angle with the field intensity $\boldsymbol{E}$ at that point, as shown in Figure 5-3 (b), the electric flux passing through the planar element d$\boldsymbol{S}$ is

$$\mathrm{d}\Phi = E\cos\theta\,\mathrm{d}S$$

Then in the electric flux passing through the whole surface should be

$$\Phi = \iint_S \mathrm{d}\Phi = \iint_S E\cos\theta\,\mathrm{d}S = \iint_S \boldsymbol{E}\cdot\mathrm{d}\boldsymbol{S} \tag{5-13}$$

where d$\boldsymbol{S}$ is a vector, its magnitude is dS, and its direction is the direction of the outer normal line n of the surface at that point.

If the surface S is a closed surface, the above formula should be rewritten as

$$\Phi = \oiint_S \boldsymbol{E}\cdot\mathrm{d}\boldsymbol{S} \tag{5-14}$$

For a closed surface, there is a mathematical rule: the positive direction of the normal n at any point on the surface is perpendicular to the surface at that point and is outward. Hence, the electric fluxes passing through all the surface elements dΦ will be possible of being positive or negative. When angle θ is acute, d$\Phi > 0$; when θ is an obtuse angle, d$\Phi < 0$.

5.2.3 Gauss' Law

Gauss' law is the theory for calculating the electric fluxes of closed surfaces. Now let's discuss the simplest case first, i.e., in an electrostatic field set up by a single point charge q. To take q as the center we imagine making a spherical surface with the radius of r, then take a surface element with the area of $d\boldsymbol{S}$ at an arbitrary point on the spherical surface, as shown in Figure 5-4 (a), the electric flux passing through $d\boldsymbol{S}$ is

$$d\Phi = \boldsymbol{E} \cdot d\boldsymbol{S} = \frac{1}{4\pi\varepsilon_0}\frac{q}{r^2}dS$$

The electric flux passing through the entire spherical surface is

$$\Phi = \oiint_{\text{sphere}} d\Phi = \oiint_{\text{sphere}} \frac{1}{4\pi\varepsilon_0}\frac{q}{r^2}dS = \frac{1}{4\pi\varepsilon_0}\frac{q}{r^2}\oiint_{\text{sphere}} dS$$

where $\oiint_{\text{sphere}} dS$ is the area of the sphere, which is equal to $4\pi r^2$, so the electric flux is expressed as

$$\Phi = \frac{q}{\varepsilon_0} \tag{5-15}$$

It shows that the electric flux passing through the spherical surface is only related to the electric quantity of the interior point charge, and independent on the radius. If the surface which encloses the point charge q is an arbitrary closed surface, as shown in Figure 5-4 (b), the number of times for any field line to penetrate through the closed surface is always an odd number as being seen from the diagram. According to the mathematical rule for the definition of the positive or negative sign of electric flux, what should merely be considered is the final time for the field line penetrating through. The contribution of the rest even number times to the flux will be canceled out each other in pairs. So it can be proved that, by calculating the electric flux passing through any closed surface, Equation (5-15) is also correct.

In the case that an arbitrary closed surface does not enclose any point charge inside, as shown in Figure 5-4 (c), the number of the field lines penetrating into the closed surface must be equal to the number of the field lines penetrating out from the closed surface. So, the total flux passing through the closed surface is zero.

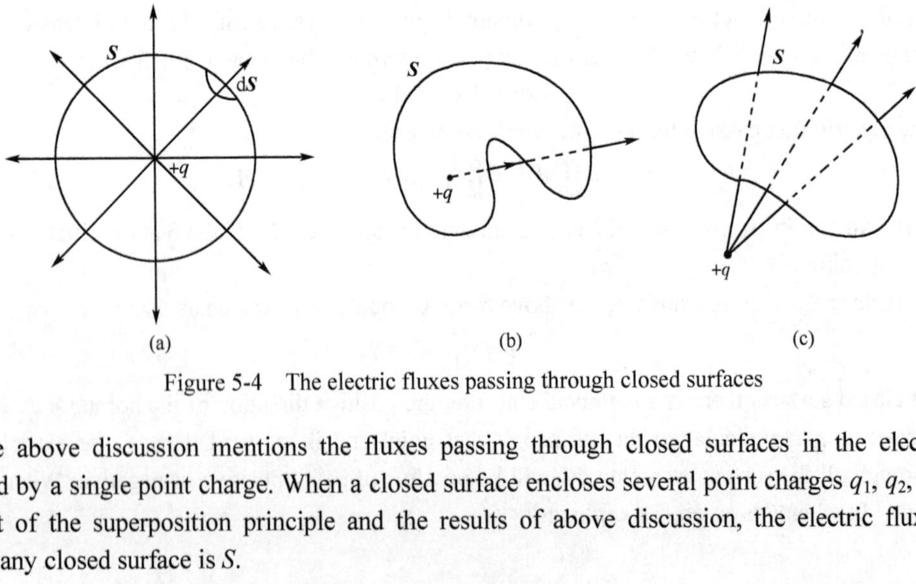

Figure 5-4 The electric fluxes passing through closed surfaces

The above discussion mentions the fluxes passing through closed surfaces in the electric field produced by a single point charge. When a closed surface encloses several point charges $q_1, q_2, \dots, q_n$, in the light of the superposition principle and the results of above discussion, the electric flux passing through any closed surface is S.

$$\Phi = \oiint_S \boldsymbol{E} \cdot \mathrm{d}\boldsymbol{S} = \oiint_S \sum \boldsymbol{E}_i \cdot \mathrm{d}\boldsymbol{S} = \sum \oiint_S \boldsymbol{E}_i \cdot \mathrm{d}\boldsymbol{S} = \sum \Phi_i$$

According to the result of Equation (5-15), we have

$$\Phi = \oiint_S \boldsymbol{E} \cdot \mathrm{d}\boldsymbol{S} = \frac{1}{\varepsilon_0} \sum q_i \tag{5-16}$$

Equation (5-16) is the **mathematical expression for Gauss' law in electrostatic field**. It is shown that **the electric flux passing through any closed surface is equal to the quotient of the algebraic sum of the charges enclosed inside the surface divided by the permittivity of vacuum ε_0, and is independent of the charges outside the closed surface**. This conclusion is called **Gauss' law in the electrostatic field**. The closed surface S is also known as Gauss' surface. When the charge distributions are of some symmetry, it is easier to determine the magnitude of the electric field intensities by using Gauss' law.

Example 5-2 Determine the electric field intensity inside and outside a uniformly charged spherical shell. Here we know the total electric quantity carried by the shell is q, and its radius is R.

Solution: First let's assume a point P outside the spherical shell discretionarily, then imagine making a spherical surface S with the radius of r ($> R$) and let it pass the point P and be a homocentric one with the charged spherical shell. We take S as Gauss' surface, as shown in Figure 5-5. According to Gauss' law we can get

$$\oiint_S \boldsymbol{E}_{\text{out}} \cdot \mathrm{d}\boldsymbol{S} = E_{\text{out}} \oiint_S \mathrm{d}S = E_{\text{out}} \cdot 4\pi r^2 = \frac{q}{\varepsilon_0}$$

so

$$E_{\text{out}} = \frac{q}{4\pi\varepsilon_0 r^2}$$

It can be seen from the above equation, the electric field intensity at any point outside a uniformly charged spherical shell is equal to the electric field intensity at the same point when all the charge on the shell looked as concentrated at the central point as an equivalent point charge.

We discuss further about the field intensity at any point inside the charged spherical shell. Imagine making a spherical surface S' with the radius of r ($< R$) and let it pass an arbitrary point inside the shell and also be a homocentric one with the charged spherical shell. We then take S′ as Gauss' surface. According to Gauss' law we can get

$$\oiint_{S'} E_{\text{in}} \mathrm{d}S = E_{\text{in}} \cdot 4\pi r^2 = 0$$

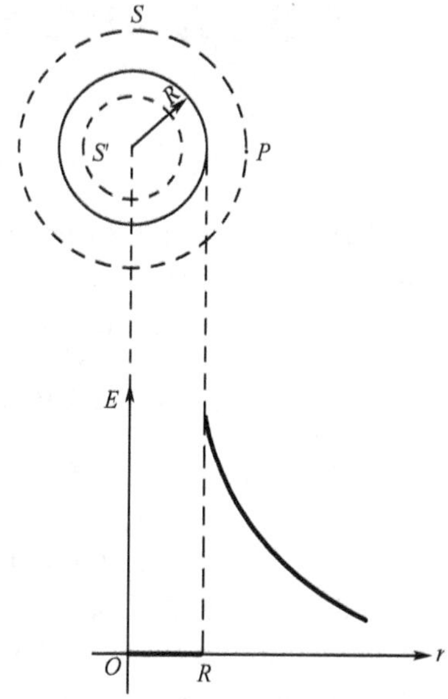

Figure 5-5 The electric field intensity of a uniformly charged spherical shell

so

$$E_{\text{in}} = 0$$

It is to say that, at any point inside a uniformly charged spherical shell, the electric field intensity is always zero. According to the above results, we can draw a function curve of the magnitude of the electric intensity E, which is changing with the distance of r from the center of spherical shell to the field point, as shown in Figure 5-5.

Example 5-3 Try to determine the electric field intensity set up by an infinitely large plane which is uniformly charged with positive charge. Here we know the surface charge density of the infinite charged plane is σ.

Solution: We imagine making a cylindrical surface as Gauss' surface. Let the cylinder's axis

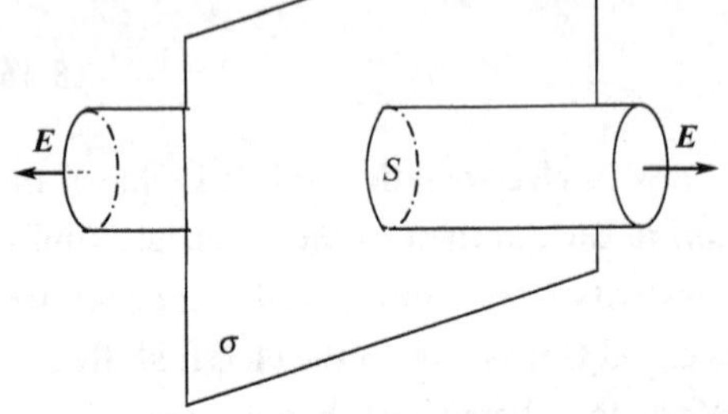

Figure 5-6 The electric field intensity of an infinitely large plane

perpendicular to the charged plane and the area of its underside be S, as shown in Figure 5-6. Then the electric flux passing through the lateral side is zero, all of the field lines penetrating through the two undersides are perpendicular to the undersides. Let $\boldsymbol{E}$ be the field intensity around the infinite charged plane, the electric flux passing through the two undersides, i.e., the electric flux passing through the whole Gauss' surface is $2ES$, meanwhile, the total charge which is enclosed by Gauss' surface is σS. By Gauss' law we have

$$2ES = \frac{\sigma S}{\varepsilon_0}$$

so

$$E = \frac{\sigma}{2\varepsilon_0}$$

It indicates that the electric field near an infinite charged plane is a uniform electric field.

5.3 Work Done by the Electric Field Force and Potential

Whenever an electric charge moves in an electrostatic field, the electric field force acting on the charge will do work to it. Studying the regularity of doing work by the electrostatic force is of great significance to understand the properties of the electrostatic field.

5.3.1 Work Done by the Electric Field Force

A test charge q_0 is assumed to move from point A to point B via any path in the electric field set up by a point charge of $+q$, as shown in Figure 5-7. We can divide the whole path into numerous displacement elements and select any displacement element $\mathrm{d}\boldsymbol{l}$ randomly. Let the electric intensity at the point where this $\mathrm{d}\boldsymbol{l}$ exists be $\boldsymbol{E}$. The work element done for the displacement element by the static electrostatic force $\boldsymbol{F}$ is

$$\mathrm{d}A = \boldsymbol{F}\cdot\mathrm{d}l = q_0\,\boldsymbol{E}\cdot\mathrm{d}\boldsymbol{l} = q_0\,E\cos\theta\cdot\mathrm{d}l$$

where θ is the angle between the direction of electric field intensity $\boldsymbol{E}$ and direction of $\mathrm{d}l$. By the geometric relation we have

$$\cos\theta\,\mathrm{d}l = \mathrm{d}r$$

where $\mathrm{d}r$ is the increment of the length of the radial vector. It is also known that, the magnitude of field intensity produced by the point charge q should be

$$\boldsymbol{E} = \frac{1}{4\pi\varepsilon_0}\frac{q}{r^2}\hat{\boldsymbol{r}}$$

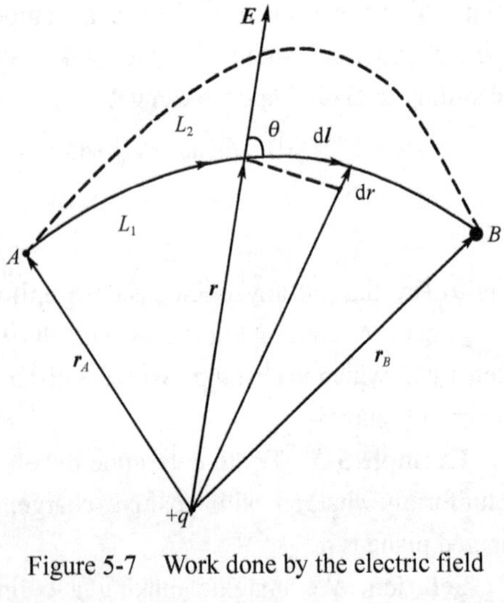

Figure 5-7 Work done by the electric field

So during the whole process for the test charge q_0 moving from point A to point B, the work done by the electric field force is

$$A_{AB} = \int \mathrm{d}A = \int_A^B q_0 E\cos\theta \,\mathrm{d}l = \frac{qq_0}{4\pi\varepsilon_0}\int_{r_A}^{r_B}\frac{\mathrm{d}r}{r^2}$$

That is

$$A_{AB} = \frac{qq_0}{4\pi\varepsilon_0}\left(\frac{1}{r_A}-\frac{1}{r_B}\right) \tag{5-17}$$

Equation (5-17) shows that, when the test charge q_0 moves in the field set up by a point charge q, the work done by the electric field force only depends on the initial and final states of the moving charge, not on the path. So **the electrostatic force is the conservative force**. This is an important property of the electrostatic field; however, the fields with this property are called the **fields of conservative force**.

The above conclusion can be extended to the case of the electric field set up by a point charge system of q_1, q_2, ⋯, q_n. When a test charge q_0 moves from point A to point B in the electric field, the total work done by the integrated electric force acting on the test charge is the algebraic sum of the works which is respectively done by the electric field force of the corresponding point charge on the test charge. That is

$$A_{AB} = \int_A^B q_0 \boldsymbol{E}\cdot\mathrm{d}\boldsymbol{l} = \int_A^B q_0 \boldsymbol{E}_1\cdot\mathrm{d}\boldsymbol{l} + \int_A^B q_0 \boldsymbol{E}_2\cdot\mathrm{d}\boldsymbol{l} + \cdots + \int_A^B q_0 \boldsymbol{E}_n\cdot\mathrm{d}\boldsymbol{l} = \sum_{i=1}^{n}\frac{q_i q_0}{4\pi\varepsilon_0}\left(\frac{1}{r_{Ai}}-\frac{1}{r_{Bi}}\right) \tag{5-18}$$

The work done by the electric field force of a system of point charges is also independent of the path.

If the test charge moves circularly along a closed path in the electrostatic field, for example, it goes from point A to point B along curve L_1, and then comes back from point B to point A along curve L_2, as shown in Figure 5-7. Based respectively on Equation (5-17) in the electric field set up by a point charge, and on Equation (5-18) in the electric field set up by a system of point charges (or by any charged body), we can get the work done by the electric field force in this case .

$$A = \oint_L q_0 \boldsymbol{E}\cdot\mathrm{d}\boldsymbol{l} = \int_A^B q_0 \boldsymbol{E}\cdot\mathrm{d}\boldsymbol{l} + \int_B^A q_0 \boldsymbol{E}\cdot\mathrm{d}\boldsymbol{l} = \sum_{i=1}^{n}\frac{q_i q_0}{4\pi\varepsilon_0}\left(\frac{1}{r_{Ai}}-\frac{1}{r_{Bi}}\right) + \sum_{i=1}^{n}\frac{q_i q_0}{4\pi\varepsilon_0}\left(\frac{1}{r_{Bi}}-\frac{1}{r_{Ai}}\right) = 0$$

That is

$$\oint_L \boldsymbol{E}\cdot\mathrm{d}\boldsymbol{l} = 0 \tag{5-19}$$

Equation (5-19) shows that, in any electrostatic field the loop integral of the electric field intensity $\boldsymbol{E}$ along any closed curve is zero. This is another important property of the electrostatic field; we call it the **circulatory theorem of the electrostatic field.**

5.3.2 Electric Potential Energy and Electric Potential

We can see from the above discussion that, **the electrostatic force is a conservative force, and the electrostatic field is a conservative force field. So we can introduce the concept of the potential energy in the electrostatic field, that is to say, an electric charge has a certain potential energy at anywhere in the electric field. We call this potential energy the electric potential energy.** The work done by the electric force on the charge is the scale to measure the change of electric potential energy. If the electric potential energy at point A or point B is expressed respectively by W_A or W_B, when the test charge q_0 moves from point A to point B in the electric field, the relationship between the work done by the electric field force on it and the change of the electric potential energy satisfies

$$A_{AB} = q_0 \int_A^B \boldsymbol{E} \cdot \mathrm{d}\boldsymbol{l} = W_A - W_B$$

Like gravitational potential energy, the electric potential energy is also a relative quantity. If we are going to define the magnitude of the electric potential energy at a point in an electric field, we must have a referential zero mark of the electric potential energy. Usually, in the case when the distribution of electric charge, which sets up the field, is in a limited range, the potential energy at the point infinitely far away is defined as zero. Therefore, the electric potential energy of the test charge q_0 at any point of A is numerically equal to the value of the work done by the electric field force on it during the process when it is removed from point A to infinity. So, according to Equation (5-17), we can determine the electric potential energy of the test charge q_0 at any point of A in the electric field set up by a point charge q.

$$W_A = \int_A^{\infty} q_0 \boldsymbol{E} \cdot \mathrm{d}\boldsymbol{l} = \frac{q q_0}{4\pi\varepsilon_0} \int_{r_A}^{\infty} \frac{\mathrm{d}r}{r^2} = \frac{q q_0}{4\pi\varepsilon_0 r_A} \tag{5-20}$$

where r_A is the distance between the field point to point charge q. From Equation (5-20) we can see that, the magnitude of electric potential energy at some point in the field is related not only with the charge which excites the field and the position of the field point, but also with the quantity of the test charge q_0. However, the ratio of W/q_0 is a quantity independent of the electric quantity of the test charge q_0, which can reflect the energy property at any given point in an electrostatic field. We use a physical quantity potential or electric potential to describe this property, and use a letter U to represent it. So the electric potential at point A is

$$U_A = \frac{W_A}{q_0} = \int_A^{\infty} \boldsymbol{E} \cdot \mathrm{d}\boldsymbol{l} \tag{5-21a}$$

Equation (5-21a) is the definition for the electric potential at point A in any electrostatic field; and the referential point of zero for potential is just the same as the point for the electric potential energy. Thus, the **potential at some point is numerically equal to the value of work done by the electric field force on a unit point charge during the process when it is removed from this point to infinity along any path**. In Equation (5-21a), although the integral path can be chosen arbitrarily, in the calculation of potential, the integral path should be actually chosen as a line along which the distribution regularity of electric field is known. The potential is a scalar, and its unit is V.

From Equation (5-20) we know that, the electric potential at some point in the electric field set up by a point charge q is

$$U = \frac{W}{q_0} = \frac{q}{4\pi\varepsilon_0} \int_r^{\infty} \frac{\mathrm{d}r}{r^2} = \frac{q}{4\pi\varepsilon_0 r} \tag{5-21b}$$

where r is the distance between the field point to point charge q.

The electric potential at some point in the electrostatic field set up by a system of point charges **equals to the algebraic sum of electric potentials at that point, and each component potential is generated by the corresponding point charge when it exists alone**. This conclusion is called the **superposition principle of electric potential.** That is

$$U = \sum_{i=1}^{n} \frac{q_i}{4\pi\varepsilon_0 r_i} \tag{5-21c}$$

This principle gives another method for the calculation of the electric potential at some point in the field produced by any charged body.

In practical instances, we often use the concept of potential difference to describe the differences of electric field's states at different points in the field. The so-called **potential difference** represents the difference of electric potentials at any two points A and B in an electric field. That is

$$\Delta U = U_{AB} = U_A - U_B = \int_A^B \boldsymbol{E} \cdot \mathrm{d}\boldsymbol{l} \tag{5-22}$$

5.4 Dielectric in Electrostatic Field

5.4.1 Dielectric and Electric Dipole

1. Dielectric and Its Classification

The dielectric, sometimes called the insulator, is a kind of material with extremely poor conductive property. Owing to the difference in the internal structure, the dielectric can also be classified into two kinds, i.e., the dielectric of polar molecules and the dielectric of non-polar molecules.

We have known that, each molecule is made of atoms, and an atom is composed of negatively charged electrons and positively charged nucleus. Positive and negative charges in each molecule are distributed to the entire volume occupied by the molecule. Looked from a point with the distance much more than the dimension of a molecule, the effect (such as the electric field) produced by an entire molecule can be approximately described by an "center model", i.e., all positive and negative charges are considered to be concentrated respectively at two geometric points, which are respectively called the positive charges' "center" of two. In this way, at that "far" place the electric field produced by an entire molecule is the same as the field produced by all of the positive and negative charges when they are concentrated respectively to the two "centers".

According to the distribution of positive and negative "centers", we classify the dielectric to two kinds: for one kind dielectric, in each of the molecules, positive and negative centers are superposed together, and this kind of molecules is called **non-polar molecules**. The dielectric which is composed of non-polar molecules is called the **dielectric of non-polar molecules**. For example, molecules such as H_2, N_2, CH_4, etc. are non-polar molecules. For another kind of dielectric, in each of the molecules, positive and negative centers are not superposed together; and this kind of molecules is called **polar molecules.** The dielectric composed of polar molecules is called the **dielectric of polar molecules**. For example, molecules such as CO, H_2O, HCl, etc. are non-polar molecules.

2. Electric Dipole

The so-called electric dipole refers to a system constructed by two point charges which carry respectively equivalent electric quantities of different signs and are very near apart. The electric quantities of the two point charges are respectively $+q$ and $-q$. The straight line connecting these two point charges is called the **axis** and the distance between them is l. The direction of the vector from negative charge to positive charge $\boldsymbol{l}$ is assumed as the positive direction of the axis. The **electric dipole moment** of the electric dipole, or the **electric moment**, is the product of the electric quantity q and l. The electric dipole moment is a vector and is represented with $\boldsymbol{p}$, and its direction is the direction of the vector $\boldsymbol{l}$, i.e.

$$\boldsymbol{p} = q\boldsymbol{l} \tag{5-23}$$

The electric dipole moment is a physical quantity to describe the overall electrical properties of electric dipole. For a non-polar molecule, because the centers of positive and negative charges are superposed together, so its electric dipole moment is $\boldsymbol{p} = 0$; for a polar molecule, the molecular electric dipole moment $\boldsymbol{p} \neq 0$. We can take a polar molecule as an electric dipole, and the dielectric as an entireness composed by numerous small electric dipoles.

5.4.2 Polarization of Dielectric and Electric Polarization Intensity

1. Polarization of Dielectric

In the case of the absence of any external electric field: for non-polar molecules, because the electric moment of every molecule is zero, the dielectric of non-polar molecules shows no electric significance to the surroundings; for polar molecules, although the electric dipole moment of each molecule is not zero, the molecules keep continuously the irregularly thermal motion, and every molecule's electric dipole moment may point stochastically to any direction, so, macroscopically, the dielectric of polar molecules shows still no electric significance to the surroundings. When a dielectric is in an external electric field, the arrangement of electric moments of either polar molecules or non-polar molecules must have some change. This change leads to the polarization of the dielectric. The polarization can be classified into two kinds: The displacement polarization and orientation polarization. Now, let's introduce them as the following.

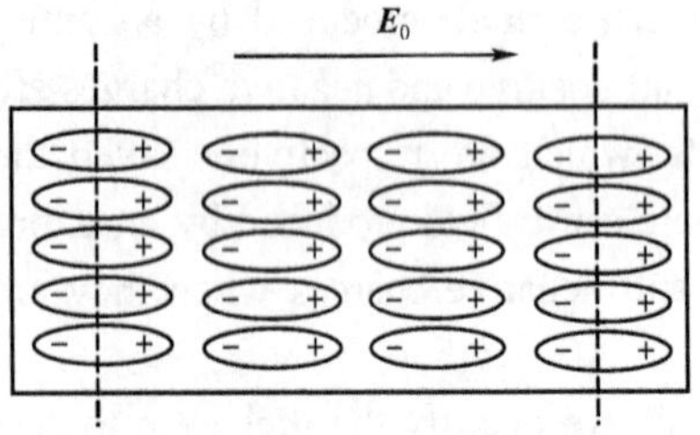

Figure 5-8 Displacement polarization of non-polar molecules

(1) Displacement polarization of non-polar molecules: under the action of the external electric field $\boldsymbol{E}_0$, the centers of positive and negative charges in a non-polar molecule will have a tiny displacement to the opposite direction, as shown in Figure 5-8. At this time, the centers of positive and negative charges in the non-polar molecule will no longer be superposed together, but form an electric dipole. For the whole piece of dielectric, because each molecule forms an electric dipole, and the direction of every electric moment of the electric dipole is the direction of the external electric field $\boldsymbol{E}_0$, being looked macroscopically, on one side of the dielectric there will be positive charges, and negative charges on the other side. These positive and negative charges cannot move freely in the dielectric, so, such charges are called the **polarization charges. Under the action of the external electric field, the polarization charges with two different signs will appear respectively on the two sides of the dielectric corresponding to the direction of the electric field. This phenomenon is called the dielectric polarization**. Due to the mass of an electron is much smaller than the mass of a nucleus, under the action of the external electric field, the displacement is mainly the change of electrons' position. This kind of polarization of non-polar molecules is called the **displacement polarization of electrons** or the **displacement polarization.**

(2) The orientation polarization of polar molecules: for the dielectric composed of polar molecules, under the action of the external electric field $\boldsymbol{E}_0$, every polar molecule will be acted by a torque of the electric forces, as shown in Figure 5-9 (a), the electric field forces make the electric moment of each molecule turn to the direction of the external electric field. Although the molecules cannot be pointed neatly to the direction of the external electric field and lined up because of the interference of the irregularly thermal motion of molecules, the overall trend is consistent. For the whole piece of dielectric, the polarization charges are also produced on the corresponding two sides. This is the polarization phenomenon of polar molecules. Because the polarization of the polar molecules depends mainly on the change of the direction of the molecules' electric dipoles themselves, this kind of polarization of the polar molecules is called the **orientation polarization**, as shown in Figure 5-9 (b).

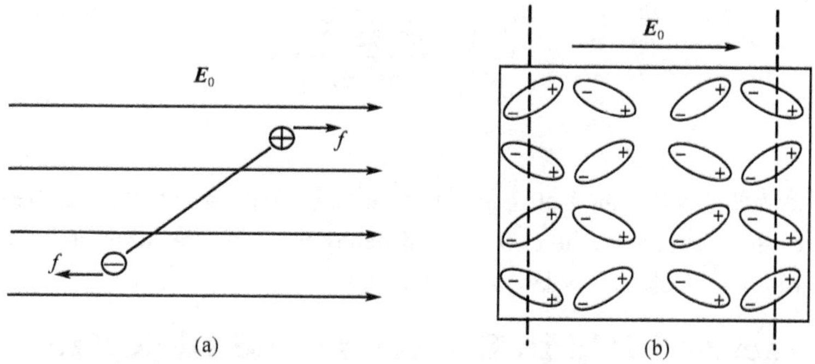

Figure 5-9 Orientation polarization of polar molecules

2. Electric Polarization Intensity

We can see from the above explanation to the mechanism of the polarization of dielectric that: when the dielectric is in the state of polarization, if we choose a small volume element ΔV in the dielectric, the vector sum of the electric dipole moments of the molecules within ΔV can not offset each other, i.e., $\sum p_i \neq 0$. When the dielectric is not polarized, because of the irregularity of the molecular motion, the result is $\sum p_i = 0$. So, in order to quantitatively describe the degree of polarization of the dielectric, we introduce a new physical quantity—the **electric polarization intensity vector**, denoted by ***P***, and it is equal to the vector sum of the molecular electric dipole moments vectors in a unit volume, i.e.,

$$\boldsymbol{P} = \frac{\sum \boldsymbol{p}_i}{\Delta V} \tag{5-24}$$

The unit of electric polarization intensity vector ***P*** is C/m^2. Now that the polarization phenomenon is caused by the electric field, there must be some corresponding relationship between the polarization intensity and the electric field intensity. It has proved theoretically and experimentally that at any point in the isotropic and uniform medium, the direction of the polarization intensity ***P*** is the same as the direction of the integrated field intensity ***E***, and its magnitude is proportional to the field intensity's, i.e.

$$\boldsymbol{P} = \varepsilon_0 \chi \boldsymbol{E} \tag{5-25}$$

where χ is called the electric polarizability of the dielectric, as a unitless digital number, and it depends on the properties of the dielectric.

Because the degrees of polarizations of the dielectric are different, the amounts of the polarization charges induced are different. Here, we are going to discuss the relationship between the polarization intensity of the dielectric and the amount of the polarization charges.

In the isotropic medium, we assume a cylindrical volume element ΔV and let the axis of ΔV be parallel to the direction of polarization P, as shown in Figure 5-10. The area of the undersides of the small cylinder are both ΔS and the length of it is Δl. The surface polarization charge density on the two undersides are respectively $+\sigma'$ and $-\sigma'$. Then the small cylinder can be looked as a bigger dipole with the electric moment's magnitude of $\sigma' \cdot \Delta S \cdot \Delta l$. In this way, the magnitude of the vector sum of electric moments vectors of all molecules in ΔV is

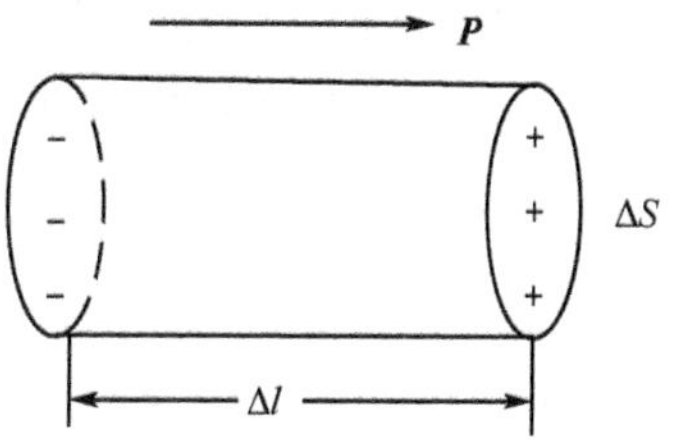

Figure 5-10 Dipole of a volume element

$$\sum p_i = \sigma' \cdot \Delta S \cdot \Delta l$$

By Equation (5-24), we know that, the magnitude of the electric polarization intensity is

$$P = \frac{\sum p_i}{\Delta V} = \frac{\sigma' \cdot \Delta S \cdot \Delta l}{\Delta S \cdot \Delta l} = \sigma'$$

That is

$$P = \sigma' \tag{5-26}$$

Equation (5-26) shows that, when the isotropic dielectric is in the polarization state, the surface density of polarization charges that appears on the two sides of being perpendicular to the external electric field is equal to the magnitude of the electric polarization intensity.

5.4.3 Electric Field in Dielectric and Dielectric Constant

Whenever there is an external electric field $\boldsymbol{E}_0$, a dielectric will be polarized and there will be polarization charges generated. These charges will also set up an additional electric field $\boldsymbol{E}'$ around the space. In the light of the superposition principle of electric field, the integrated field intensity $\boldsymbol{E}$ at some point inside the dielectric should be the vector sum of external electric field $\boldsymbol{E}_0$ and the additional electric field $\boldsymbol{E}'$, i.e.

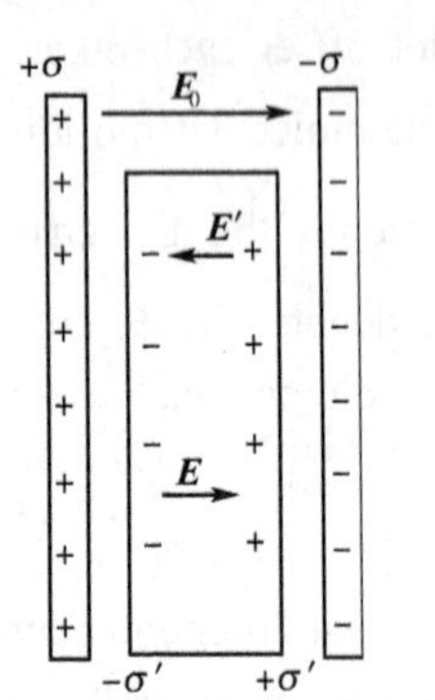

Figure 5-11 The electric intensity in the dielectric

$$\boldsymbol{E} = \boldsymbol{E}_0 + \boldsymbol{E}'$$

In order to describe quantitatively the field inside the dielectric, let's imagine filling the space between the two plates of an "infinite" parallel-plate capacitor with an isotropic dielectric, as shown in Figure 5-11. The surface charge densities on the two parallel plates of the capacitor are $+\sigma$ and $-\sigma$, and the field intensity produced is $\boldsymbol{E}_0$; the surface polarization charge densities resulted from the polarization of the dielectric are $+\sigma'$ and $-\sigma'$, and the additional electric field produced is $\boldsymbol{E}'$. $\boldsymbol{E}_0$ and $\boldsymbol{E}'$ have just the opposite directions, so the magnitude of the integrated field intensity $\boldsymbol{E}$ in the dielectric is

$$E = E_0 - E'$$

Because $E' = \dfrac{\sigma'}{\varepsilon_0}$ and $P = \sigma' = \chi\varepsilon_0 E$, by taking them into the above equation, we get

$$E = E_0 - \frac{\chi\varepsilon_0 E}{\varepsilon_0} = E_0 - \chi E$$

Further more we have

$$E = \frac{E_0}{1+\chi} = \frac{E_0}{\varepsilon_r} \tag{5-27a}$$

We call $\varepsilon_r = 1 + \chi$ in the above equation the **relative permittivity** (or relative dielectric constant) of the dielectric. Its value is dependent on the property of the dielectric, in vacuum $\varepsilon_r = 1$, and in any other dielectric $\varepsilon_r > 1$. The relative permittivity is also a unitless digital number. Equation (5-27a) shows that the field intensity in the dielectric is $\dfrac{1}{\varepsilon_r}$ times of the original field intensity.

Considering $E_0 = \dfrac{\sigma}{\varepsilon_0}$, we can also rewrite the electric field in the dielectric as

$$E = \frac{\sigma}{\varepsilon_0\varepsilon_r} = \frac{\sigma}{\varepsilon} \tag{5-27b}$$

In physics, $\varepsilon = \varepsilon_0 \cdot \varepsilon_r$ is also called the **dielectric constant of some dielectric material.**

Example 5-4 The liquids inside and outside the membrane of a nerve cell are both supposed to be the electrically conductive electrolyte, and the membrane of the cell is an excellent insulator with the relative dielectric constant of being about 7. In the resting state, a layer of positive charges is distributed on the outer side of the membrane, and on the inner side of the membrane is a layer of negative charges. If the transmembrane potential differential is –70 mV, and the thickness of the membrane is 6 nm, determine: (1) The electric field intensity within this cell membrane; (2) the surface charge densities on both sides of the membrane.

Solution: (1) The electric field intensity within the membrane

$$E=\frac{U}{d}=\frac{70\times10^{-3}}{6\times10^{-9}}\approx1.2\times10^{7}\ \mathrm{N/C}$$

(2) Referencing the formula of calculating the electric field intensity when there is dielectric between two parallel plates

$$E=\frac{\sigma}{\varepsilon}=\frac{\sigma}{\varepsilon_0\varepsilon_\mathrm{r}}$$

Hence, we can get the theoretical value of the charge density on both sides of the membrane.

$$\sigma=\varepsilon_\mathrm{r}\varepsilon_0 E=7\times8.85\times10^{-12}\times1.2\times10^{7}=7.4\times10^{-4}\ \mathrm{C/m^2}$$

5.5 Bioelectrical Phenomena

Bioelectrical phenomena are common electrical phenomena existing among all kinds of organism. They are closely related with the states of lives, and happen along with all the processes of lives' activities. Many routine clinical examinations in modern medicine such as electrocardiogram (ECG), electroencephalogram (EEG), electromyogram (EMG), etc. are the records of human bioelectrical phenomena in different forms, and these records are regarded as important indexes to judge the physiological or pathological states of activities of organs. The research to bioelectrical phenomena will help us to understand the essences of life states. The basic knowledge of the bioelectrical phenomena and electrical characteristics of neural conduction will be introduced as the following.

5.5.1 Nernst Equation

The cell membrane is a semi permeable membrane. There are some different ions in different concentrations in the electrolytes on both sides of the membrane (Table 5-1), and those more important are K^+, Na^+ and Cl^-. The state in which a cell is not stimulated by any kind of physical and chemical factors (such as heat, cold, light, sound and smell, and so on) is known as the **resting state**. In the resting state, the outer side of the membrane is positively charged, and the inner side is negatively charged. Alarge number of Na^+ and Cl^- exist on the outer side of the cell membrane, and a larger number of K^+ exists on the inner side of the membrane. Because there are differences of the ions' concentrations on both side of the cell membrane, there will be a certain potential difference ΔU between the inner and outer sides of the cell membrane. It is called the **membrane potential** (or the **transmembrane potential**). Now let's explain the reasons of the formation of the cell membrane potential.

Table 5-1 Ions' concentrations in the electrolytes inside and outside a cell membrane (Unit: mol/L)

Ion type	Intracellular concentration C_1	Extracellular concentration C_2
Na^+	0.010	0.142
K^+	0.141	0.005
Cl^-	0.004	0.103
Other negative ions	0.147	0.044
Total	0.151	0.147

Suppose the concentrated ① and the dilute ② solutions of some kind of **electrolyte** are separated by a semipermeable membrane; and the concentrations of the solutions are respectively C_1 and C_2, $C_1 > C_2$, as shown in Figure 5-12 (a). It is assumed that, the semipermeable membrane can only allow positive ions to pass through, while the negative ions are not allowed. So, the positive ions will diffuse from left with higher concentration to right with lower concentration, however, because of the attraction from the excess negative ions on the left, the positive charges can not go farther. The result is: positive and negative ions will accumulate respectively on both sides of the membrane, and the polarization phenomenon is formed. An electric field E which counterworks the further diffusion of positive ions is set up. Finally, a homeostasis is achieved, and a potential difference between both sides of the membrane is formed, too, as shown in Figure 5-12 (b). The formation of the cell membrane potential must have two conditions: **firstly, there must be an ions' concentration difference on inner and outer sides of the membrane; secondly, the cell membrane has a selecting permeability to ions.** The theoretical calculations can give the equation for calculating the membrane potential.

$$\varepsilon = \pm\frac{kT}{Ze}\ln\frac{C_1}{C_2} = \pm 2.3\frac{kT}{Ze}\lg\frac{C_1}{C_2}(\mathrm{V}) \tag{5-28}$$

Equation (5-28) is called **Nernst's equation**, and $\varepsilon = U$ is also called **Nernst electric potential**. Where k is Boltzmann constant mentioned in Chapter 3; T is the thermodynamic temperature of the solution; e is the electric quantity of electronic charge; Z is the number of charges of the ion, i.e., the number of valences of the ion; C_1 and C_2 are respectively the concentrations of the solution on two sides of the membrane. The minus sign in the equation is for the permeation of positive ions, and the plus sign is for the permeation of negative ions.

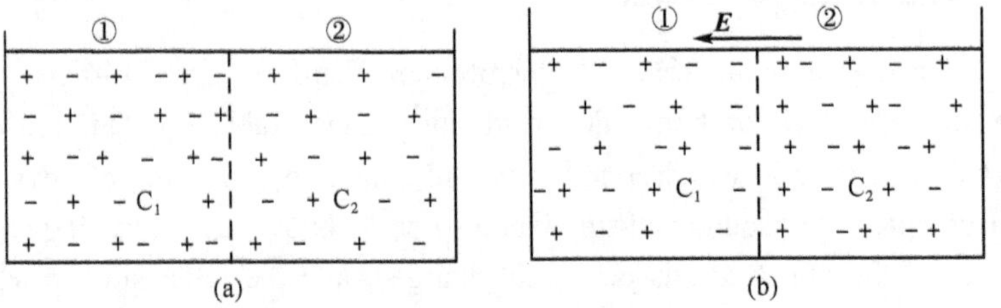

Figure 5-12 The formation of the membrane resting potential

When a cell is in the resting state, and the temperature is T = 300 K (27 ℃), by taking the data including concentrations of sodium, potassium, chloride ions from Table 5-1, k, T, e and others into the equation, we can get the membrane potentials generated by these ions: ε_{K^+}= −89 mV, ε_{Na^+}=70 mV, ε_{Cl^-} = −86 mV.

Comparing the calculated results with the membrane potential measured actually i.e., −85 mV, we can see that, ε_{Cl^-} is just in the state of balance; this means the numbers of Cl^- diffusing in and out of the cell through the membrane are in equilibrium. The numerical value of ε_{K^+} is slightly lower than that actually measured value; this means there is still a small amount of K^+ diffusing from the inside to the outside through the membrane. Although the numerical value of ε_{Na^+} differs from that actually measured value very much, because the permeability of cell membrane to Na^+ is very small in the resting state, there is only a small amount of Na^+ that can diffuse from the outside with higher concentration to the inside with lower concentration through the membrane.

5.5.2 Resting Potential and Action Potential

When a cell is not disturbed by the environment, the potential difference between the inside and the outside of the cell membrane is called the **resting potential**. The membrane resting potential corresponds to the state that the inner side of the cell membrane is negatively charged, and the outer side is positively charged. It is caused by the differences of ions' concentrations inside and outside the cell membrane and also by the permeability of the cell membrane which is different for different ions. **We usually take the potential on the outer side of a cell membrane as the zero reference point**. The potential value inside the membrane people often talk about, is actually the potential difference between both sides of the membrane.

In the resting state, K^+ and Cl^- can permeate through the cell membrane, and the permeability of the membrane to Na^+ is very small. However, the permeability of cell membrane to Na^+ can be adjusted. When a cell is stimulated and excited, the permeability of the cell membrane to Na^+ increases rapidly. The membrane potential will have a rapid and brief change on the basis of the resting potential, and the change of potential can spread around. This potential change is known as the process of the **action potential**. The process for an action potential can be divided into two parts: **depolarization process** and **repolarization process**.

When the permeability of a cell membrane to Na^+ increases rapidly, because the concentration of Na^+ on the outer side of the membrane is much higher than that inside, meanwhile, the potential inside the membrane is lower than the potential outside, there is a influx of Na^+ into the cell. This causes a rapid increase of the numerical value of the positive ions and a rapid increase of the potential on the inner side of the membrane. This increase of the potential on the inner side of the membrane then blocks the further diffusion of Na^+ toward the inside of the membrane and builds up a homeostasis, the inner side of the membrane will be positively charged and the outer side of the membrane will be negatively charged, the polarization state of the membrane is reversed, and the membrane potential increases rapidly from the original -85 mV to about $+60$ mV. This is the process of depolarization. Later, the permeability of cell membrane to Na^+ is restored, and the permeability to K^+ suddenly increases, so that a large number of K^+ diffuse through the membrane to the outside. In this way, the membrane potential decreases rapidly from a positive to a negative, until the original state of polarization is achieved. This is the process of repolarization. The relationship between action potential and time is shown in Figure 5-13.

During the action potential process of the cell membrane responding to an external stimulation, a large number of Na^+ and K^+ diffuse respectively from the regions of their higher concentrations into the regions of lower concentrations. However, the concentrations of ions in the resting state remain unchanged. How to explain this problem? The hypothesis of potassium pump and sodium pump is provided, and the cell membrane is assumed to have a mechanism similar to the function of a water pump, which is called the **sodium pump** (or **Na pump**). The pump plays the role of bringing Na^+ or K^+ back to the higher concentration region from the lower concentration region against the concentration difference, so that the normal distribution of ions on both sides of the membrane is maintained. The corresponding study has found the sodium pump is a special protein, which is studded in the lipid bilayer of the membrane. In addition to the function of transporting Na^+ and K^+, it has also the activity of enzyme for adenosine triphosphate (ATP), and it can decompose ATP to release its energy.

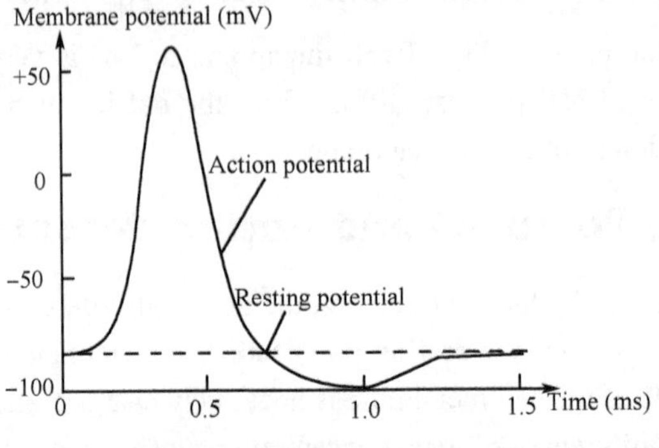

Figure 5-13 The action potential

Under normal physiological conditions, accompanying with the decomposition of 1 ATP molecule, three sodium ions can be transported out through the membrane, at the same time, two potassium ions will be transported to the inner side of the membrane, and a current to the outside of the membrane will be formed. It was this current that could cause the hyperpolarization of the cell membrane, and maintain the resting potential of a cell.

5.6 The Basic Principle of the Formation of ECG Waves

5.6.1 The Potential in the Electric Field of Electric Dipole

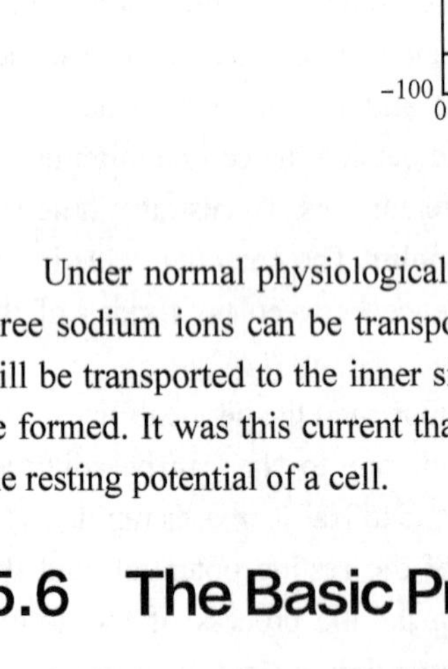

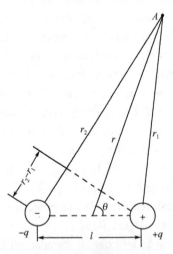

Figure 5-14 The potential in the electric field of a dipole

As we have mentioned previously, the concept of electric dipole means a system constructed with two point charges which have the equal electric quantity and different signs, and are separated near apart. The electric quantities of the two point charges of the electric dipole are respectively $+q$ and $-q$, and the distance between them is l. Now we are going to discuss the potential status at some field point A in the space around such an electric dipole, as shown in Figure 5-14. Assume that the distances to the field point A from $+q$ and from $-q$ are respectively r_1 and r_2. According to Equation (5-21c), if $K=\dfrac{1}{4\pi\varepsilon_0}$, at point A, the potential generated by the electric dipole is

$$U=U_+ + U_- = K\left(\frac{q}{r_1}-\frac{q}{r_2}\right)=Kq\frac{r_2-r_1}{r_1 r_2} \tag{5-29}$$

Let r be the distance from the central point of the electric dipole's axis to point A, the angle between the line of r and the electric dipole moment of $\boldsymbol{p}$ be θ. Because r_1, r_2 and r are much greater than l, so it can be considered approximately that $r_1 \cdot r_2 \approx r^2$ and $r_2 - r_1 \approx l\cos\theta$. Taking these two results into Equation (5-29), we have

$$U = Kq\frac{l\cos\theta}{r^2} = K\frac{p\cos\theta}{r^2} \tag{5-30}$$

In Equation (5-30), $p = ql$ is the magnitude of the electric dipole moment. We can see from this equation that, at some point with the distance of r from the midpoint of electric dipole's axis, such as point A, the potential is proportional to the electric dipole moment p, and is inversely proportional to the square of the distance r, and it is also associated with the angle θ. If point A is on the extended line of the axis ($\theta = 0$, or π), the potential of point A is $U = \pm K\frac{p}{r^2}$; if point A is on the plane which is perpendicular to the axis of the electric dipole ($\theta = \pi/2$, or $3\pi/2$), the potential of point A is $U = 0$. Because in the first or the fourth quadrants $\cos\theta$ is positive, and in the second and third quadrants, it's negative, the space of the potential distribution corresponding to the field of electric dipole is divided into two regions which are symmetric for positive and negative. The potential in the region where $+q$ exists is positive; and the potential in the region where $-q$ exists is negative. This is the distribution character of the potential produced by the electric dipole. Knowing this distribution will be very helpful for understanding the formation of ECG waves.

5.6.2 Electrocardiovector and Ring of Electrocardiovector

The heart consists of a large number of myocardial cells. These cells have an elongated shape. A typical myocardial cell has the length of about 100 μm and the width of about 15 μm. Each cell is surrounded by a layer of cell membrane with the thickness of 8-10 nm. Inside the cell, there is the conductive intracellular fluid, outside the cell, there is the conductive intercellular fluid, and they are both electrolytes. If there is not any stimulation received, these myocardial cells are in the resting state, then, the outer side of a cell membrane is positively charged and the inner side is negatively charged. This state is also called the **polarization state**, as shown in Figure 5-15 (a).

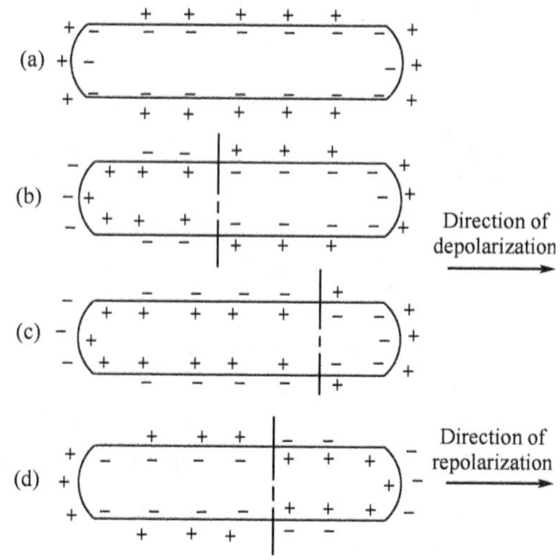

Figure 5-15 The depolarization and repolarization in a myocardial cell

When a myocardial cell, which is originally in the polarization state, is stimulated and becomes excited, the cell membrane's permeability to ions will have a change; this will cause an action potential. Accompanying with the action potential of the myocardial cell, the electric potentials on the inner side and the outer side of the membrane will change inevitably, so that the original polarization state will be destroyed. We call this phenomenon the **depolarization phenomenon**. The depolarization starts at the point of excitement and spreads around along the cell. As shown in Figure 5-15 (b) and Figure 5-15 (c), it spreads from the left to the right. In the process of depolarization, the myocardial cell is equivalent to an electric dipole; the direction of the electric moment is the same as the spreading direction. Depolarization process is a very short process. After that, the cell gradually restores to the original state, i.e., the outside is positive and the inside is negative, as shown in Figure 5-15 (d). This process is called the **repolarization process**. Here, the cell is also equivalent to an electric dipole, but the direction of the electric moment is opposite to the direction of the electric moment when the depolarization happens. When the repolarization finishes, the whole cell returns to the original polarization state. In conclusion, during the myocardial cell's depolarization and repolarization processes, it will form a changing electric moment, thus, it will cause a potential change in the surrounding space.

Because a myocardial cell can be regarded as an equivalent electric dipole during the processes of the depolarization and the repolarization, when an external stimulation transfers from one cell to another, this transfer can be considered equivalently as the transfer of an electric dipole. For a piece of myocardial muscle composed of numerous myocardial cells, its depolarization and repolarization processes can also be regarded as the transferring processes of many electric dipoles of this kind.

Each electric dipole has a corresponding physical quantity electric moment $\boldsymbol{p}_i$. By using the method of vector superposition, we can compose an integrated dipole moment vector with several vectors of electric moments. In a piece of myocardial tissue, the spreading process of depolarization is expressed as the manner of the depolarization front's extending forward (the depolarization front is the interface of the part depolarized and part not depolarized), as shown in Figure 5-16. We can see from the figure above, during the process of the depolarization in a piece of myocardial tissue, the directions of electric moments of those small dipoles are not all the same. We integrate all the electric moments of these many small electric dipoles according to the method for calculating vector sum at any time, and finally, get an integrated vector. We call this integrated vector $\boldsymbol{p}$, which is composed at some moment, the **transient integrated electrocardiovector**, or the **electrocardiovector** for short. Here in Figure 5-16 $\boldsymbol{p}=\sum \boldsymbol{p}_i$.

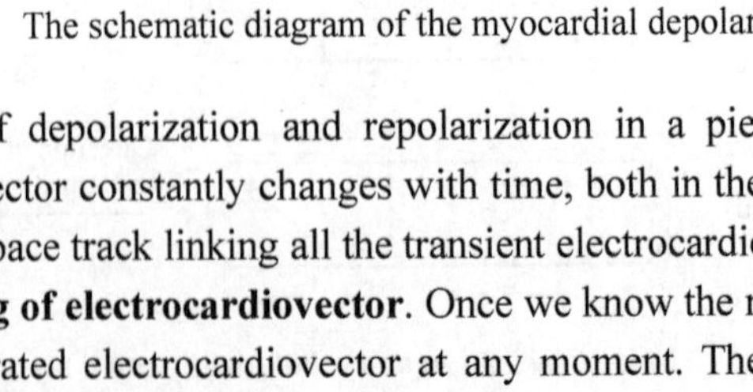

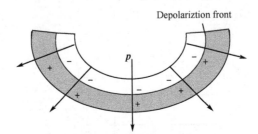

Figure 5-16 The schematic diagram of the myocardial depolarization front

During the processes of depolarization and repolarization in a piece of myocardial tissue, the corresponding electrocardiovector constantly changes with time, both in the direction and the magnitude. In a period of heartbeat, the space track linking all the transient electrocardiovectors' arrow points forms a ring. We call this ring the **ring of electrocardiovector**. Once we know the ring of electrocardiovector, we will have the transient integrated electrocardiovector at any moment. The heart electrical activity in a heartbeat period can be theoretically represented with a series of transient integrated electrocardiovectors. Nowadays, the VCG (vectorcardiogram) diagnostic instrument used in clinics can measure the diagrams of the rings of electrocardiovectors. During the process of depolarization in the atrial region, at any moment there will be the corresponding transient integrated electrocardiovector produced, thus, the corresponding space vector ring of P is formed; during the process of depolarization in the ventricular region, the QRS vector ring is formed; during the process of repolarization in the ventricular region, the T ring is formed, as shown in Figure 5-17. Figure 5-17 only shows the planar diagrams, and they are the projections of spatial vector rings in a plane. A practical VCG diagnostic instrument can draw the projecting planar diagrams in three-dimensional planes.

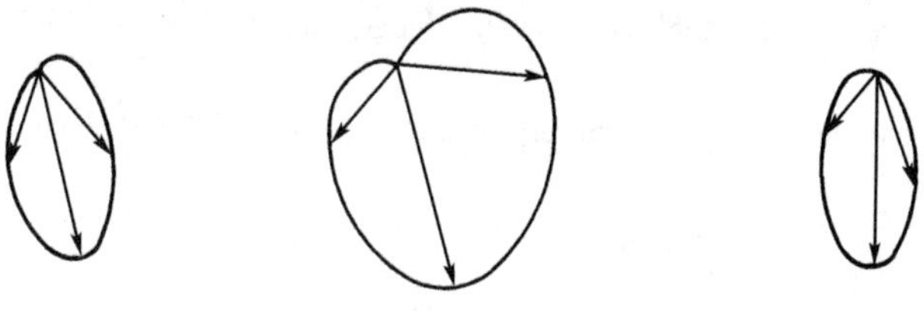

(a) P-ring (b) QRS-ring (c) T-ring

Figure 5-17 Rings of the electrocardiovectors

5.6.3 The Formation of the Electrocardiogram Waves

When myocardial muscle is excited, there will be electrocardiovectors generated at any moment. We can take the transient integrated electrocardiovector equivalently as an electric dipole moment of an electric dipole. The change of this electric dipole moment will cause the change of potential on body surface. According to Equation (5-30), we can get this potential change.

$$U = K\frac{p\cos\theta}{r^2}$$

where p is the magnitude of the transient integrated electrocardiovector (the electric moment of the equivalent electric dipole), r is the distance from the central point of the electric dipole to the detected point. This body surface potential, which keeps on varying with the heartbeat period, is called the **electrocardiogram** (ECG), when it is expressed by a planar diagram. As shown in Figure 5-18, the vertical axis represents the potential value, the horizontal axis represents time, and the curve shows the potential value at every moment at some point on the body surface. In practice, ECG is one of the important physical diagnostic indexes to examine whether the generation of the heart's excitement, the spread of the heart's excitement, and the recovery process are in normal state or not. It has been playing an important role in the diagnosis of heart diseases.

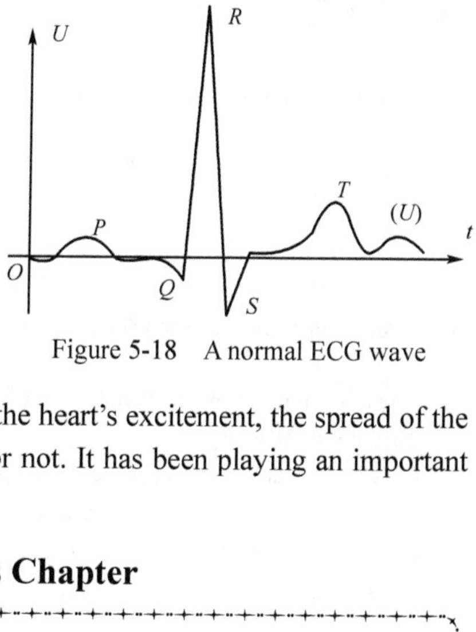

Figure 5-18 A normal ECG wave

A Brief Summarization of This Chapter

(1) The vectorial expression of Coulomb's law: $\boldsymbol{F} = \dfrac{1}{4\pi\varepsilon_0}\dfrac{q_1 q_2}{r^2}\hat{\boldsymbol{r}}$

(2) The definition of the electric field intensity vector: $\boldsymbol{E} = \dfrac{\boldsymbol{F}}{q_0}$

(3) The superposition principle of electric field intensity: $\boldsymbol{E} = \boldsymbol{E}_1 + \boldsymbol{E}_2 + \cdots + \boldsymbol{E}_n = \sum \boldsymbol{E}_i$

(4) The calculation of field:

1) The electric field intensity of a field set up by a point charge: $\boldsymbol{E} = \dfrac{1}{4\pi\varepsilon_0}\dfrac{q}{r^2}\hat{\boldsymbol{r}}$

2) The electric field intensity of a field set up by a system of point charges: $\boldsymbol{E}=\sum_{i=1}^{n}\boldsymbol{E}_i=\frac{1}{4\pi\varepsilon_0}\sum_{i=1}^{n}\frac{q_i}{r_i^2}\hat{\boldsymbol{r}}_i$

3) The electric field intensity of a field set up by any charged body: $\boldsymbol{E}=\frac{1}{4\pi\varepsilon_0}\int\frac{\mathrm{d}q}{r^2}\hat{\boldsymbol{r}}$

(5) The electric flux passing through an arbitrary surface S: $\Phi=\iint_S \mathrm{d}\Phi=\iint_S E\cos\theta\,\mathrm{d}S=\iint_S \boldsymbol{E}\cdot\mathrm{d}\boldsymbol{S}$

(6) Gauss' law: $\Phi=\oiint_S \boldsymbol{E}\cdot\mathrm{d}\boldsymbol{S}=\frac{1}{\varepsilon_0}\sum q_i$

(7) The circulatory theorem of the electrostatic field: $\oint_L \boldsymbol{E}\cdot\mathrm{d}\boldsymbol{l}=0$

(8) The electric potential at point A in an electric field: $U_A=\frac{W_A}{q_0}=\int_A^{\infty}\boldsymbol{E}\cdot\mathrm{d}\boldsymbol{l}$

(9) The calculation of the potential of a point charge: $U=\frac{W}{q_0}=\frac{q}{4\pi\varepsilon_0}\int_r^{\infty}\frac{\mathrm{d}r}{r^2}=\frac{q}{4\pi\varepsilon_0 r}$

(10) The superposition principle of the electric potential: $U=\sum_{i=1}^{n}\frac{q_i}{4\pi\varepsilon_0 r_i}$. It shows the electric potential at some point in the electric field set up by a system of point charges is equal to the algebraic sum of the component electric potentials at that point, and each component potential is generated by the corresponding point charge when it exists alone.

(11) The potential difference between any two points A and B in the electric field: $\Delta U=U_{AB}=U_A-U_B=\int_A^B \boldsymbol{E}\cdot\mathrm{d}\boldsymbol{l}$

(12) The electric polarization intensity of a dielectric in an external electric field $\boldsymbol{E}_0$: $\boldsymbol{P}=\frac{\sum \boldsymbol{p}_i}{\Delta V}$

Exercises 5

5-1. According to the formula for calculating the electric field around a point charge $\boldsymbol{E}=\frac{1}{4\pi\varepsilon_0}\frac{q}{r^2}\hat{\boldsymbol{r}}$ someone may conclude the following statement: when $r\to 0$, $E\to\infty$. However, the field intensity can not be infinite. Try to explain the reason.

5-2. Give a brief description for the polarization processes of the dielectrics which are respectively composed of polar molecules and non-polar molecules.

5-3. Give a brief description for the mechanism of the human ECG waves.

5-4. There is a uniformly charged straight wire AB with the length of l =15 cm, and positive linear charge density $\lambda = 5\times 10^{-9}$ C/m. Determine:

(1) The field intensity at point P with a distance of 5 cm from one end of the wire B and on the extensional line of the wire;

(2) The field intensity at point Q with a distance of 5 cm from the center of the wire and on the perpendicular bisector of the wire.

5-5. A small charged ball with the mass of 1×10^{-6} kg and the electric quantity of 2.0×10^{-11} C, is hanging by a string at the lower end, now, put it near to a huge uniformly charged plate which is placed vertically; and then the thread makes an angle of 30° with the charged plate. Try to determine the surface charge density of the charged plate.

5-6. (1) There is a uniformly charged ring with the radius of R, and the linear charge density of λ. Determine the electric field intensity at point P that is on the central axis of the ring and has a distance of x from the ring's center.

(2) By using the result from (1), try to determine the electric field intensity at point P that is on the central axis of a uniformly charged disc which has a radius of R and a surface charge density of σ. The distance from point P to the disc's central point O is x.

5-7. Determine the magnitude of the field intensities inside and outside an infinitely long straight electric charged tube, which has a radius of R, and a surface charge density of σ.

5-8. Determine the magnitude of the field intensity around a uniformly charged infinitely long straight fine stick with the linear charge density of λ.

5-9. Suppose a circular hole with the radius of R and the center of O is digged on a uniform charged infinitely large plate, which has a surface charge density of σ. Determine the magnitude of the field intensity at point P, which has a distance of x from the central point O. Here, the line segment PO is perpendicular to the plate.

5-10. Determine the field intensity at point P, which is on the extensional line of the axis of an electric dipole and has a distance of r from the center of the dipole. The situation is shown in Figure for Exercise 5-10 (Here, the distance between two point charges $\pm q$ of the electric dipole is l).

5-11. There is a sphere of radius R, which is uniformly charged with the electric quantity of q, and its volume charge density is ρ. Determine the field intensities at any points inside and outside the sphere.

5-12. As shown in Figure for Exercise 5-12, there is a test charge q_0 moving in the electric field set up by two point charges q_1 and q_2. The known quantities are: r = 8 cm, a = 12 cm, $q_1 = q_2 = 1.3 \times 10^{-8}$ C, $q_0 = 10^{-9}$ C. Determine:

(1) The work done by the electric field force on q_0, during the process when q_0 moves from point A to point B;

(2) The work done by the electric field force on q_0, during the process when q_0 moves from point C to point D.

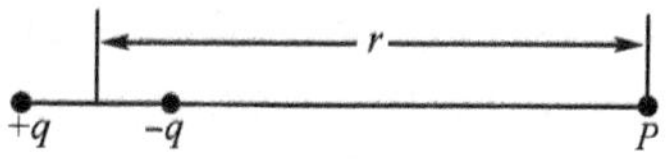

Figure for Exercise 5-10

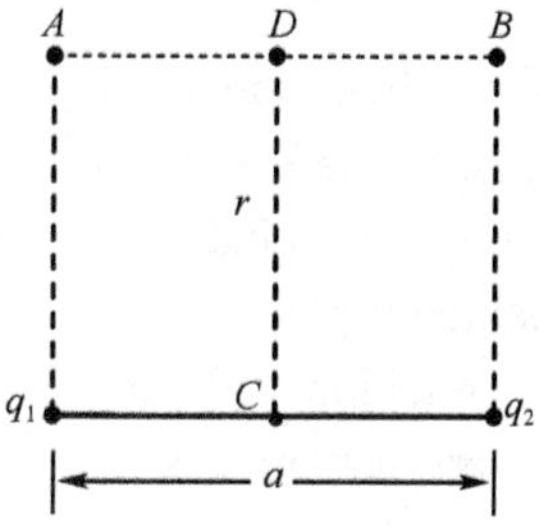

Figure for Exercise 5-12

Chapter 6 Direct Current Circuit

The application of electric current is extremely wide. Electric current can be used for energy transportation and also for information convection. Wherever in modern science and technology or in our routine lives we have close relations with electric current. Meanwhile, electric current also plays important roles in the living processes of human beings. The electric current is formed by the directional motion of electric charges in the electric field. If the direction of the current does not change with time, the current is called the direct current. In this chapter, we will discuss the conditions to form the direct current and Ohm's law in a section of circuit with sources of emf; based on these, we will introduce Kirchhoff's rules and the corresponding applications for solving problems of complicated circuits; and finally, we will introduce some knowledge about the applications of electrotherapy.

6.1 Current Density

6.1.1 Current Intensity

In an electric field, the moving direction of positive charges is always opposite to the direction of negative charges. We define the moving direction of positive charges as the direction of a current. So, it is not difficult for us to conclude that, in a conductor the direction of a current always points from a place of higher potential to the place of lower potential along the direction of the electric field.

There are conditions only on which a current can exist in the conductor: firstly, there is the existence of charge carriers that moves freely in the conductor; secondly, there is the existence of potential difference between the two terminals of the conductor, i.e., there is an electric field in it.

We define the **current intensity** as the net electric quantity passing through any cross-sectional area in a unit time. As a physical quantity, current intensity is used to describe the strength of a current, and it is denoted by I. Thus, if a net electric quantity passing through the area in a time interval of Δt is Δq, the current intensity flowing through the area is defined as

$$I = \frac{\Delta q}{\Delta t} \tag{6-1}$$

If both the magnitude and the direction of a current are not varying with time, the current is called a **steady current**. When the magnitude of a current varies with time, the current intensity is then expressed as

$$I = \lim_{\Delta t \to 0} \frac{\Delta q}{\Delta t} = \frac{dq}{dt} \tag{6-2}$$

The unit of current intensity in SI system is ampere. It is denoted by A, and 1 A = 1 C/s. Other common units of current intensity are mA and μA.

6.1.2 Current Density (Vector)

In the case of calculation for a general circuit, what we need to know is merely the current intensity flowing through the cross section in each branch of the circuit, and we needn't to consider whether the distribution of the current is uniform or not in the cross-sectional area. When a current is flowing in a big block of the conductor (such as the trunk or limbs of the human body, or the electrolyte in a container), generally, at different points inside the conductor, the magnitudes and the directions of the current intensities are different. This kind of conductor is called the volume conductor. It is obvious that we should introduce a new physical quantity for describing the distribution of the current inside a volume conductor exactly. This quantity is the **current density**.

At some point inside the conductor, assume to take a cross section with the area of ΔS, which is perpendicular to the direction of the field intensity at that point. We define the limit of the ratio of the current flowing through this cross section (ΔI) to the area (ΔS) as the magnitude of the current density at that point, i.e.

$$j = \lim_{\Delta S \to 0} \frac{\Delta I}{\Delta S} = \frac{dI}{dS} \tag{6-3}$$

The current density is a vector denoted as $\boldsymbol{j}$; its direction is the same as the direction of the field intensity there. It is a physical quantity for describing the current distribution inside a conductor; its unit is A/m^2.

For ease of applying, let's derive another expression of the current density vector. As shown in Figure 6-1, assume that a cross section with the area of ΔS is put perpendicularly to the direction of the field intensity. The charge carriers (those a large number of charged particles can move freely in the conductor) flow along the direction of being perpendicular to ΔS. Suppose the number of the charge carriers in the unit volume i.e. the numeral density of the charge carriers is n; the average drift velocity of them is $\bar{v}$; the electric quantity of every charge carrier is Ze (here, Z is the valence of the charge carrier). The distance that the charge carriers traveled during a time interval Δt is

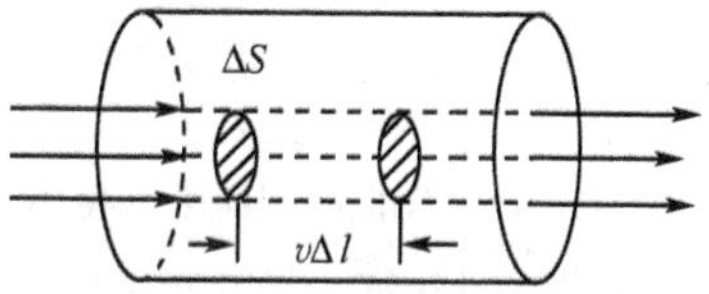

Figure 6-1 The relationship between the current density and the average drift velocity

$$\Delta l = \bar{v}\Delta t$$

The electric quantity passing through the cross section will be

$$\Delta q = nZe\Delta l\Delta S = nZe\bar{v}\Delta t\Delta S$$

The current intensity flowing through the cross section is

$$\Delta I = \frac{\Delta q}{\Delta t} = nZe\bar{v}\Delta S$$

According to Equation (6-3), we can get the magnitude of the current density

$$j = \lim_{\Delta S \to 0} \frac{\Delta I}{\Delta S} = nZe\bar{v} \tag{6-4}$$

Equation (6-4) shows that the magnitude of the current density is the product of the three quantities: n means the numeral density of the charge carriers in the conductor; Ze means the electric quantity of each charge carrier; $\bar{v}$ means the average drift velocity of charge carriers.

In the case of a piece of metal as the conductor, there are numerous free electrons moving irregularly inside it. If an electric potential difference is put on the two terminals of it, the electrons will drift along the opposite direction of the electric field intensity $\boldsymbol{E}$, and form an electric current of directional motion. The average drift velocity of the free electrons is very slow in the metal. In a piece of metal conductor with the numeral density of the free electrons n and with their average drift velocity of $\bar{v}$, we assume to take a cross section with the area of ΔS. The electric quantity of an electron is known as e, so, the electric quantity passing through the cross section ΔS in a time interval of Δt is $\Delta q = ne\bar{v}\Delta t\Delta S$; the current intensity flowing through it is $\Delta I = \dfrac{\Delta q}{\Delta t} = ne\bar{v}\Delta S$; here, the magnitude of the current density will be

$$j = \frac{\Delta I}{\Delta S} = ne\overline{v} \tag{6-5}$$

Example 6-1 The electric current with the intensity of 200 mA is flowing in a piece of copper wire with the diameter of 0.15 cm. There are 8.5×10^{28} free electrons in a volume of 1 m^3 of the wire. Determine the average drift velocity of the free electrons in the wire.

Solution:

$$j = \frac{\Delta I}{\Delta S} = ne\overline{v},\ \Delta S = \pi r^2$$

$$\overline{v} = \frac{j}{ne} = \frac{\Delta I}{ne\Delta S} = \frac{\Delta I}{ne\pi r^2} = \frac{200\times10^{-3}}{8.5\times10^{28}\times1.6\times10^{-19}\times3.14\times\left(\frac{0.15\times10^{-2}}{2}\right)^2} = 8.3\times10^{-6}\ \text{m/s}$$

We can see from the result of Example 6-1: the average drift velocity of directional motion of free electrons in the wire is much lower than the speed of the current (i.e. the light speed). As soon as the potential difference is put on the two terminals of a circuit, the electric field will be set up in the whole circuit; at nearly the same moment, the free electrons in the conductor will start the directional motion and form an electric current.

In the case of an electrolyte solution as the conductor, the charge carriers are positive and negative ions. If the solution is put in an electric field, the positive ions in it will drift along the direction of the field intensity to form an electric current and the negative ions will drift conversely to form another electric current. Here, the total current density is the sum of the current densities formed by the positive ions and negative ions, i.e.

$$\boldsymbol{j} = \boldsymbol{j}_+ + \boldsymbol{j}_- = Zen\overline{\boldsymbol{v}}_+ + Zen\overline{\boldsymbol{v}}_- \tag{6-6}$$

where Z represents the valence of the ions. For a certain kind of electrolyte, under a certain temperature, $\boldsymbol{j}$ is proportional to $\boldsymbol{E}$, and they have the same direction.

6.2 Ohm's Law in a Section of Circuit with Sources

6.2.1 Electromotive Force (emf) of a Source

To form a current in a conductor, the conductor should be on two conditions: one is that there must be numerous free charges inside; the other is that there must be a potential difference on the two terminals of it. The function of a source is to set up and maintain a potential difference by the non-electrostatic force. If the potential difference is maintained, a steady current will be obtained.

In different sources the work done by the non-electrostatic force will be different. The **electromotive force** of a source is a physical quantity to describe the ability of the non-electrostatic force to do work inside the source. **The electromotive force of a source is equal to the work done by the non-electrostatic force on a unit positive charge during the process when the charge is transported from the cathode to the anode via the inside of the source.** If the electric quantity of the charge being transported is q, and the work is W, the emf will be

$$\varepsilon = \frac{W}{q} \tag{6-7}$$

The electromotive force is a scalar; it has the same unit as potential's, i.e., volt (V). For applying conveniently, an emf is defined to have a direction; its direction is commonly regulated as the direction from the cathode to the anode via the inside of the source.

The magnitude of the emf is only dependent on the properties of the source itself and independent on the constructing forms of outer circuit. The resistance inside a source is called its inner resistance. When an electric current flows inside the source the current will also be resisted. The drop of the potential on the outer circuit is called the **terminal voltage**. If the outer circuit is an open circuit, the terminal voltage is equal to the source's emf.

There are so many kinds of sources, such as dry batteries, storage batteries, solar cells, generators, etc.; for different sources, the corresponding manners to generate non-electrostatic forces are different and the forms to consume energy are also different. But the hypostasis for all kinds of non-electrostatic forces to do work is to transform energies of other forms to the electric energy. So, a source (sometimes called an emf source or a source of emf) is a kind of transducer.

6.2.2 Ohm's Law in a Section of Circuit with emf Sources

Now let's discuss the case of a section of circuit which contains emf sources. In calculations for this kind of circuits, it is very convenient to analyze and solve problems from the view of potential drop.

As shown in Figure 6-2, *ACB* is a section of some closed circuit, and this section contains sources. Let's calculate the potential difference between point *A* and point *B*. Here, E_1, E_2 and E_3 represent three sources; their electromotive forces and inner resistances are respectively ε_1, r_1, ε_2, r_2 and ε_3, r_3. The directions of the currents are assumed as those shown in the figure. First, we take the direction from *A* to *B* as our rounding direction; then, determine the potential drop in every part between *A* and *B*; finally, calculate the algebraic sum as the potential difference between point *A* and point *B*. Now let's define that along the rounding direction, if the potential decreases, then the value of the potential drop is positive; just oppositely, if the potential increases, then the value is negative. In the part *AC*, because the rounding direction is from *A* to *C* and it is just the direction of the current I_1, the potential drop on R_1 is I_1R_1; on the source E_1 the rounding direction is from the anode to the cathode, the potential drop is ε_1, and the potential drop on r_1 is I_1r_1. In the part *CB*, on the source E_2 the rounding direction is from the cathode to the anode, the potential gets a rise of ε_2; on the source E_3 the rounding direction is from the anode to the cathode, the potential drop is ε_3; because the rounding direction from *C* to *B* is the opposite direction of the current I_2, the potential drop on R_2 is $-I_2R_2$; and the potential drops on r_2 and r_3 are respectively $-I_2r_2$ and $-I_2r_3$. So, the potential difference between point *A* and point *B* is

$$U_{AB} = U_A - U_B = I_1R_1 + \varepsilon_1 + I_1r_1 - \varepsilon_2 - I_2r_2 - I_2R_2 + \varepsilon_3 - I_2r_3$$

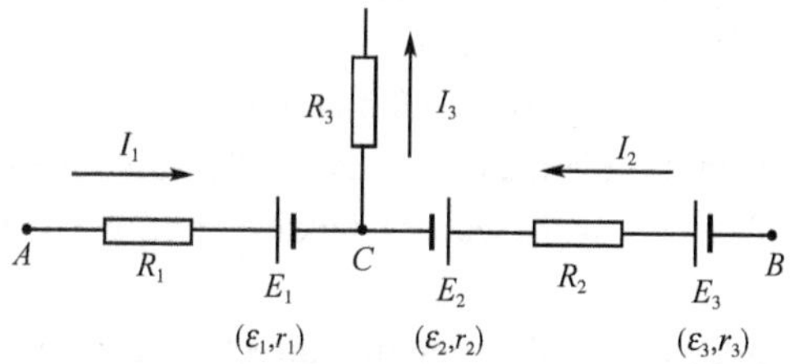

Figure 6-2 A section of circuit with emf sources

If the algebraic sum of the potential drops on all resistors is expressed as ΣIR, and the algebraic sum of the potential drops on all sources is expressed as $\Sigma\varepsilon$, we will get the conclusion from the above equation: **the potential difference between the two terminals of a section of circuit containing sources is equal to the algebraic sum of the potential drops on all resistors and all sources.** Rewritten as the general form, the conclusion will be expressed as

$$U_{AB} = U_A - U_B = \Sigma IR + \Sigma\varepsilon \tag{6-8}$$

This is **Ohm's law in a section of circuit with emf sources.** Here, we emphasize that the rounding direction is chosen randomly. For ease of calculating, we define the positive and negative signs in Equation (6-8) as follows.

(1) If the direction of the current intensity is the same as the designate rounding direction, the potential drop on a resistor will be positive, IR is looked as a positive; if the directions are contrary, IR is a negative.

(2) If the designate rounding direction chosen is from the anode to the cathode of a source, the potential drop contributed by it will be positive, ε is looked as a positive; if contrarily, ε is negative.

We can see from Equation (6-8): if $U_A - U_B > 0$, the potential at point A is higher than that at point B; if $U_A - U_B < 0$, the potential at point A is lower than that at point B; well, if points A and B are superposed, a closed circuit is constructed and the equation becomes

$$U_{AB} = U_A - U_B = \Sigma IR + \Sigma\varepsilon = 0$$

If the current intensity has the same magnitude and direction in a closed circuit, i.e., the circuit is a simple loop, we will have

$$I = \frac{\sum \varepsilon}{\sum R} \tag{6-9}$$

This is **Ohm's law in a closed circuit**. In this case, it should be noted that in Equation (6-9) $\Sigma\varepsilon$ represents the algebraic sum of the **potential increments** caused by all electromotive forces.

Example 6-2 A closed circuit is as shown in Figure 6-3. Determine (1) the current intensity in the circuit; (2) the terminal voltage U_{AB} on the source E_2; (3) the terminal voltage U_{BC} on the source E_1.

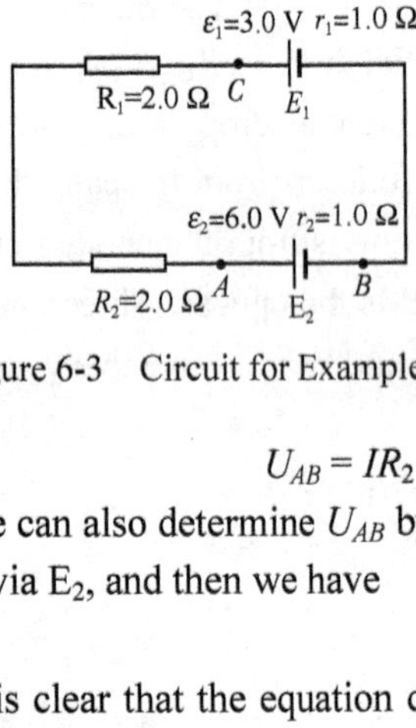

Figure 6-3 Circuit for Example 6-2

Solution: (1) Because $\varepsilon_2 > \varepsilon_1$, the direction of the current in the circuit is designated in clockwise. According to Ohm's law in a closed circuit we have

$$I = \frac{\varepsilon_2 - \varepsilon_1}{R_1 + R_2 + r_1 + r_2} = \frac{6-3}{2+2+1+1} = \frac{3}{6} = 0.5\ \text{A}$$

(2) For determining U_{AB}, we designate the rounding direction as clockwise, from point A to point B via R_2, R_1 and E_1, and then we have

$$U_{AB} = IR_2 + IR_1 + Ir_1 + \varepsilon_1 = 0.5\times2.0 + 0.5\times2.0 + 0.5\times1.0 + 3.0 = 5.5\ \text{V}$$

We can also determine U_{AB} by choosing the rounding direction as counterclockwise, from point A to point B via E_2, and then we have

$$U_{AB} = -Ir_2 + \varepsilon_2 = -0.5\times1.0 + 6.0 = 5.5\ \text{V}$$

It is clear that the equation derived by this method is easier. To solve the practical problems, we should use Ohm's law in a section of circuit with sources flexibly, and make the calculations as simple as possible.

(3) For determining U_{BC}, we designate the rounding direction as counterclockwise, i.e., from point B to point C via E_1, and we have

$$U_{BC} = -\varepsilon_1 - Ir_1 = -3.0 - 0.5\times1.0 = -3.5\ \text{V}$$

Because

$$U_{CB} = -U_{BC} = 3.5\ \text{V}$$

i.e., the value of voltage U_{CB} between the two terminals of the source E_1 is bigger than its emf ε_1, which means the direction of the current in the circuit is just opposite to the direction of the imagined current that the source should have supplied. There, the source E_1 will not supply any energy but consume some energy.

6.3 Kirchhoff's Rules

For simple circuits, no matter how complicated they may seem to be, they can be simplified as simple loops with the calculating regulations for serial and parallel circuits, and the corresponding problems can be solved by different forms of Ohm's law. But in practical calculations, the majority of circuits are often more complicated. They can not be simplified as simple loops by the calculating regulations for serial and parallel circuits; for solving the corresponding problems, merely applying Ohm's law will not reach satisfied. It was in 1847 that a German physicist Kirchhoff published two rules for analyzing networks (or **complicated circuits**), they are both called **Kirchhoff's Rules**. They are the derivations of Ohm's law and have been playing important roles in solving problems of complicated circuits.

In a complicated circuit, a point where three or more branches are joined is called a **junction** (or **branch point**). And a **branch** is a section of circuit between any two branch points; it can be constructed by one or a series of electrical pieces; at any points in a branch, the current is consistent. Any closed path composed with several branches in the circuit is called a **loop**. The circuit shown in Figure 6-4 has three branches, two junctions and three loops.

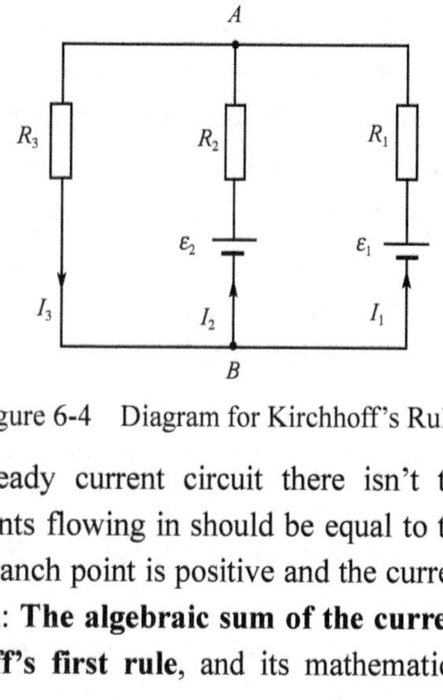

Figure 6-4 Diagram for Kirchhoff's Rules

6.3.1 Kirchhoff's First Rule

Kirchhoff's first rule is also called Kirchhoff's **junction rule of current**. It confirms the relationships between the currents at any branch point. According to the principle of the continuity of the current, we know that, at any point in a steady current circuit there isn't the accumulation of charges. So, for any branch point the sum of currents flowing in should be equal to the sum of currents flowing out. If we define the current flowing in a branch point is positive and the current flowing out of the branch point is negative, we have the conclusion: **The algebraic sum of the current intensities meeting at a branch point is zero**, this is **Kirchhoff's first rule**, and its mathematical expression is

$$\sum_{i=1}^{n} I_i = 0 \qquad (6\text{-}10)$$

where n is the number of the currents meeting at the branch point.

For the branch point A in the circuit shown in Figure 6-4, the corresponding equation is

$$I_1 + I_2 - I_3 = 0$$

For the branch point B, the corresponding equation is

$$I_3 - I_1 - I_2 = 0$$

The equations corresponding to Kirchhoff's first rule are called junction equations of current. From the above results we can see that, corresponding to the two branch points in the circuit there are two junction equations, but only one is independent. We can prove that if there are n branch points in a circuit, we can only obtain $n-1$ independent junction equations. In practical application, if the directions of currents can not be confirmed beforehand, the directions could be assumed randomly first. By the calculating results the exact directions can be finally confirmed. If the calculating result of a current intensity I is calculated as a positive, it means that, the exact direction of the current is the same as the direction of being assumed; if the current intensity I is negative, it means that, the exact direction of the current is opposite to the direction of being assumed.

6.3.2 Kirchhoff's Second Rule

Kirchhoff's second rule is also called the **loop rule of voltage**. It confirms the relationships between potential differences on any sections in a loop.

According to the conclusions of previous section, if the rounding path starts at any point in a loop, and forms a round along the loop then comes back to the original point, the algebraic sum of potential drops is zero. The mathematical expression is

$$\Sigma IR + \Sigma \varepsilon = 0 \tag{6-11}$$

Equation (6-11) shows that, **after taking a round along a loop, the corresponding algebraic sum of potential drops is zero**. This is **Kirchhoff's second rule**.

When applying Kirchhoff's second rule, the rounding direction can be designated randomly. It is similar to the case of Ohm's law in a section of circuit with sources: if the rounding direction is the direction of the current, the potential drop on a resistor is positive, i.e., the sign of IR is taken as a positive; if the directions are contrary, it is a negative; if the rounding direction is from the anode to the cathode of a source, the potential drop contributed by it will be positive, the sign of ε is taken as positive; contrarily, the sign of ε is negative.

In the circuit shown in Figure 6-4, there are three loops: $AR_3B\varepsilon_2R_2A$, $AR_2\varepsilon_2B\varepsilon_1R_1A$ and $AR_3B\varepsilon_1R_1A$; if the rounding directions are all designated to be clockwise, we get three equations. These equations corresponding to Kirchhoff's second rule are called the loop equations of voltage.

Corresponding to the loop $AR_3B\varepsilon_2R_2A$, we have

$$I_3R_3 + I_2R_2 - \varepsilon_2 = 0$$

Corresponding to the loop $AR_2\varepsilon_2B\varepsilon_1R_1A$, we have

$$-I_2R_2 + \varepsilon_2 - \varepsilon_1 + I_1R_1 = 0$$

Corresponding to the loop $AR_3B\varepsilon_1R_1A$, we have

$$I_3R_3 - \varepsilon_1 + I_1R_1 = 0$$

For any two of the equations above, by doing plus or minus operations we can get the third one. This means there are only two independent equations. When we choose the loops for setting up the equations, we should pay attention to the independence of the loops. If there are n branch points and m branches in a circuit, $m - (n-1)$ independent equations can be gotten. We commonly choose the single loops (or net holes) for setting up the independent equations, because the number of the single loops is just $m - (n-1)$.

Example 6-3 In the network shown in Figure 6-5, $\varepsilon_1 = 6.0$ V, $\varepsilon_2 = 2.0$ V, $R_1 = 3.0\ \Omega$, $R_2 = 1.0\ \Omega$, $R_3 = 10\ \Omega$. Determine the current intensities in the three branches.

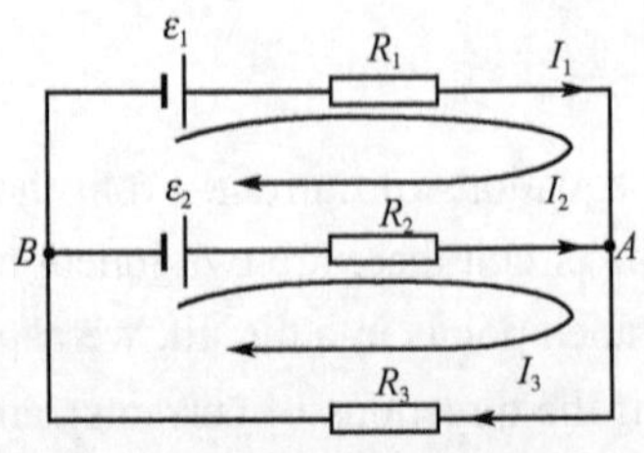

Figure 6-5 Circuit for Example 6-3

Solutions: Assume the directions of currents in the branches are shown in Figure 6-5, according to Kirchhoff's first rule, for the junction A, we have the junction equation of current

$$I_1 + I_2 - I_3 = 0$$

According to Kirchhoff's second rule, we can get the loop equations of voltage. The rounding directions for the two single loops are both designated to be clockwise as shown in the figure. In this way, we have two independent loop equations.

Corresponding to the loop $B\varepsilon_1R_1AR_2\varepsilon_2B$, there is

$$-\varepsilon_1 + I_1R_1 - I_2R_2 + \varepsilon_2 = 0$$

Corresponding to the loop $B\varepsilon_2R_2AR_3B$, there is

$$-\varepsilon_2 + I_2R_2 + I_3R_3 = 0$$

Substituting the quantities in the equations with the values known, we can get the results

$$I_1 = \frac{46}{43} \approx 1.1\ \text{A}, \quad I_2 = -\frac{34}{43} \approx -0.8\ \text{A}, \quad I_3 = \frac{12}{43} \approx 0.3\ \text{A}$$

In the results, I_1 and I_3 are positive, this means the assumed directions of currents are the same as the exact directions; I_2 is negative, it shows the assumed direction of the current is opposite to the exact one. By analyzing this example, we should understand the meaning of positive or negative sign of a current intensity more correctly, and the different functions of the sources in different situations. In solving practical problems those are what we should pay close attention to.

Generally speaking, when we analyze and calculate a complicated circuit with Kirchhoff's rules, we should firstly assume the direction of the current in each branch and assume the rounding direction for every independent loop, then set up the $n-1$ independent branch points equations of current and $m-(n-1)$ corresponding loop equations of voltage, then solve these simultaneous equations correctly, finally, decide the exact directions of these currents.

6.4 Wheatstone's Bridge

The applications of Kirchhoff's rules are extremely wide. Here in this section we are going to discuss one of these applications, i.e., the analysis for Wheatstone's bridge.

Wheatstone's bridge is a widely practical instrument for the accurate measurement of the resistance. Its structure is shown in Figure 6-6.

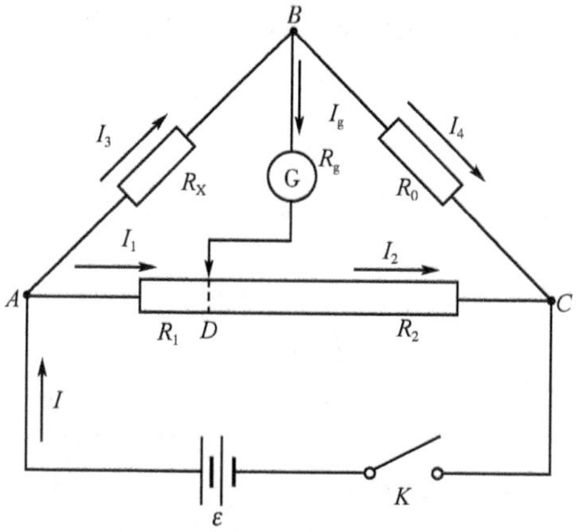

Figure 6-6 A Wheatstone's bridge

Where R_x and R_0 are respectively the resistance to be measured and the resistance known. The section between points A and C is a piece of uniform wire-formed resistor with the resistance of R_1+R_2. R_g is the inner resistance of the sensitive galvanometer, and D is the sliding end. The emf of the source is ε, and K is a switch. The directions of currents are assumed as those shown in Figure 6-6.

There are four branch points A, B, C, and D in this network, so, we can set up three independent junction equations

Corresponding to point A, there is

$$I - I_1 - I_3 = 0$$

To the point B,

$$I_3 - I_g - I_4 = 0$$

To the point D,

$$I_1 + I_g - I_2 = 0$$

There are three single net holes in this network; so, there will be three independent loop equations of voltage. The rounding directions for them are all assumed to be clockwise.

Corresponding to the loop $AR_1R_2C\varepsilon A$, we have

$$I_1R_1 + I_2R_2 - \varepsilon = 0$$

To the loop $BCDB$, we have

$$I_4R_0 - I_2R_2 - I_gR_g = 0$$

To the loop $ABDA$, we have

$$I_3R_x + I_gR_g - I_1R_1 = 0$$

In a normal bridge, if the emf of the source and the resistances corresponding to the resistors are known, the current intensity in each branch can be determined by solving the above 6 simultaneous equations; as one of the results, the current intensity in R_g is

$$I_g = \frac{(R_1R_0 - R_xR_2)\varepsilon}{R_xR_0(R_1 + R_2) + R_1R_2(R_x + R_0) + R_g(R_x + R_0)(R_1 + R_2)} \tag{6-12}$$

According to Equation (6-12), when $R_1R_0 = R_xR_2$, $I_g = 0$, and in this operating situation the bridge is called the **balanced bridge**. By using its condition, we can measure the resistance of R_x. The process is to adjust the position of the sliding end D for changing the ratio of resistances R_1 and R_2 till $I_g = 0$, here, $R_1R_0 = R_xR_2$, and R_0, R_1, R_2 are all known quantities, then to calculate the resistance of R_x with

$$R_x = \frac{R_1}{R_2}R_0 \tag{6-13}$$

In general cases, AC is a piece of uniform thickness wire of resistor, so

$$\frac{R_1}{R_2} = \frac{l_1}{l_2}$$

The ratio of resistances R_1 and R_2 can be substituted by the corresponding ratio of lengths $\frac{l_1}{l_2}$, so we have

$$R_x = \frac{l_1}{l_2}R_0 \tag{6-14}$$

If $R_1R_0 \neq R_xR_2$, $I_g \neq 0$, and the bridge in this operating situation is called the **unbalanced bridge**. It can also be used in the measurement of resistance. In normal applications, R_0, R_1, R_2, R_g and ε should be constant. As an unknown resistance, R_x is a variable quantity, which can be measured by the value of I_g according to Equation (6-12). If the scale on the panel of a galvanometer is replaced directly by the value of resistance, this restructured unbalanced bridge can be used to measure the resistance. Unlike the case in a balanced bridge, it is not necessary to adjust the balance point and to calculate the value of R_x according to the equation. While, in practical measurement, it is very difficult to keep R_0, R_1, R_2, R_g and ε as constants; so, its precision is lower than the precision of the balanced bridge.

An unbalanced bridge can also be restructured as a thermometer to measure the temperature.

Generally, the thermosensitive semiconductors are chosen to manufacture different forms of thermal resistors, such as drop-formed or slice-formed ones. The essential electrical character of this kind of resistors is that their resistances vary evidently with the change of temperature. When the temperature becomes higher, their resistances decrease; when the temperature becomes lower, their resistances increase; and their reactions are so sensitive that this kind of resistors are called the thermosensitive resistors. If we replace the resistor R_x in a bridge with a thermosensitive resistor, and let the resistor contact to the object to be measured, when the temperature of the object changes, the resistor will respond by the varying of the resistance's value; and I_g will get a corresponding change, too. This means the varying I_g will correspond with the varying temperature, so we may print the scale of temperature on the panel of the galvanometer directly. The normally used semiconductor thermal meters are manufactured on the principles of the unbalanced bridge. In addition to this, the unbalanced bridge can also be used in measurement and automatic controlling systems.

6.5 Electrophoresis and Electrotherapy

6.5.1 Electrophoresis

In the interstitial fluid of human body, besides the cationic ions and anionic ions, which are produced after the electrolysis of inorganic salts, there are also charged and uncharged organic molecules or colloidal particles, such as protein, and so on. These particles such as cells, viruses, globulin molecules or synthesized particles will drift under the influence of electric field. This phenomenon is called electrophoresis.

For different particles, their molecular weights, volumes and the amount of charges are all different, hence, under the influence of electric field the drifting speeds of different particles will not be the same. To explore their drifting speeds in the electric field, or to separate different components in the sample by using the difference of the drifting speeds has become a commonly used method in biochemistry investigations, pharmacy researches and clinical examinations. Taking plasma for instance, under the influence of electric field, several proteins in it, such as serum albumin, globulin, fibrinogen and other ingredients can be separated for further researches. More precise electrophoresis technology can distinguish more than 40 kinds of proteins in human plasma.

Figure 6-7 shows a schematic diagram of a simplest electrophoresis device, in which two electrodes (made of carbon rods or sheets of platinum) are respectively put in two containers with some buffer solution. Then immerse both ends of a filter paper strip in the buffer solution. After it is fully soaked, drop a little bit of sample for measuring on the strip. Then turn the switch on. Charged particles start to swim in the electric field. After a period of time, because the drifting speeds of different components are different,

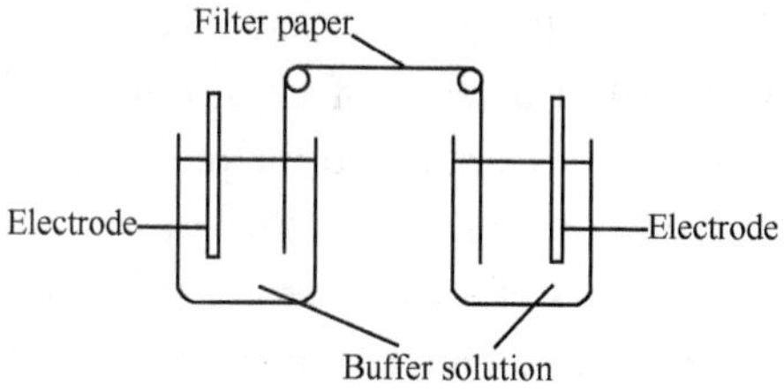

Figure 6-7 Equipment of electrophoresis on paper

the distances among them will be increased gradually. Finally, dry and dye the strip for analyzing.

Sometimes, an ultraviolet light is also applied for fluorescent analysis.

6.5.2 Electrotherapy

The DC electrotherapy is a treatment for curing diseases by leading direct electric current penetrating into human body, which has obvious effects on the treatment of venous thrombosis and the healing of bone fractures. Meanwhile, it is also the basis of iontophoresis. Human body is an intricate conductor that contains over fifty elements, such as carbon, hydrogen, oxygen, potassium and sodium. Those elements construct five main substances of the organism, i.e., water, protein, saccharide, fat, mineral salts, and others, among which water occupies 60%-70% of the body weight. The elements mentioned above also exist in water as the form of ions to compose body fluids. As a matter of fact, the body fluid is a kind of electrolyte solution, which is the basis of the electric conduction in the organism. The conductivity of human tissues is directly related to the content of water. If the tissue contains more water, it has the stronger conductivity. But there are individual differences of the conductivity; in addition to that, even for the same person there are also differences of the conductivity by the influence of various environmental factors such as the season, the age and the health condition etc.

As a direct current passes across the human skin and flows into the organism, a series of complicated physical and chemical reactions will be aroused. In human body the content of sodium chloride is comparatively higher. There will be the electrolyte under the influence of direct current, thus, the Na^+ move towards cathode of the DC source, while, the Cl^- towards the anode. Thus sodium hydroxide will accumulate at the cathode to form the alkaline reaction; and chlorine hydride will accumulate at the anode to form the acidic reaction. So it should be noted during the electrotherapy treatments that don't contact the electrodes directly to patients' skin. The proper method is to add a wet cushion between the skin and the electrode. In this way, the acid or alkali produced below the electrode can be diluted and absorbed by the wet cushion to preserve the skin from damaged by the stimulation of acid or alkali. Moreover, the wet cushion can also reduce the resistance of skin, so as to enable the current distribute uniformly and flow into the organism.

When a direct current is acting on the human organism, the ions in the tissue should move toward the corresponding electrodes opposite to their signs, but the resistant force exerted on ions by the cellular membrane is comparatively great. As positive and negative ions move reversely and arrive at the membrane, there will be the accumulations of ions on both sides. This is what we called polarization phenomenon. Polarization not only impedes the further enlargement of the electric current, but also sets up a potential difference opposite to polarity of the original electric field as the result of the accumulation of more and more ions with time. Therefore, during the practical process of DC electrotherapy, the current intensity may decrease sharply. After 1 ms operating time the current intensity may drop to 0.1-0.01 of its original value. That is caused by ionic accumulation under the external electric field.

As a direct current flowing in the body, there will be the drifts of various ions inside the organism. Besides, different ions have different drift velocity, and this will cause the changes of the ions' concentrations. These changes will lead to a series of physiological effects. Although there are ionic diffusions from the points with higher concentration to the points with lower concentration inside and outside the cell membrane, the diffusions are so slow that they can not counteract the changes of the ions' concentrations caused by the accumulations of ions under the action of the external electric field. So in the process of electrotherapy treatment, the current must be increased gradually to avoid patients' feeling of electric shock.

The concentration changes of potassium, sodium, calcium and magnesium ions will cause some physiological responses. Under the effect of electric field brought by the direct current, the drifting rates of potassium ions and sodium ions are greater than that of calcium's and magnesium's. Therefore, the ions' concentrations of potassium and sodium near the cathode are relatively higher; this will increase the solubility of colloid, and lead to the cellular membranes loosened. Thus, the cellular membranes will become more permeable for ions, and allow some more substances to enter the cells; as a result, the cells' function will be affected, expressed as an increase of physiological excitement. Meanwhile, the densities of calcium ions and magnesium ions around the anode will increase relatively; the result is that, the cellular membranes become denser and the permeability becomes lower. Thus, the metabolism is lessened and the excitement is weakened. And that will help ease pains and diminish inflammation. Some concepts and applications about electrotherapy are as follows.

(1) Impedances of acupoints in human bodies: researches for the electric conductivity on meridians and acupuncture points in human bodies are accelerating the study of the mechanics of acupuncture treatment. Since 1958, experiments have shown that the impedances at different points on the skin are different. At many points the impedances are relatively lower, which are called good conducting points. The distribution of these points is quite similar to that of acupuncture points mentioned in the meridian theory of traditional Chinese medicine. Moreover, it has been discovered in clinic that, besides the influences of skin's type and moisture condition the impedance at each point is also related with the physiological activities. Thereupon, by using the technology for detecting the variation of the conductivity at acupoints, people have developed some instruments for medical diagnoses such as "main and collateral channels determinator" "ear acupuncture points determinator", "apparatus of biological electronic shock guide balance method" and other apparatuses.

(2) Iontophoresis: the method to transport medication ions into the organism by applying direct currents to human body is called DC iontophoresis. The specific steps are as follows: soaking the filter paper or gauze cushion with medicine solution, which are ready to transport into the body; putting it on the relevant part and according to the polarity of the medicine, insuring the cushion below the corresponding electrode, i.e., putting the cushion of medicine with positive ions under cathode, or putting the cushion of medicine with negative ions under anode; putting another medicine free cushion under the other electrode; after that, getting the direct current through. So that the medication ions will be transported into the body and permeated by body fluids so as to fulfill the treatment.

Generally, the determination for the polarity of a medicine is in accordance with its chemical structure formula or is analyzed with the application of electrophoresis.

The characteristics of iontophoresis are: it not only enables the medicine to be transported directly into superficial locations under body skin, but also ensures a high concentration of the medicine to be kept there, thus, the treatment is effectively enhanced, especially for the locations where medicines are difficult to reach by oral dosing; the medication ions accumulate in dermis and permeate gradually into deeper parts, therefore, its active time in the organism is longer; furthermore, it won't cause any damage or pain to the skin and any stimulation to gastrointestinal system; besides, it has integrated effect of electrotherapy and medication treatment. The species, concentrations, polarities, functions and indications of several practical medication ions for iontophoresis are given in Table 6-1.

(3) To accelerate the cicatrization of wound: it has proved by the animal experiments and clinical applications that direct currents can expedite the hyperplasia of epithelium and accelerate the cicatrization of wound with the suitable choices of polarities and other parameters.

(4) To cure the atrium tremors: the synchronization DC rhythm resuming treatment is a simple, safe and effective method to cure the atrium tremors. It is still an indispensable treatment for rhythm's rapidly resuming, for preventing cardiac reconstruction and for more patients' benefits.

Table 6-1 Species, concentrations, polarities, functions and effects of several medication ions for iontophoresis

Active ingredient	Name of medicine solution	Concentration	Polarity	Main effects	Indications
berberine	*Berberine* solution	0.5%-1%	+	Bacteriostatic and bactericidal effects	Pyogenic infections, dysentery, prostatitis, mastitis
schisandra chinensis	*Schisandra chinensis* solution	15%-50%	–	Stimulating central nerves, regulating cardiovascular function, inhibiting bacillus	Neurasthenia, somnolence, night sweat, cough, spermatorrhea, skin infection
rhizoma chuanxiong	*Ligustrazine*	0.8%-3%	+	Dilating blood vessels	Hypertension, coronary heart disease
corydalis rhizoma	*Corydalis rhizome injection*	10%(1-2 ml each time)	+	Sedative effect	All kinds of pain (neuralgia, dysmenorrheal, lumbago, headache, et al.)
rhizoma polygoni cuspidati	*Polygoni cuspidati* liquid	30%	–	Inhibiting bacillus and coccus	Infection of skin, mucosa and surface tissue, prostatitis, etc.
datura stramonium Linn	*Flos daturae* total alkaloids	0.5%	+	Dilating the smooth muscle of bronchus	Bronchial asthma
aconitum kusnezoffii reichb	*Aconitum kusnezoffii reichb total* alkaloids	0.1%-0.3%	+	Analgesics	Superficial nerve neuralgia, superficial arthralgia
Chloroamphenicol	*Chloroamphenicol*	0.25%	+	Bacteriostasis	Eye conjunctivitis, keratitis, superficial tissue inflammation
Strepolin	*Streptomycin sulfate*	0.1 g	+	Bacteriostatic and bactericidal effects	Tuberculous disease

A Brief Summarization of This Chapter

(1) Current intensity: The electric quantity passing through any cross section of the conductor in a unit time, i.e.

$$I = \frac{dq}{dt}$$

(2) Current density: The current density is a vector expressed by $\boldsymbol{j}$; its direction is the direction of the electric field intensity at that point. At some point in the conductor, assume to take a cross section with the area of $dS_\perp$, which is perpendicular to the direction of the field intensity $\boldsymbol{E}$ at that point. We define the ratio of the current flowing through this cross section (dI) to the area ($dS_\perp$) as the magnitude of the current density at that point, i.e.

$$j = \frac{dI}{dS_\perp}$$

(3) Ohm's law in a section of circuit with emf sources: The potential difference between the two terminals of a section of circuit containing sources is equal to the algebraic sum of the potential drops on all sources and all resistors. Rewritten as general form

$$U_{AB} = U_A - U_B = \Sigma I_i R_i + \Sigma \varepsilon_i$$

(4) Kirchhoff's Rules:

1) Kirchhoff's first rule: The algebraic sum of the current intensities meeting at a branch point is zero, and its mathematical expression is

$$\sum_{i=1}^{n} I_i = 0 \tag{6-10}$$

2) Kirchhoff's second rule: After taking a round along a loop, the corresponding algebraic sum of potential drops is zero, i.e.

$$\Sigma I_i R_i + \Sigma \varepsilon_i = 0$$

Exercises 6

6-1. If the current densities at different points inside a conductor are different, is it possible or not that the current flowing in the conductor is a steady current?

6-2. An electric current with the current intensity of 2 A is flowing through a piece of copper wire with the diameter of 2 cm. Suppose the numeral density of free electrons in the copper wire is $8.5\times10^{28}\ \mathrm{m^{-3}}$, and the electric quantity of an electron is known as 1.6×10^{-19} C. Determine the magnitude of current density and average drift velocity of electrons.

6-3. In the circuit shown in Figure for Exercise 6-3, we know that $\varepsilon_1 = 24$ V, $r_1 = 2\ \Omega$, $\varepsilon_2 = 6$ V, $r_2 = 1\ \Omega$, $R_1 = 2\ \Omega$, $R_2 = 1\ \Omega$, and $R_3 = 3\ \Omega$. Determine

(1) the magnitude and the direction of the current intensity;

(2) the potentials at point A and point B;

(3) U_{AD} and U_{CD}.

6-4. In the circuit shown in Figure for Exercise 6-4, we know that $\varepsilon_1 = 6$ V, $\varepsilon_2 = \varepsilon_3 = 3$ V, $R_1 = R_2 = R_3 = 2\ \Omega$. Determine U_{AB}, U_{AC} and U_{BC}.

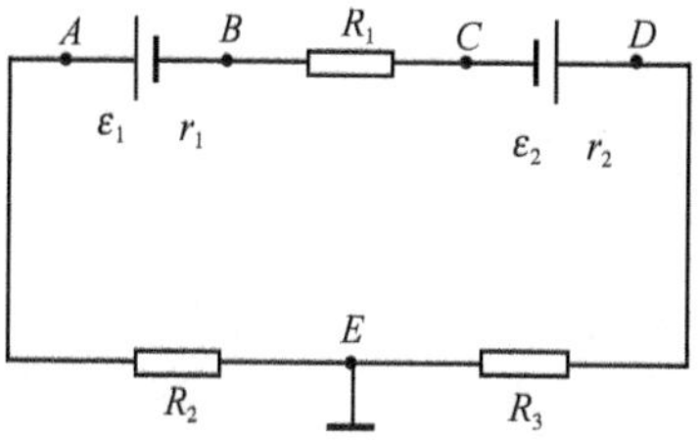

Figure for Exercise 6-3

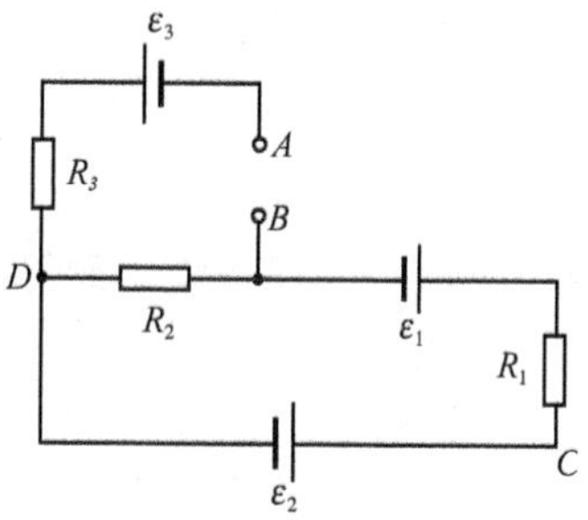

Figure for Exercise 6-4

6-5. In the circuit shown in Figure for Exercise 6-5, we know that $\varepsilon_1 = 6$ V, $\varepsilon_2 = 2$ V, $R_1 = 6\Omega$, $R_2 = 2\ \Omega$, and $R_3 = R_4 = 4\ \Omega$. Determine

(1) the current intensity flowing through each resistor;

(2) the potential difference U_{AB} between point A and point B.

6-6. In the circuit shown in Figure for Exercise 6-6, we know that $\varepsilon_1 = 2$ V, $\varepsilon_2 = 1$ V, $R_1 = 4\ \Omega$, $R_2 = 2\ \Omega$, and $R_3 = 3\ \Omega$. Determine

(1) the current intensity flowing through each resistor;

(2) the potential difference between point A and point B.

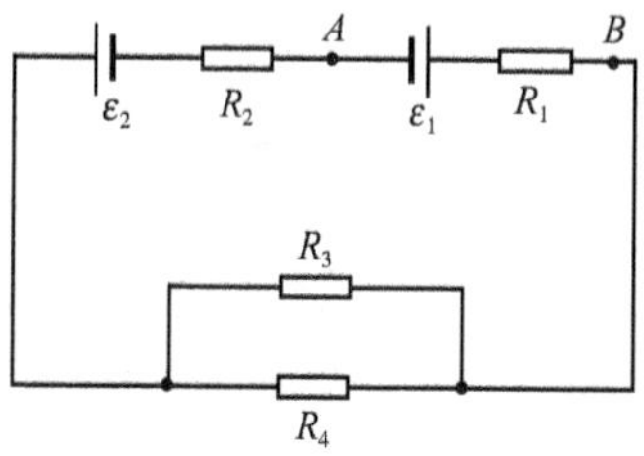

Figure for Exercise 6-5

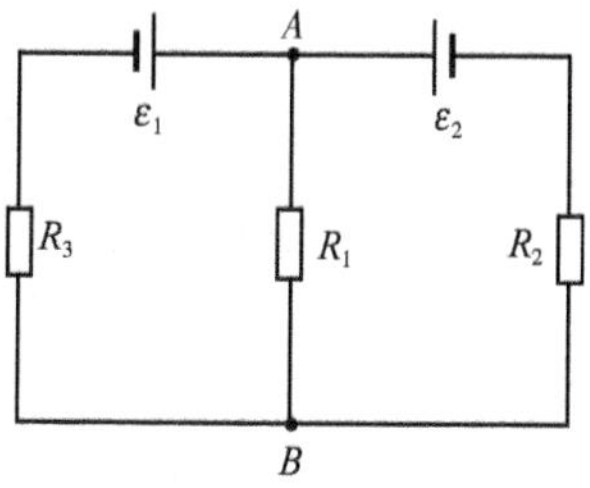

Figure for Exercise 6-6

6-7. In the circuit shown in Figure for Exercise 6-7, we know that $\varepsilon_1 = 12$ V, $\varepsilon_2 = 9$ V, $\varepsilon_3 = 8$ V, $r_1 = r_2 = r_3 = 1\ \Omega$, $R_1 = R_2 = R_3 = R_4 = 2\ \Omega$, and $R_5 = 3\ \Omega$. Determine

(1) the potential difference between point A and point B;

(2) the potential difference between point C and point D;

(3) the current intensity flowing through R_5 when point C and point D are connected to form a short circuit.

6-8. In the circuit shown in Figure for Exercise 6-8, we know that $\varepsilon_1 = 2$ V, $\varepsilon_2 = \varepsilon_3 = 4$ V, $R_2 = 2\ \Omega$, $R_1 = R_3 = 1\ \Omega$, and $R_4 = R_5 = 3\ \Omega$. Determine

(1) the current intensity flowing through each resistor;

(2) the potential difference between point A and point B.

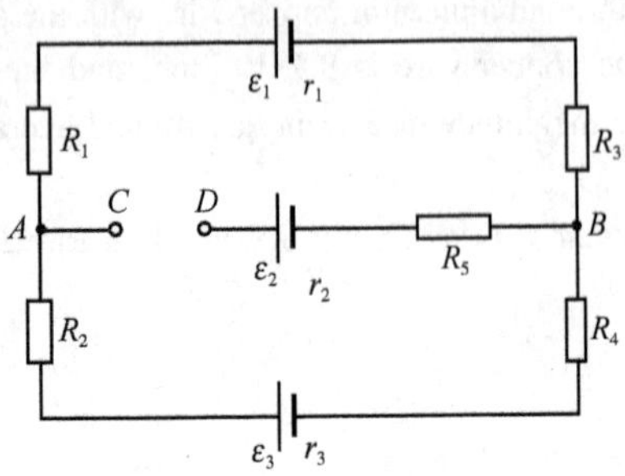

Figure for Exercise 6-7

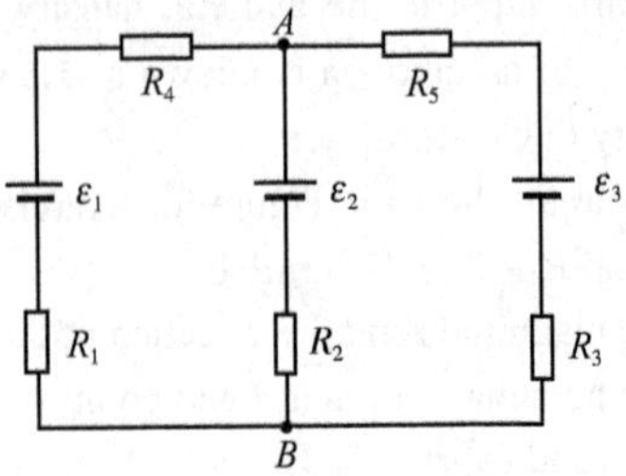

Figure for Exercise 6-8

Chapter 7 Electromagnetic Phenomena

Electromagnetic motion is one of the basic motion forms of substances. Over the years, electric phenomena and magnetic phenomena had been considered independent with each other. The relationship between electricity and magnetism was not noticed until Hand Christian Oersted discovered that there was an effect acted on a compass needle by an electric current in 1819; and André-Marie Ampère discovered that there was also an effect on a current by a magnet in 1820. Electromagnetic inducement was first observed by Michael Faraday, which not only enabled people to have a deeper understanding of the relationship of electricity and magnetism, but also set up the foundation for modern electric technique. Furthermore, it paved the way for the wide utilization of electric energy and promoted the development of social productivity.

In this chapter, we will explain the properties of magnetic field more explicitly in terms of theoretical studies and practical applications. We'll mainly focus on the discussion of Ampère's circuital law, the formula for Lorentz force, and so on. Finally, we will give a brief introduction of bio-magnetism and magnetic therapy.

7.1 Magnetic Fields Produced by Electric Currents

7.1.1 Magnetic Field and Magnetic Induction

In the space around any moving electric charges or currents, there will be the electric field similar to the one set up by stationary charges; besides, there is another special substance—the **magnetic field**. The interactions between magnets are passed on by the magnetic field. A magnetic field exerts magnetic forces on moving charges (or currents) in it; the interactions between moving electric charges, or currents, or between a current and a magnet can be regarded as the result that the magnetic field produced by any one of them exerts an acting force on the other. As electric field the magnetic field is another existing form of substance, it has also got mass, energy and momentum.

In principle, we could take any one of them—a moving charge, a piece of current carrying wire, or a piece of permanent magnet as a "test charge", and give the magnetic field a quantified description by introducing the intensity of the magnetic field according to the characteristics of the force on it in the magnetic field. An element of current carrying wire is taken as a test unit to introduce **magnetic induction *B*** (i.e., a physical quantity to describe the intensity of the magnetic field) in the discussion of this chapter. In order to determine the property at each point and make sure that the measurements are accurate, it is required that the original characteristics of the field won't be affected after the current carrying wire element was put in. Meanwhile, the dimension of the current carrying wire element must be very small. This current carrying wire element is what we called test current carrying wire unit.

Experimental results show that if a test current carrying wire element is put at any point in a magnetic field, there will be an specific direction along which the current is flowing, and there isn't any magnetic force exerted on the current carrying wire element, i.e., $\boldsymbol{F} = 0$. If the direction turns an angle of $\pi/2$, the magnetic force on the element is maximum, and the magnitude of this force is not only associated with the position in the magnetic field, but also proportional to the length of the current carrying wire unit dl and the current intensity I, i.e., $F_{max} \propto Idl$. Moreover, the direction of magnetic force is perpendicular to the plane which is determined by that specific direction and Idl. The experimental results also prove that at the same point in the magnetic field, the ratio of F_{max}/Idl is a constant for any different value of Idl. So this ratio reflects the nature of the magnetic field itself. Hence, we define the ratio as the magnitude of magnetic induction $\boldsymbol{B}$, i.e.

$$B = \frac{F_{max}}{Idl} \tag{7-1}$$

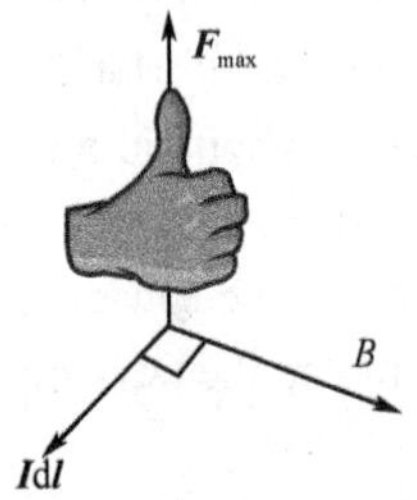

Figure 7-1 Right-handed screw rule

From the discussion above, we come to the conclusion that at each point in a magnetic field, the magnetic induction $\boldsymbol{B}$ is numerically equal to the maximum magnetic force on per unit current carrying wire element; and its direction is that: along which there will not any magnetic force exerted on the wire element, and it points towards the orientation determined uniquely by right-handed screw rule, as shown in Figure 7-1.

The unit of magnetic induction is T in the SI system. In practice, Gs is also a commonly used unit of $\boldsymbol{B}$, 1 T = 10^4 Gs.

In a magnetic field if the magnetic induction $\boldsymbol{B}$ has the same magnitude and the same direction at any points, the field is called a uniform magnetic field; otherwise, it is called the nonuniform magnetic field.

The magnetic induction on the surface of the earth is 0.3×10^{-4} T (equator)-0.6×10^{-4} T (two poles); the magnetic induction of the permanent magnet in a normal instrument is about 10^{-2} T; the magnetic induction of the large-scale electromagnetic object can be 2 T; the electromagnetic object made from superconductive materials can produce the magnetic induction of 10^2 T; in the microscopic field, it has been found that the magnetic fields around some atomic nuclei can reach the magnetic induction of 10^4 T.

7.1.2 Magnetic Flux and Gauss' Law for Magnetism

1. Magnetic Field Lines

In order to describe the magnetic field graphically, we shall introduce the idea of the magnetic field lines. The cases shown in Figure 7-2 are some specific distributions of magnetic field lines detected by experiments. As shown by the distributions of these magnetic field lines, they are all closed curves encircling the currents or the lines coming from infinity and going to infinity, without starting and terminal points. We can perceive from the characteristic of these closed curves that the magnetic field and the electric field are different in nature. What we need to notice is that the magnetic field lines are some imagined curves for graphically describing the magnetic field, while, the magnetic field is an objective real substance.

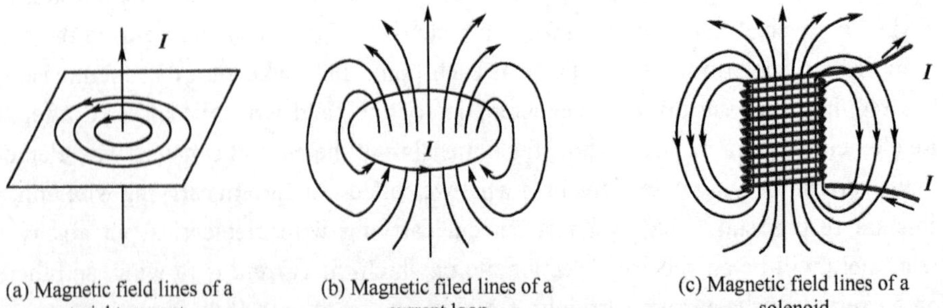

(a) Magnetic field lines of a straight current (b) Magnetic filed lines of a current loop (c) Magnetic field lines of a solenoid

Figure 7-2 The distribution of magnetic field lines

The magnetic field lines can not only describe the direction of a magnetic field but also express the intensity of the magnetic field. Everywhere in the field, the tangential direction of the line is the same to the direction of magnetic field $\boldsymbol{B}$ at that point; the number of the magnetic field lines penetrating through per unit area which is perpendicular to the direction of the magnetic induction $\boldsymbol{B}$ is the magnitude of the magnetic induction. So, where the magnetic field is more intense the magnetic field lines are denser; otherwise, where the magnetic field lines are sparse, the magnetic field is less intense.

2. Magnetic Flux

The total number of magnetic field lines penetrating through a given surface is called the **magnetic flux** through that surface, denoted by Φ. If there is a plane with the area of S in a uniform magnetic field, and the angle between its normal direction and the direction of the magnetic induction $\boldsymbol{B}$ is θ, as shown in Figure 7-3, we can get the corresponding magnetic flux

$$\Phi = BS\cos\theta$$

If the magnetic field is not uniform, in evaluating magnetic flux through any curved surface, we can assume an element dS on the surface, and the magnetic field in the region of the element can be looked as a uniform one. If the angle between the normal direction of the element dS and the direction of magnetic induction $\boldsymbol{B}$ at that point is θ, as shown in Figure 7-4, the magnetic flux through the element dS is

$$\mathrm{d}\Phi = B\cos\theta \mathrm{d}S$$

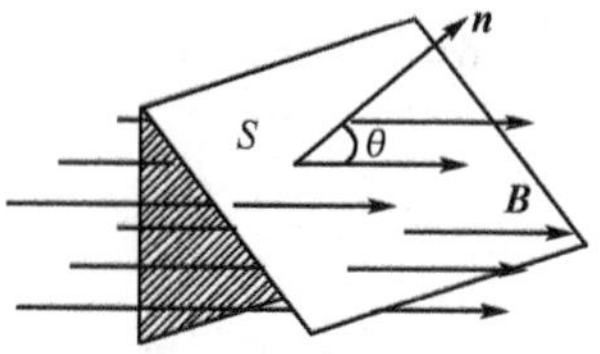

Figure 7-3 Magnetic flux of uniform magnetic field

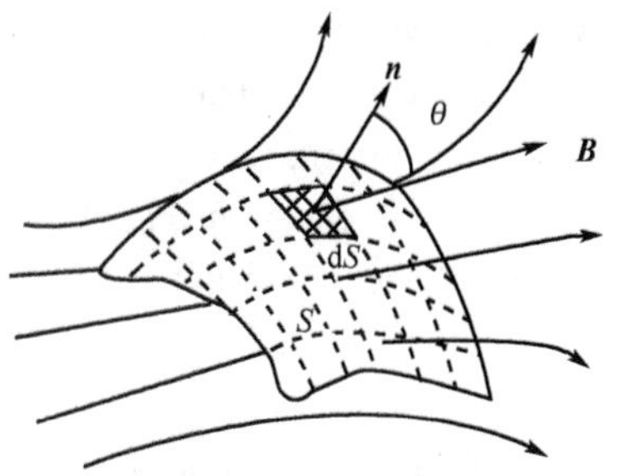

Figure 7-4 Schematic diagram of magnetic flux

So the magnetic flux through a limited curved surface S is

$$\Phi = \iint_S B\cos\theta \mathrm{d}S = \iint_S \boldsymbol{B}\cdot \mathrm{d}\boldsymbol{S} \tag{7-2}$$

The SI unit of magnetic flux is Wb.

3. Gauss' Law for Magnetism

For a closed curve surface, because the magnetic field lines produced by currents are always closed or coming from infinity and going to infinity, the number of magnetic field lines entering the closed surface must be equal to that exiting the surface. The angle between a magnetic field line penetrating into the surface and its outer normal direction is an obtuse angle, so it corresponds to a negative flux; on the contrary, the angle between a magnetic field line penetrating from the inside of the surface and its outer normal direction is an acute angle, and it corresponds to a positive flux, as shown in Figure 7-5; these two parts will cancel out. So the net magnetic flux through any closed surface in a magnetic field is always zero, i.e.

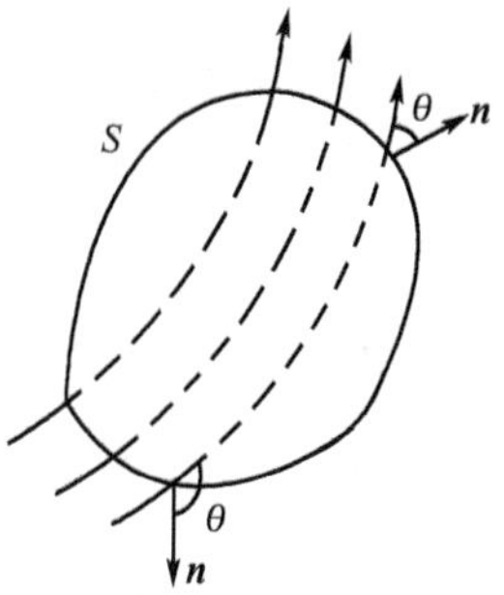

Figure 7-5 Magnetic flux of a closed curve surface

$$\oiint_S \boldsymbol{B}\cdot \mathrm{d}\boldsymbol{S} = 0 \tag{7-3}$$

Equation (7-3) is called **Gauss' law in magnetism**. It is similar to Gauss' law in electrostatics, but they have the material differences. In an electrostatic field, the electric flux may not be zero, due to the fact that there are free independent charges in the nature. It indicates that an electric field is a field with origins starting at positive charges and ending at negative charges. While in a magnetic field, there are not independent magnetic poles with the single sign in the present nature, so the net magnetic flux through any closed surface must be zero, which demonstrates that magnetic field is a field without the origin. In other words, the magnetic field and the electrostatic field are different in nature. So Gauss' law in magnetism is exactly one of the most important theorems to describe the characteristics of the magnetic field.

7.1.3 Ampère's Circuital Law

In the study of electric field, we have proved that the integral of electric field intensity $\boldsymbol{E}$ along a closed path L is zero, denoted by $\oint_L \boldsymbol{E} \cdot d\boldsymbol{l} = 0$. The conclusion means the electrostatic field is a conservative force field. Whether the magnetic field is a conservative field or not? What is the integral of the magnetic induction $\boldsymbol{B}$ along a closed path L $\oint_L \boldsymbol{B} \cdot d\boldsymbol{l}$ in a magnetic field? What characteristics of the magnetic field can be expressed by the integral? These are the main issues to be discussed in this section.

Therefore, our discussion starts from the distributing situation of the magnetic field around current carrying wires. Experimental results show that the magnetic field distribution around current carrying wires is associated with the shapes, current intensities, and the distribution of medium there. Firstly, we are going to study the magnetic field produced by an infinitely long straight current carrying wire. Suppose the current intensity through the wire is I, according to what we have learnt in high school, we can get the magnetic induction at any point in space

$$B = K\frac{I}{r} \tag{7-4}$$

where r is the distance from that point to the wire, and K is a proportional coefficient, and its value is related with the choice of its unit. In SI system, K is conventionally expressed as $\frac{\mu_0}{2\pi}$, μ_0 is called the permeability of the vacuum and its value is

$$\mu_0 = 4\pi \times 10^{-7}\ \text{T·m/A}$$

In this way, Equation (7-4) can be rewritten as

$$B = \frac{\mu_0}{2\pi}\frac{I}{r} \tag{7-5}$$

The direction of magnetic induction $\boldsymbol{B}$ is perpendicular to the plane determined by the wire and that point, and it is towards the direction determined by the right-handed screw rule.

Secondly, in the following cases we will calculate the value of the integral $\oint_L \boldsymbol{B} \cdot d\boldsymbol{l}$ along any closed loop L on the plane perpendicular to the infinitely long current carrying wire. L is the so-called Ampère loop.

1. There Is a Current Encircled in the Ampère Loop

As shown in Figure 7-6, L is a random Ampère loop. Let's consider any linear element $dl = \overline{KM}$ in the loop; and on the plane with L, let's take the point at which the current appears as the centre O to draw an arc with the radius of $r = \overline{OK}$, the arc contacts to $\overline{OM}$ at point N. The triangle $\triangle KMN$ is approximately a right triangle, and the angle $\angle NKM = \theta$ is the angle made by $\boldsymbol{B}$ and $d\boldsymbol{l}$. So we have

$dl\cos\theta = \overline{KN}$. On the other hand, suppose the central angle corresponding to dl at point O is $d\phi$, then, the length of arc is $\overline{KN} = r\,d\phi$, therefore

$$dl\cos\theta = r\,d\phi$$

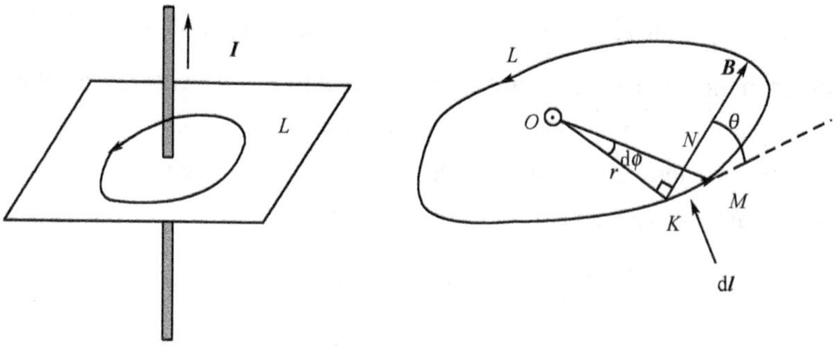

(a) Space diagram (b) Vertical view

Figure 7-6 The proof of Ampère's law

So

$$\oint_L \boldsymbol{B}\cdot d\boldsymbol{l} = \oint_L B\,dl\cos\theta = \int_0^{2\pi}\frac{\mu_0}{2\pi}\frac{I}{r}r\,d\phi = \frac{\mu_0 I}{2\pi}\int_0^{2\pi}d\phi = \mu_0 I$$

Obviously, if the direction of I is reversed, the direction of $\boldsymbol{B}$ will be reversed too, and θ will be an obtuse angle, $d\boldsymbol{l}\cos\theta = -r d\phi$. The mere difference with the above integral will be the negative sign. It is suggested that in calculating the integral if the direction of Ampère circulation and the current is in conformity with the right-handed screw rule, the sign of current is positive, otherwise, it is negative.

2. There Isn't Current Encircled in the Ampère Loop

In the case shown in Figure 7-7, there is another linear element $d\boldsymbol{l}'$ corresponding to each $d\boldsymbol{l}$. They have the same central angle respecting to the point O. But the magnetic induction $\boldsymbol{B}$ at the point of dl makes an acute angle θ with $d\boldsymbol{l}$; while, the magnetic induction $\boldsymbol{B}'$ at the point of $d\boldsymbol{l}'$ makes an obtuse angle θ' with $d\boldsymbol{l}'$. If the distance from point O to dl is r, and the distance to point $d\boldsymbol{l}'$ is r', we have

$$dl\cos\theta = r\,d\phi,\ dl'\cos\theta' = -r'\,d\phi$$

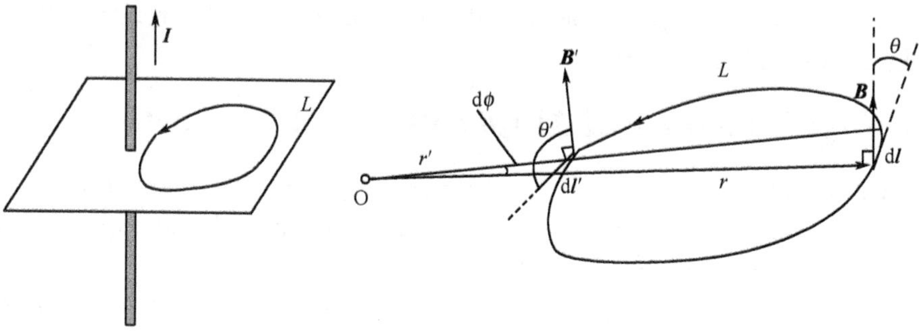

(a) Space diagram (b) Vertical view

Figure 7-7 The proof of Ampère's law

The magnitudes of the magnetic inductions at those two points are respectively $B = \frac{\mu_0}{2\pi}\frac{I}{r}$ and $B' = \frac{\mu_0}{2\pi}\frac{I}{r'}$, so we have

$$\boldsymbol{B}\cdot \mathrm{d}\boldsymbol{l}+\boldsymbol{B}'\cdot \mathrm{d}\boldsymbol{l}' = B\mathrm{d}l\cos\theta + B'\mathrm{d}l'\cos\theta' = \frac{\mu_0}{2\pi}\frac{I}{r}r\mathrm{d}\phi - \frac{\mu_0}{2\pi}\frac{I}{r'}r'\mathrm{d}\phi' = 0$$

It suggests that the contributions of the two linear elements to the integral cancel out in pairs, so we can get the illation that the integral along the whole closed loop is zero.

From the calculations in the above two cases, we know that the value of $\oint_L \boldsymbol{B}\cdot\mathrm{d}\boldsymbol{l}$ is only related to the currents encircled in the Ampère loop, and is independent of the currents outside the loop. If there are many straight current carrying wires with the current intensities of I_1, I_2, $\cdots$, I_n, I_{n+1}, $\cdots$, I_k, and among them only I_1, I_2, $\cdots$, I_n pass through the Ampère loop, according to the principle of the superposition of the magnetic field intensity, we can generalize the above results and get

$$\oint_L \boldsymbol{B}\cdot \mathrm{d}\boldsymbol{l} = \mu_0 \sum_{i=1}^{n} I_i = \mu_0 \sum_{(L\mathrm{in})} I_i \tag{7-6}$$

The sign for some current intensity is dependent on the direction of the current and the rounding direction of integral circulation. If they are accordant with the right-handed screw rule, the current intensity is positive; otherwise, if they are not accordant with the right-handed screw rule, the corresponding current intensity is negative.

Although the above result is derived from the case in which the magnetic field is produced by infinitely long straight current carrying wires, in the static magnetic field produced by steady currents, it can be proved that, no matter how the current distributions are and to any closed integral path shape, Equation (7-6) is always valid. In other words, in a static magnetic field, the line integral of $\boldsymbol{B}$ along any closed path is equal to the μ_0 times of the algebraic sum of all currents through the loop. This conclusion is called **Ampère's circuital law**.

According to Ampère's circuital law, it is known that magnetic fields are distinct with electric fields in characteristics, and the line integral of a magnetic field does not necessarily be zero. Therefore, the magnetic force is not conservative, i.e., the magnetic field is not a field with potential.

From the above derivation we should pay attention to understanding the meanings of each physical quantity in the equation of Ampere's law. The sum of currents ΣI_i on the right side of Equation (7-6) only includes the currents passing through the Ampère loop, but on the left side, $\boldsymbol{B}$ represents the vector sum of magnetic inductions produced by all the currents in this space, including the magnetic field caused by the currents which do not pass through the loop L. But the total effect of the integral of latter magnetic inductions along the closed path is zero.

7.1.4 Applications of Ampère's Circuital Law

Ampère's circuital law can be used in the calculation of some special distributions of magnetic fields produced by certain symmetric current carrying wires. Taking the calculation of magnetic field induction produced by a long uniform solenoid as our following example.

Suppose there is a long uniform closely winded solenoid with a current intensity of I flowing through. Due to its length, the magnetic field at the internal middle range of the solenoid is approximately uniform, and the direction is parallel to the axis of the solenoid which can be determined by the right-handed screw rule. While outside the solenoid, the magnetic field is so feeble that can be negligible. As shown in Figure 7-8, in order to determine the magnetic induction at point P in the internal middle range of the solenoid, we can draw a closed rectangle path $ABCDA$ via P. The line segment CD and parts of BC and DA are outside of the solenoid, where $\boldsymbol{B} = 0$. Though the other parts of BC and DA are inside the solenoid, where $\boldsymbol{B}\neq 0$, the $\mathrm{d}l$ there is perpendicular to $\boldsymbol{B}$, that is, $B\cdot\mathrm{d}l = 0$. So we get the integral of $\boldsymbol{B}$

along this closed path

$$\oint_L \boldsymbol{B}\cdot d\boldsymbol{l}=\int_A^B \boldsymbol{B}\cdot d\boldsymbol{l}+\int_B^C \boldsymbol{B}\cdot d\boldsymbol{l}+\int_C^D \boldsymbol{B}\cdot d\boldsymbol{l}+\int_D^A \boldsymbol{B}\cdot d\boldsymbol{l}=\int_A^B \boldsymbol{B}\cdot d\boldsymbol{l}=B\cdot\overline{AB}$$

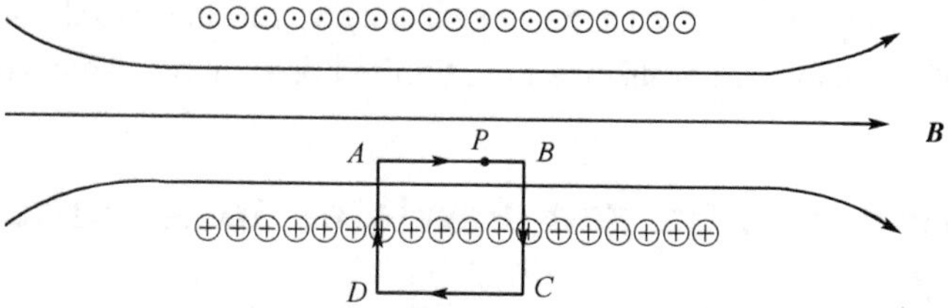

Figure 7-8 To determine the magnetic field inside a long straight solenoid with Ampère's circuital law

It is supposed that the length of the solenoid is L and it consists of N turns, there will be $N/L = n$ turns per unit length. If all the turns carry the same current I, the sum of currents encircled in the closed path $ABCDA$ is $\overline{AB}\,nI$. According to the right-handed screw rule, the sign of the currents I is positive, and by applying Ampère's law we can get

$$\oint_L \boldsymbol{B}\cdot d\boldsymbol{l}=B\cdot\overline{AB}=\mu_0\,\overline{AB}\,nI$$

Therefore,

$$B=\mu_0 n I \tag{7-7}$$

Form the above calculation we can realize a method for calculating magnetic induction with the application of Ampère's circuital law. This method is convenient only on some special situations (e.g. the magnetic fields are uniform and symmetrical), so we can also use Ampère's circuital law for calculating the magnetic field inductions near an axis-symmetric current carrying conductor or near an infinite current carrying plane.

7.2 Magnetic Force on Moving Charges

7.2.1 Lorentz Force

Force exerted on a moving charge by the magnetic field is called **Lorentz force**. We've already learnt in high school that when a positive charge q is moving with the velocity of $\boldsymbol{v}$, which makes an angle θ with the magnetic field $\boldsymbol{B}$, the magnitude of Lorentz force exerted on the moving charge f is

$$f=q\,v\,B\sin\theta \tag{7-8}$$

The direction of the force is perpendicular to the plane determined by the velocity $\boldsymbol{v}$ of the moving charge and the magnetic field $\boldsymbol{B}$, moreover, the relationship among the directions of $\boldsymbol{v}$, $\boldsymbol{B}$ and $\boldsymbol{f}$ submits to the right-handed rule, that is to say, when the four fingers of right hand turn to $\boldsymbol{B}$ from $\boldsymbol{v}$ via the included angle less than 180°, then the thumb direction represents the direction of Lorenz force $\boldsymbol{f}$; if the charge is negative, the direction is opposite, as shown in Figure 7-9. So that, the formula can be written in vector expression

$$\boldsymbol{f}=q\,\boldsymbol{v}\times\boldsymbol{B} \tag{7-9}$$

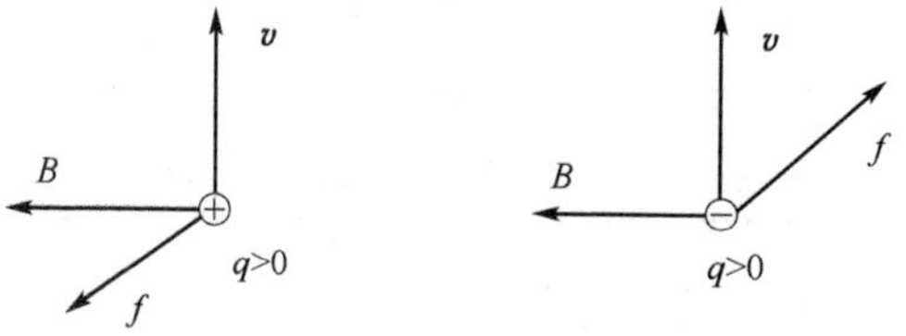

Figure 7-9 The directions of Lorenz forces

Equation (7-8) shows that, when $\sin\theta = 0$ or $\boldsymbol{v} = 0$, the force $\boldsymbol{f} = 0$. It indicates that: ① when $\boldsymbol{v}$ is parallel or anti-parallel to $\boldsymbol{B}$, a moving charge is free from the magnetic force; and ② so is the charge at stationary, which means magnetic forces act only on moving charges. From Equation (7-9), we can see that, Lorenz force $\boldsymbol{f}$ *is* always perpendicular to the velocity $\boldsymbol{v}$. In other words, Lorenz force can only change the direction of the velocity, not its direction. So the Lorenz force can never do work on moving charges.

7.2.2 Motion of Charged Particles in a Uniform Magnetic Field

As we have learnt in high school, if a charged particle with the mass of m and the electric quantity of q enters into a uniform magnetic field with the velocity of $\boldsymbol{v}$ perpendicular to the magnetic induction $\boldsymbol{B}$, the particle will perform a uniform circular motion in the magnetic field, and the radius of its circular orbit, i.e., the radius of gyration is

$$R = \frac{mv}{qB} \tag{7-10}$$

The time required for one revolution of the particle's gyration, that is, the period of gyration is

$$T = \frac{2\pi R}{v} = \frac{2\pi m}{qB} \tag{7-11}$$

Revolutions of the charged particle performed per unit time, that is, the frequency of gyration is

$$\nu = \frac{1}{T} = \frac{qB}{2\pi m} \tag{7-12}$$

Equation (7-11) and Equation (7-12) indicate that the period T and frequency ν are independent of the magnitude of particle's velocity $\boldsymbol{v}$ and the radius of gyration R. In other words, a particle with higher velocity will move along a circle with the bigger radius, and vice versa; time for a circular gyration to the same kind of particles are the same. This is a very important conclusion. It is the fundamental principle of the mass spectrometer, the circular accelerator and the magnetic focus technology.

Generally, when the velocity $\boldsymbol{v}$ isn't perpendicular to the magnetic field $\boldsymbol{B}$, the velocity will be decomposed into two components $\boldsymbol{v}_{//} = v\cos\theta$ and $v_{\perp} = v\sin\theta$, as shown in Figure 7-10, which are parallel and perpendicular to the magnetic field respectively. It is the perpendicular component of the velocity $v_{\perp}$ that assists the charged particle moving in uniform circular motion on the plane perpendicular to $\boldsymbol{B}$, and the parallel component $v_{//}$ assists the charged particle moving in uniform linear motion with or opposite to the direction of $\boldsymbol{B}$. The result of composition of these two motions is an integrated motion of the particle along a helical path. Its screw pitch h, which is the distance traveled along the helix axis per revolution, is determined as

$$h = v_{//}T = \frac{2\pi m v_{//}}{qB} \tag{7-13}$$

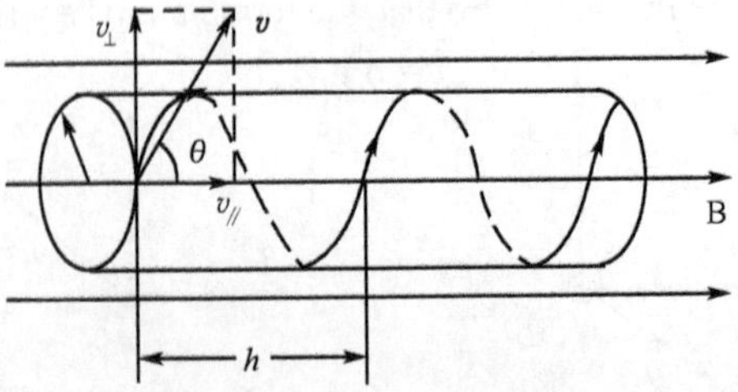

Figure 7-10 Helix motion of a moving charge in a magnetic field

It is independent of the perpendicular component of the velocity $v_{\perp}$.

The result shown above gives the simplest principle of the magnetic focusing technology. Suppose that a very narrow stream of charged paticles is emitted from a point A in the magnetic field, their speeds v are nearly the same, and the angles between their moving directions and magnetic induction $\boldsymbol{B}$ are all very small, as shown in Figure 7-11, so we have

$$v_{/\!/} = v\cos\theta \approx v$$

$$v_{\perp} = v\sin\theta \approx v\theta$$

Particles with different perpendicular components of velocity $v_{\perp}$ will move along different helixes with different radiuses under the actions of magnetic forces. But as their parallel components of the velocity $v_{/\!/}$ are approximately equal, after travelling a distance of $h = v_{/\!/}T \approx \dfrac{2\pi mv}{qB}$, they will meet again at another point. This is similar to the phenomenon of light focus after passing through a lens, so it is called the phenomenon of **magnetic focusing**.

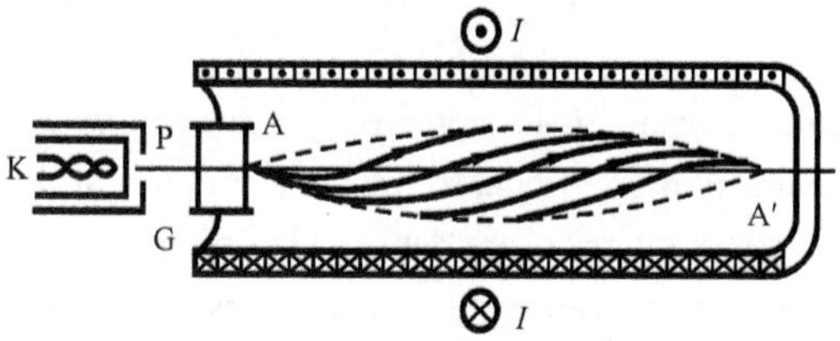

Figure 7-11 Magnetic focusing

What we discussed above is the phenomenon of magnetic focusing in a uniform magnetic field, which could be realized by a long solenoid. While, in practical applications, what we use most is the magnetic focus in the non-uniform magnetic field produced by short coils. Here, a short coil plays the similar role as an optical focusing lens, so it is called a **magnetic lens**. This technology is widely used in many kinds of vacuum systems, e.g., the electron microscope, etc.

7.2.3 Hall Effect

In 1879 Edwin Herbert Hall discovered that when an electrical current passes through the both ends of a thin sample of conductor placed in a uniform magnetic field, which is perpendicular to the planes of the sample, a weak potential difference is developed across the material on the other two sides of the sample. This effect is known as **Hall effect**, and the corresponding potential difference is called **Hall voltage**.

Hall effect can be explained with the principle of the Lorenz force acting on the charged particles. The particles, which take part in conducting electric currents (also called current carriers) in metal conductors, are free electrons. As shown in Figure 7-12, there is a conductor with the width of b and the thickness of d; and a current I is flowing through it. When the current is flowing in the metal, it means the electrons are moving in the opposite direction inside the metal. If the average drift velocity of the electrons is v, the magnitude of the Lorenz force acting on an electron will be $f = evB$, and its direction is downward. So the electrons turn downward and accumulate on the bottom surface, at the same time there will be extra positive charges accumulated on the top surface; across the metal material there will be an electric field between the two sides. This electric field will become more intense as the process of the charges' accumulation. When the electrostatic force acting on an electron is balanced by the Lorenz force on it the accumulation of charges reaches steady. The potential difference at that state is just Hall voltage. Experiments show that, in a magnetic field of not so intense, Hall voltage is directly proportional to the current intensity and the magnetic induction, and inversely proportional to the thickness of the metal piece, i.e.,

$$V_{\mathrm{H}} = k\frac{IB}{d} \tag{7-14}$$

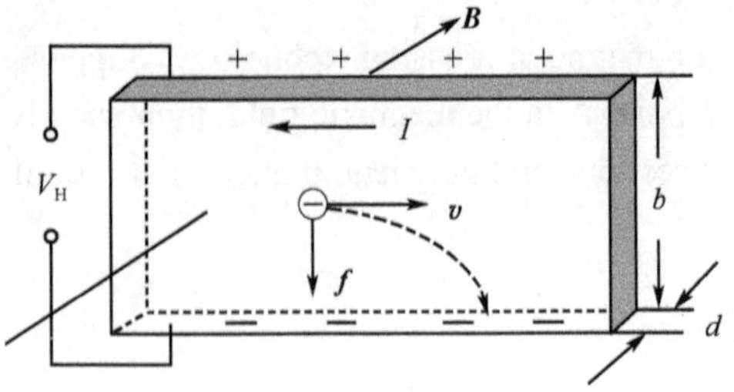

Figure 7-12 Hall effect

where $k = \frac{1}{nq}$ is a constant called Hall coefficient, which is related with the concentration of the current carriers in the metal n.

Besides metals, semiconductors are the materials in which Hall effect can take place. Semiconductors can be divided into two types — n-type semiconductors and p-type semiconductors, the current carriers in the former are mainly electrons and in the latter are mainly holes. A hole corresponds to a positively charged particle with the electric quantity e. Because Hall coefficient is inversely proportional to the concentration of the current carriers, in general metals the concentrations of the current carriers are denser, Hall effect is not obvious; while, in the semiconductors the concentrations of the current carriers are not so dense, Hall effect is more obvious, as the other conditions are the same. Therefore, the common Hall pieces are made of semiconductors.

In the study of semiconductors, the types of current carriers can be determined with the polarities of the Hall voltage; according to the relationship between Hall voltage and B, I, and the concentration of the current carriers, it can be used for measuring magnetic field, strong electric current (of thousands of amperes), and the concentrations of current carriers. The magnetohydrodynamic generators can also be designed with the principle of Hall effect.

One of the important applications of Hall effect in medicine is the electromagnetic flow meter. It is an instrument for measuring the quantity of blood flow by using Hall effect. Suppose that the diameter of a tube is D, inside which the blood is flowing with the average velocity of v. A magnetic field $\boldsymbol{B}$ is applied in the direction perpendicular to the axis of the tube, then, the positive and negative ions will turn under the actions of Lorenz forces and form a Hall voltage v_H. When the Lorenz force is balanced with the electrostatic force, i.e.

$$qE = qvB$$

The electric field intensity is

$$E = \frac{V_H}{D}$$

So that, the flow rate

$$Q = Sv = \frac{\pi D^2}{4}\frac{E}{B} = \frac{\pi D V_H}{4B} \tag{7-15}$$

In the measurement of the quantity of blood flow inside a section of blood vessel with an electromagnetic flow meter, it is necessary to peel up the vessel by operation and to put it in the magnetic space of the flow meter. This is a damaged measurement of flow rates and is commonly used in animal experiments and the operations of hearts and arteries.

In the industry and agricultural productions the electromagnetic flow meter has its wide applications, it is mainly used in the measurement of the volume flow rates of conductive liquids or seriflux in a closed tube including the corrosive liquids, such as acid, alkali, salt and so on. It is also used in the fields such as petroleum industry, chemical engineering, metallurgy, textile manufacture, food, pharmacy, paper making and environmental protection, municipal administration, water conservancy, etc.

7.2.4 Mass Spectrometer

The mass spectrometer is an apparatus for analyzing the isotopes of chemical elements, and measuring their masses and their contents. The principle of the mass spectrometer has been mentioned in high school, so, it is not necessary to repeat the statement. Because the isotopes of one kind element have the same chemical properties, we can not distinguish them by chemical methods; instead, we can merely take advantage of physical methods to distinguish them. The mass spectrometers used nowadays are very precise apparatuses. They can not only distinguish the particles with the same charges and different masses, but also detect the ratios of any isotopes in some kind of element.

7.3 Magnetic Force on a Current Carrying Conductor

7.3.1 Ampère Force

As we know that in a magnetic field a moving electric charge is acted by the Lorenz force. Since a current is formed when charges perform directional motion, each moving charge inside the current carrying conductor in a magnetic field will be acted by the Lorenz force. Due to the restraints exerted by the conductor, these charges will convey the corresponding forces to the conductor, and the integrated result is that the conductor as a whole experiences a magnetic force, which is called **Ampère force**.

Now let's derive the expression of Ampère force from the Lorenz force acted on each moving charge. Assume that there is a current element Idl with the current intensity of I and length of $\mathrm{d}l$, and with the cross-sectional area of S, as shown in Figure 7-13. On average, the Lorenz force acting on each charge performing the directional motion inside the current element is

$$\boldsymbol{f} = -e\,\boldsymbol{v} \times \boldsymbol{B}$$

where $\boldsymbol{v}$ is the directional drift velocity of the electrons, which is in the opposite direction with current density vector $\boldsymbol{j}$, i.e., $\boldsymbol{j} = -ne\boldsymbol{v}$; and n is the number of the free electrons in per unit volume, so the integrated magnetic force on all the directionally moving electrons in this element is

Figure 7-13 The derivation of Ampère force

$$\mathrm{d}\boldsymbol{F} = N(-e\,\boldsymbol{v} \times \boldsymbol{B}) = S\,\mathrm{d}l\,(-n\,e\,\boldsymbol{v} \times \boldsymbol{B}) = S\,\mathrm{d}l\,\boldsymbol{j} \times \boldsymbol{B}$$

On the condition of current element, the direction of current density is represented by $\mathrm{d}\boldsymbol{l}$, and the current intensity $I = j\,S$, so the equation above is rewritten as

$$\mathrm{d}\boldsymbol{F} = I\mathrm{d}\boldsymbol{l} \times \boldsymbol{B} \tag{7-16}$$

Equation (7-16) is the expression of the integrated magnetic force on all charges performing directional motion inside this element, i.e., the force transmitted to the current carrying conductor; and the current element or the current carrying conductor segment as a whole experiences a magnetic force with the magnitude

$$\mathrm{d}F = I\mathrm{d}l\,B\sin\theta \tag{7-17}$$

where θ is the angle between the current element $I\mathrm{d}\boldsymbol{l}$ and magnetic induction $\boldsymbol{B}$. The direction of the force is given by the right-handed screw rule as shown in Figure 7-14, and the vector expression Equation (7-16) is called the **equation of Ampère force**. For the Ampère force on a finite length straight current carrying conductor L, it is equal to the vector superposition of all Ampère forces acted on all current elements, i.e.

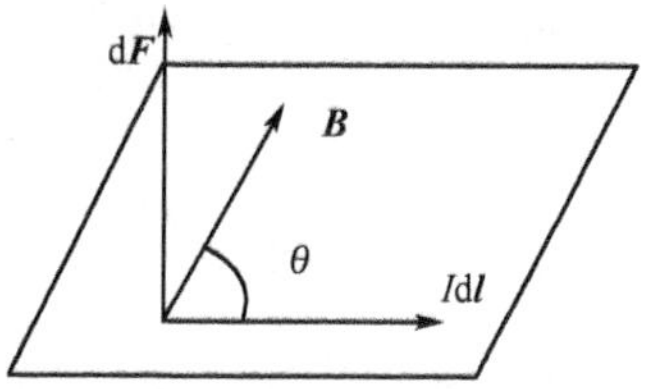

Figure 7-14 Direction of Ampère force

$$\boldsymbol{F} = \int_L \mathrm{d}\boldsymbol{F} = \int_L I\mathrm{d}\boldsymbol{l} \times \boldsymbol{B} \tag{7-18}$$

Example 7-1 Try to analyze the force acted on a semi-circle current carrying conductor in a uniform magnetic field.

Solution: As shown in Figure 7-15, a semi-circle-typed wire with the radius of R carrying a current I. The magnetic field is perpendicular to the plane of the wire and the coordinate system Oxy is selected corresponding to the plane. By the known conditions we can get the magnitude of Ampère force exerted on each current element is $\mathrm{d}F=BI\mathrm{d}l$, radially and the direction is outward from the centre. So the force on the whole wire is equal to the vector superposition (integral) of all Ampère forces acted on all current elements

$$\boldsymbol{F} = \int_L \mathrm{d}\boldsymbol{F}$$

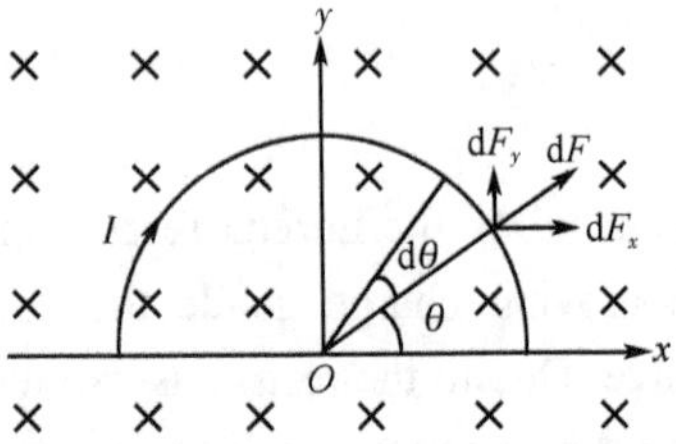

Figure 7-15 Analysis of the force exerted on a semi-circle current carrying conductor in a uniform magnetic field

For calculating this vector integral, we should decompose the force acted on each current element $\mathrm{d}\boldsymbol{F}$ into components along the two directions of x and y, i.e., $\mathrm{d}F_x$ and $\mathrm{d}F_y$. Because of the symmetrical distribution of the current, the x-component of the integrated force is zero, and the y-component of the force on an element is

$$\mathrm{d}F_y = \mathrm{d}F \sin\theta = B\, I\mathrm{d}l \sin\theta$$

So, the direction of the integrated force is the direction of y axis, because $\mathrm{d}l = R\mathrm{d}\theta$, its magnitude is

$$F = \int_L \mathrm{d}F_y = \int_L BIR\sin\theta\,\mathrm{d}\theta = 2BIR\int_0^{\frac{\pi}{2}} \sin\theta\,\mathrm{d}\theta = 2BIR$$

Obviously, as the integrated force $\boldsymbol{F}$ acts on the center of the semi-circle and its direction is upward.

7.3.2 Action Exerted on a Current Carrying Loop by Magnetic Field

As shown in Figure 7-16, a rectangular coil $ABCDA$ with the area of S carrying a current of I is put in a uniform magnetic field with magnetic induction $\boldsymbol{B}$. When the angle between the plane of the coil and the direction of the magnetic field is θ, and the sides AB and CD are both perpendicular to the magnetic induction, we can get the formula to calculate the magnitude of the torque acted on the coil by the magnetic field

$$M = BIS\cos\theta$$

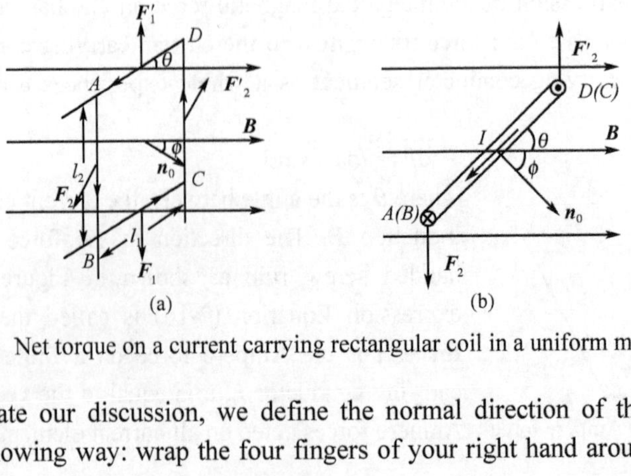

Figure 7-16 Net torque on a current carrying rectangular coil in a uniform magnetic field

In order to facilitate our discussion, we define the normal direction of the plane of the current carrying coil in the following way: wrap the four fingers of your right hand around the perimeter of the coil along the direction of the current, then extend your thumb, the direction of the thumb pointing to is the normal direction of current carrying coil plane, denoted by the unit vector $\boldsymbol{n}_0$; since $\theta+\phi = \pi/2$, the equation above can be rewritten as

$$M = BIS \sin\phi$$

If there is N turns in the coil, then the magnitude of the torque on the current carrying coil is

$$M = BINS\sin\phi = mB\sin\phi \tag{7-19}$$

where $m=INS$ is called the magnitude of **magnetic moment**. It is a vector determined by the characteristic of current carrying coil itself. Its direction is the same as the normal of the current carrying coil.

$$\boldsymbol{m}=INS\boldsymbol{n}_0 \tag{7-20}$$

Apparently, the torque on a current carrying coil is equal to the cross product of magnetic moment $\boldsymbol{m}$ and $\boldsymbol{B}$, represented as

$$\boldsymbol{M} = \boldsymbol{m} \times \boldsymbol{B} \tag{7-21}$$

Equation (7-20) and Equation (7-21) are not only valid for rectangle current carrying coils, but also for current carrying planar coils of any shapes in uniform magnetic fields; even for the magnetic moments formed by charged particles as their rotating along closed paths or as their spinning, the magnetic moments and the torques can be described respectively by the two equations. Later, in the discussion of atomic spectrum and nuclear magnetic resonance, the concept of magnetic moment will be mentioned again.

We can draw a conclusion from Equation (7-19) that the magnitude of the torque is not only dependent on the magnitudes of $\boldsymbol{m}$ and $\boldsymbol{B}$, but also on the angle between $\boldsymbol{m}$ and $\boldsymbol{B}$. The torque is the greatest when $\phi = \pi/2$; and it is zero when ϕ is 0 or π, which corresponds to the two equilibrium positions of coil. The case when $\phi = 0$ corresponds to the stable equilibrium position; while, the case when $\phi = \pi$ corresponds to an unstable equilibrium state in which the resultant torque tends to rotate the coil back to the equilibrium state of $\phi = 0$, whenever the coil is deflected slightly to form this position. It is clear that, when a current carrying coil is in a magnetic field, under the action of the magnetic force, its direction will always be accordant with the direction of the external magnetic field; then the current carrying coil will be in a stable equilibrium state. The regularity of the torque exerted on a current carrying coil by the magnetic field is one of the basic principles for manufacturing electric motors and electric meters.

In the applications of this torque equation, if the unit of the magnetic induction $\boldsymbol{B}$ is T and the unit of the magnetic moment $\boldsymbol{m}$ is $A{\cdot}m^2$, the unit of magnetic torque will be N·m.

7.3.3 Energy of a Magnetic Moment in an External Magnetic Field

In the discussion of the action exerted on a current carrying coil by a magnetic field, we can conclude that, when the direction of the magnetic moment of a current carrying coil is changed in an external magnetic field $\boldsymbol{B}$, the magnetic field (or the external force) will do work on it, this means there is a corresponding potential energy. The zero potential point can be selected arbitrarily. If the potential energy is defined as zero at the position that the magnetic moment is perpendicular to the external magnetic field, i.e., at the position of $\phi = \pi/2$, we can define the potential energy of a current carrying coil at any position of ψ as: the potential energy is equal to the work done by the magnetic torque during the process of turning the coil from the position of zero potential energy to that position of ψ, i.e.

$$E_m = A = \int_{\frac{\pi}{2}}^{\psi} mB \sin\phi \, d\phi = mB\int_{\frac{\pi}{2}}^{\psi} \sin\phi \, d\phi = -mB\cos\psi$$

Its vector form is

$$E_m = -\boldsymbol{m}\cdot\boldsymbol{B} \tag{7-22}$$

Equation (7-22) is the expression of the potential energy of a current carrying coil at any position in a magnetic field.

7.4 Law of Electromagnetic Induction

7.4.1 Law of Electromagnetic Induction

Since the discovery of the magnetic effect of the electric current, there had been people engaging in the experimental study on producing electric current with magnetism. It was not until the year 1831 that Faraday first discovered the phenomenon of electromagnetic induction and got an explicit conclusion: When the magnetic flux passing through the area encircled by a closed loop experiences a change, there will be current emerging in the loop. This phenomenon is called the **electromagnetic induction** and that current is called the **induced current**.

In 1833, based on the investigations of Faraday, Heinrich Friedrich Ernie Lenz summed up a rule from experiments for determining the direction of induced current. The direction of an induced current in a closed loop always makes the new magnetic field aroused by the current impede the change of the magnetic flux which causes the induced current. This conclusion is called **Lenz's law**. We can determine the direction of the induced current by this law.

There is an induced current in a closed loop caused by the change of magnetic flux means there is an electromotive force in the loop. This emf caused by the change of magnetic flux in a closed circuit is called **induced electromotive force**. In fact, it is independent of the structure of the circuit and of the situation whether the circuit is closed or not; so, it can reflect the nature of electromagnetic induction phenomenon more clearly. Faraday summarized the relationship between induced emf and the change of magnetic flux from experiments, which is called **Faraday's law of electromagnetic induction**. It indicates that the magnitude of induced emf in a closed circuit is proportional to the ratio of the increment of magnetic flux and the corresponding time interval $\frac{\mathrm{d}\Phi}{\mathrm{d}t}$ passing through the circuit. Its mathematical expression is

$$\varepsilon_\mathrm{i} = -\frac{\mathrm{d}\Phi}{\mathrm{d}t} \tag{7-23}$$

where, the negative sign "–" expresses that the induced emf is impeding the change of the magnetic flux, so, it is also the mathematic expression of Lenz's law.

We should notice that Equation (7-23) is for the case of a single loop i.e. the coil with only one turn. If the circuit is consist of a coil of N turns, when the magnetic flux is changing, each turn of the coil will produce an induced emf, so the total emf of N turns will be

$$\varepsilon_\mathrm{i} = -N\frac{\mathrm{d}\Phi}{\mathrm{d}t} \tag{7-24}$$

We will explain Faraday's law of induction and Lenz's law with the example of the following case in which a part of a closed circuit moves in a uniform magnetic field.

Example 7-2 There is a uniform magnetic field with magnitude of the magnetic induction of B = 0.22 Wb/m^2, and its direction is pointing into the page perpendicularly, as shown in Figure 7-17. Now, the side CD of the rectangle loop is sliding to the right with a constant speed v = 0.5 m/s, the length of side

CD is $l = 10$ cm. Find the induced emf in this rectangle loop.

Solution: As shown in Figure 7-17, the magnetic flux passing through the loop ABCDA at any time is

$$\Phi = B\,l\,x$$

where $x = \overline{AD} + vt$.

As *CD* sliding towards right, the magnetic flux increases, so $\frac{d\Phi}{dt} = Bl\frac{dx}{dt} = Blv > 0$, that is,

$$\varepsilon_i = -\frac{d\Phi}{dt} = -Blv = -0.22 \times 0.10 \times 0.50 = -0.011\ \text{V}$$

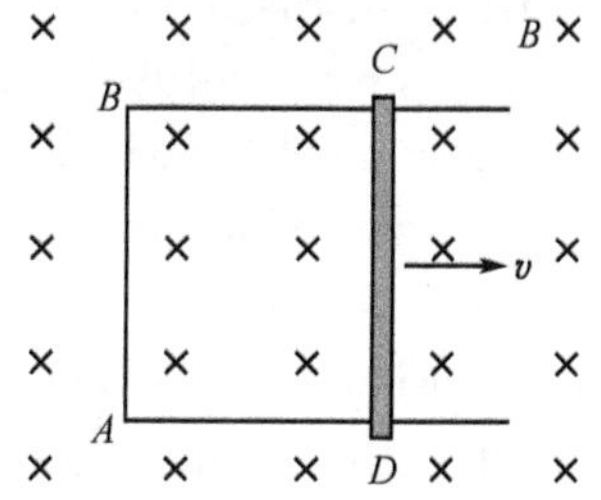

Figure 7-17 Induced emf produced by the sliding side of a wire frame

Here, the negative sign means the direction of ε_i is from *D* to *C*. The direction of the induced current is the same as the direction of the induced emf. That is the magnetic field produced by the induced current directs oppositely to that of the original magnetic field. In other words, it impedes the increase of the magnetic flux. For sure, the direction of the induced current can be determined directly by Lenz's law.

7.4.2 Nature of Electromagnetic Induction

Faraday's induction law indicates whenever there is a change of the magnetic flux in a closed loop there will be a corresponding induced emf. There are only two reasons to cause the changes of the magnetic flux. One is the case that the magnetic field is fixed but the conductor (which may be a part of the circuit or the entire circuit) is moving; the other one is that the circuit is fixed but the magnetic field is changing with time. The induced emf in the circuit produced by the first reason is called **motional electromotive force**; and the induced emf in the circuit produced by the second reason is called **induced electromotive force**.

1. Motional Electromotive Force

As described in Example 7-2, there, the magnetic field is stationary, the only reason to cause the change of magnetic flux is the motion of the metal rod *CD*, and an induced emf is produced in the rod *CD*, that is, motional emf. The reason to cause the motional emf can be regarded as being caused by Lorenz Force. When the conductor rod *CD* moves to the right with a constant velocity ***v***, the free electrons inside the conductor also move with the same velocity to the right. Therefore, every free electron will accumulate towards the end *D* under the action of Lorenz Force $\boldsymbol{f} = -e(\boldsymbol{v} \times \boldsymbol{B})$, as a result, the end *D* is negatively charged while the end *C* is positive. If we take this moving conductor part as a source, then the end *D* is cathode and *C* is anode. The non-electrostatic force in the source is exactly the Lorenz Force on a unit positive charge:

$$\boldsymbol{E}_k = \frac{\boldsymbol{f}}{-e} = \boldsymbol{v} \times \boldsymbol{B}$$

Therefore, the motional emf is equal to

$$\varepsilon_i = \int_{-}^{+} \boldsymbol{E}_k \cdot d\boldsymbol{l} = \int_D^C (\boldsymbol{v} \times \boldsymbol{B}) \cdot d\boldsymbol{l}$$

where $d\boldsymbol{l}$ represents a small displacement in the process in which the unit positive charge moves from point D to C. The cross product of ***v*** and ***B*** is the magnitude and direction of force acting on per unit positive charge, and in this case ***v*** is perpendicular to ***B***, that means the cross product of ***v*** and ***B*** is in the same direction with $d\boldsymbol{l}$, so the integral above is equal to

$$\varepsilon_i = \int_D^C (\boldsymbol{v} \times \boldsymbol{B}) \cdot d\boldsymbol{l} = \int_D^C vB\,dl = Bvl$$

This result is consistent with the conclusion of Example 7-2, which is derived by the ratio of the change of magnetic flux passing through the loop to the time interval.

We've discussed the special case of a straight wire in a uniform magnetic field, and in which the wire moves perpendicularly to the magnetic field. For a wire L of any shape moving or reformatting in any magnetic field, it will also give rise to a motional electromotive force. Then we can divide the wire into numerous infinitesimal elements $\mathrm{d}\boldsymbol{l}$, and the motional emf produced by an element $\mathrm{d}\boldsymbol{l}$ is

$$\mathrm{d}\varepsilon_i = (\boldsymbol{v} \times \boldsymbol{B})\cdot \mathrm{d}\boldsymbol{l}$$

where $\boldsymbol{v}$ denotes the velocity of the element $\mathrm{d}\boldsymbol{l}$, and $\boldsymbol{B}$ is the magnetic induction of the point where the element is. So the total motional emf produced by the whole wire is

$$\varepsilon_i = \int_L (\boldsymbol{v} \times \boldsymbol{B})\cdot \mathrm{d}\boldsymbol{l} \tag{7-25}$$

Equation (7-25) provides another way to calculate induced emf. In the case that the circuit is not closed, Faraday's induction law can't be applied directly but the equation above is still valid.

From the above discussion, we see that motional emf can only exist in the moving part of the conductor in magnetic field, while there is no emf in the stationary part of the conductor. The stationary part only provides a passageway for current to complete the circuit. In the case there is only a section of wire moving in the magnetic field, not a closed circuit, though there is no induced current, there may still exists motional emf in this wire. As for the case in which there must be a motional emf produced in a moving wire section depends on the manner of how the wire moving in the magnetic field. There are only the two conditions which there will be motional emf produced: One is the angle between the velocity of the wire $\boldsymbol{v}$ and $\boldsymbol{B}$ is not zero, and the other is the angle between the cross-product of $(\boldsymbol{v} \times \boldsymbol{B})$ and $\mathrm{d}\boldsymbol{l}$ is not $\pi/2$.

Lorenz force does no work on electric charges, but the above description indicates that the motional emf is the production of Lorenz force. Are these two statements contradicted? Actually, they are not at all. In the previous discussion only one part of the Lorenz forces is taken into account. If we consider totally, we will find that the electrons in the conductor move not only with a velocity $\boldsymbol{v}$ (the same as the velocity of the moving conductor), but also with another directional velocity $\boldsymbol{u}$ relative respect to the conductor, as shown in Figure 7-18. It is exactly the latter motion of the electrons that produces the induced current. In integrate, the Lorenz force exerted on an electron is

$$\boldsymbol{f} = -e(\boldsymbol{v} + \boldsymbol{u}) \times \boldsymbol{B}$$

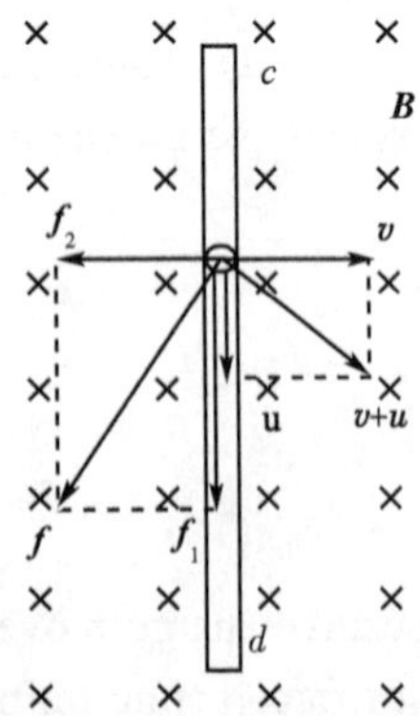

Figure 7-18 Lorenz force does no work

where the force $\boldsymbol{f}$ is perpendicular to the resultant velocity$(\boldsymbol{v} + \boldsymbol{u})$, so the integrated Lorenz force does no work on electrons. However, the force $\boldsymbol{f}_1 = -e(\boldsymbol{v} \times \boldsymbol{B})$ as a component of force $\boldsymbol{f}$ does do positive work on electrons and produces a motional emf; while the other component $\boldsymbol{f}_2 = -e(\boldsymbol{u} \times \boldsymbol{B})$ whose direction is opposite to the velocity $\boldsymbol{v}$ is an impediment to the motion of the conductor, thus its work is negative. It can be proved that the total work done by these two components is zero. Therefore, Lorenz force doesn't provide energy but merely transmits energy, which means that the work done by the external force in overcoming a component of Lorenz force turns into the energy of induced current via another component.

Example 7-3 There is a copper rod AB with the length of L in a uniform magnetic field. It rotates about point A in the plane perpendicular to the magnetic field with the angular velocity ω, as shown in

Figure 7-19. Find the electric potential difference between the two ends of the copper rod.

Solution: (1) solve the problem by applying the equation $\varepsilon_i = \int_L (\boldsymbol{v} \times \boldsymbol{B}) \cdot \mathrm{d}l$:

Let's select an element $\mathrm{d}\boldsymbol{l}$ arbitrarily on the copper rod and assume the distance between point A and this element $\mathrm{d}\boldsymbol{l}$ is l. Then the magnitude of its velocity respect to the magnetic field is $v = \omega\, l$, and the direction is as shown in Figure 7-19. Since $\boldsymbol{v} \perp \boldsymbol{B}$, the direction of $(\boldsymbol{v} \times \boldsymbol{B})$ is consistent with $\mathrm{d}\boldsymbol{l}$, the electric potential on the element is

$$\mathrm{d}\varepsilon_i = (\boldsymbol{v} \times \boldsymbol{B}) \cdot \mathrm{d}\boldsymbol{l} = v\, B\, \mathrm{d}l = \omega\, B\, l\, \mathrm{d}l$$

So, the emf produced by the whole copper rod is

$$\varepsilon_{AB} = \int_A^B \omega B l \mathrm{d}l = \omega B \int_0^L l \mathrm{d}l = \frac{1}{2}\omega B L^2$$

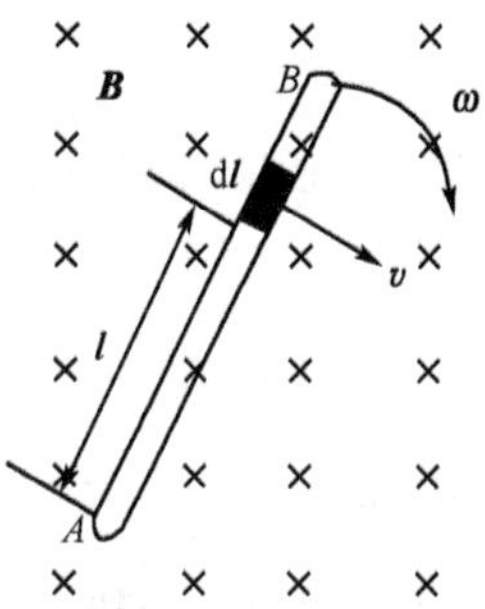

Figure 7-19 The potential difference between two ends U_{AB}

We can know from the right-hand rule for motional emf that the direction of the emf directs from A to B, and the potential difference is

$$U_{AB} = -\varepsilon_{AB} = -\frac{1}{2}\omega B L^2$$

The negative sign means the electric potential at point B is greater than that at A.

(2) We leave the solution by the application of Faraday's law to the readers.

2. Induced Electromotive Force

Experiments show that the induced emf in a loop caused by the change of magnetic field has nothing to do with the category and character of the conductor, and it is only related to the situation of the change of magnetic flux. This indicates that the induced emf is produced by the change of the magnetic field itself. After analyzing some of the phenomena about electromagnetic induction, Maxwell came up with the hypothesis that there is an electric field in the shape of vortex around the changing the magnetic field, which is called **rotational electric field or induced electric field**. The induced emf in a conductor is exactly the result of this electric field force exerted on free charges inside it.

Both the rotational electric field and the static electric field have a common characteristic that they both exert forces on electric charges. Meanwhile, there are also differences: On the one hand, the rotational electric field isn't produced by electric charges, instead, it is produced by the changing magnetic field; on the other hand, the electric field lines describing the rotational electric field are all closed, so this kind of field is not conservative. The mathematical expression for this is

$$\oint_L \boldsymbol{E}_\mathrm{r} \cdot \mathrm{d}\boldsymbol{l} \neq 0$$

While, the non-electrostatic force to produce the induced emf is just this rotational electric field, i.e.

$$\varepsilon_\mathrm{i} = \oint_L \boldsymbol{E}_\mathrm{r} \cdot \mathrm{d}\boldsymbol{l} \tag{7-26}$$

Generally, the total electric field in the space $\boldsymbol{E}$ is the superposition of the electrostatic field $\boldsymbol{E}_\mathrm{p}$ and rotational field $\boldsymbol{E}_\mathrm{r}$. That is

$$\boldsymbol{E} = \boldsymbol{E}_\mathrm{r} + \boldsymbol{E}_\mathrm{p}$$

Amidst it, $\oint_L \boldsymbol{E}_\mathrm{p} \cdot \mathrm{d}\boldsymbol{l} = 0$, so, induced emf can be rewritten as

$$\varepsilon_\mathrm{i} = \oint_L (\boldsymbol{E}_\mathrm{r} + \boldsymbol{E}_\mathrm{p}) \cdot \mathrm{d}\boldsymbol{l} = \oint_L \boldsymbol{E} \cdot \mathrm{d}\boldsymbol{l}$$

On the other hand, according to Faraday's induction law we have

$$\varepsilon_\mathrm{i} = -\frac{\mathrm{d}\Phi}{\mathrm{d}t} = -\frac{\mathrm{d}}{\mathrm{d}t}\iint_S \boldsymbol{B} \cdot \mathrm{d}\boldsymbol{S}$$

The range of surface integral S in the equation is a curved surface encircled by the closed path L. If the closed path is fixed, we can transpose the order of the derivative to time with the surface integral on the surface in the above equation, and get:

$$\oint_L \boldsymbol{E} \cdot \mathrm{d}\boldsymbol{l} = -\iint_S \frac{\partial \boldsymbol{B}}{\partial t} \cdot \mathrm{d}\boldsymbol{S} \tag{7-27}$$

The equation above expresses that the line integral of electric field intensity along a closed path is equal to the negative value of changing rate of the magnetic flux in the surface encircled by the path.

In a stationary case, every quantity won't change with time, then, $\frac{\partial \boldsymbol{B}}{\partial t} = 0$, $\boldsymbol{E}_r = 0$, so Equation (7-27) turns into $\oint_L \boldsymbol{E} \cdot \mathrm{d}\boldsymbol{l} = 0$, this is the circuital theorem in the electrostatic field. As you see that, it is a special case of Equation (7-27).

Here, we should indicate that the motional emf and induced emf can not be partitioned absolutely from each other. From different coordinate systems, an emf may be a motional one or an induced one. But it is not in all the cases that we can convert the conceptions of motional emf and induced emf by means of the changes of coordinate systems. The self-induction phenomenon is an example. In addition, we should notice that the original expression of Faraday's induction law is suitable only for the closed circuits structured by conductors; but Maxwell's hypothesis is suitable for various situations, no matter where there are conductors or not, it is in the mediums or in the vacuum.

3. Self Induction

Whenever the electric current in a current carrying coil changes, the magnetic flux passing through the coil will change with it, so that, an induced emf will be aroused in the coil. This kind of electromagnetic induction phenomenon caused by the coil's own change of the current is called **self induction**, and the corresponding emf is called the **self induced electromotive force.**

In practical utilizations, people find the value of self induced emf is closely related with the characters of the coil itself. So a physical quantity called the **coefficient of self induction** or the **inductance** is introduced to describe these characters of the coil. The inductance is denoted by L, in the SI system its unit is H. After introducing the inductance, we can express the magnetic flux passing through the coil with

$$\Phi = LI$$

By applying Faraday's induction law we can get the self induced emf in a closed circuit

$$\varepsilon_i = -\frac{\mathrm{d}\Phi}{\mathrm{d}t} = -L\frac{\mathrm{d}I}{\mathrm{d}t} \tag{7-28}$$

We see from Equation (7-28) that the value of the self induced emf is proportional to the ratio of the change of current to corresponding time interval; in the case that this ratio is fixed, the bigger is the coefficient L, the bigger the self induced emf will be, and the more intensive the function to impede the change of the current will be.

7.5 Magneto-biology and Magneto Therapy

Bio-magnetism is also called magneto-biology. It is a discipline which set up to investigate the correlations between the magnet of materials or magnetic field and activities of lives, along with the applications of magnetism in biomedicine. In this section we will only introduce some main concepts.

7.5.1 Bio-magnetic Fields

Similar to generating the bioelectricity any creatures can also generate bio-magnetism, meanwhile, there are magnetic fields produced with the activities of lives, these magnetic fields are bio-magnetic fields. The sources of the bio-magnetic fields are mainly in the following cases: ① The magnetic field is generated by bioelectric currents. The moving charges can arouse corresponding magnetic field. Anywhere inside the organism if there is a bioelectric phenomenon there must be a bio-magnetic field accompanied with, like the magnetic fields in the heart, brain, and muscles. ② The magnetic field is set up by bio-magnetic materials. Some materials to compose the organisms of the creatures are magnetic, so, under the effect of the external magnetic field they will have the induced magnetic fields. The tissues composing the organs such as the liver, the spleen and so on are this kind of bio-magnetic materials. ③The magnetic field is set up by intensive magnetic materials in side the organisms. Some particles of intensive magnetic materials may be taken into the lung or along with foods into the stomach and intestines and deposited there. After being magnetized by external magnetic field, these particles would stay in the body as small magnetite pieces which will magnetize the organisms around and set up bio-magnetic fields. The magnetic fields in lungs and in abdomens are this kind of bio-magnetic fields.

The bio-magnetic fields are very feeble. The magnetic fields of lungs are most intensive, the corresponding magnetic inductions are at the level of 10^{-11}-10^{-8} T; the magnetic field of heart is about 10^{-10} T; the spontaneous magnetic field of brain is merely about 10^{-12} T; the induced magnetic field of brain and magnetic field of retina are weaker. The interference of magnetic fields of surroundings and magnetic noise are much stronger. The induction of the geomagnetic field is nearly the level of 0.5×10^{-4} T, and magnetic fields of alternating current magnetic noises in modern cities can reach to the level of 10^{-8}-10^{-6} T. So to measure the magneto-biological signal is rather difficult. In recent years, many kinds of magnetic measuring apparatuses have been developed in succession, such as superconducting quantum interference device, SQUID for short. With a higher resolution about 10^{-15} T, this kind of systems can measure almost any magnetic fields of the organisms inside human body. It is the main approach of measuring the bio-magnetic fields at present.

7.5.2 Biological Effects of Magnetic Field

The influences on life activities made by external magnetic field are called biological effects of magnetic field, which is one of the significant research subjects in magneto-biology.

1. Biological Effect of Geomagnetic Field

The earth is a huge magnet and the geomagnetic field is a long-standing environmental physical factor, relying on which the living creatures could subsist. Many biologic phenomena are relevant to the geomagnetic field. For examples, pigeons can fly back from the distance of several thousand kilometers away; sea turtles will perform their thousand kilometers' breeding migration; migrant birds complete their yearly migrations on courses; in addition, some bacteria are able to swim along the direction of geomagnetic field and so on. Some scientific researches have found that inlayed in the organisms of some creatures, there are some natural magnet pieces as compasses, which can perceive the geomagnetic field and navigate for them. Researches also reveal that the circadian rhythms of human beings and animals are relevant to the alteration of geomagnetic field. So, just as the air, sunlight, water, and suitable temperature, geomagnetic field is one of the important factors for lives.

2. Biological Effects of Constant Magnetic Field

Biological effects of constant magnetic field are variable due to the differences of intensity, gradient and acting time. If a laboratory rat is raised in a uniform magnetic field of 4×10^{-1} T, the activity of oxidase in its liver may have some changes, the contents of sodium and potassium in urine may increase sharply, and pathological changes may also happen in adrenal glands. But when a laboratory rat is put into a stronger magnetic field, there is not distinct abnormal change. Experiments show that biological effect is dependent on the intensity and acting time, so we adopt the product of the intensity and acting time as the dose of the action of the magnetic field to express the extent of its biological effect.

Research data show that when exposed in the magnetic fields of 50×10^{-4} T, 400×10^{-4} T, 5000×10^{-4} T, the erythrocyte agglutination velocity of human being will increase by 21%, 25% and 30% respectively. And some of the people working long time in high-intensity magnetic field for 3-5 years would suffer from vegetosis symptoms such as the increase of hand perspiration, headache, insomnia, inappetence and vestibular dysfunction.

3. Biological Effects of Extremely Weak Magnetic Field

Extremely week magnetic fields acting on different living creatures have different influences, for example, if the tissue of chicken embryo is in a magnetic field of 5×10^{-9} T for 4 days' fostering, there is no influence on the embryo. But if a laboratory rat is put into a magnetic field of 10^{-7} T, after 1 year's fostering, the rat's life may be shortened for 6 months and it may lose the ability of giving any birth. As the developments of aerospace technology and science of cosmos, researches in this field are of great significance, for the magnetic fields in cosmos space are much weaker than the geomagnetic field.

4. Biological Effect of Alternation Field

Because there are accessional effects of bioelectric currents produced by electromagnetic induction, the biology effects caused by alternating magnetic fields are more complicated than which by constant magnetic fields. Constant magnetic field plays a suppressive role in the regeneration and healing of the tissues, yet alternating and pulse magnetic fields can help promote the healing of bone fractures well. The alternating and rotational magnetic field can influence the lymphocyte transformation, and boost the immunity of organisms as well.

7.5.3 Applications of Magneto-biological Effect in Medicine

1. Magnetic Diagnostics Techniques

The curve of the relationship that human body's magnetic field varies with time is called human body magnetic diagram. Similar to the electrocardiogram diagnosing, by the method of comparing the abnormal diagrams with the normal ones, the human body magnetic diagram is a kind of evidence to diagnose diseases.

The magnetic probe for measuring the human magnetic graph shouldn't contact to the organisms so as to avoid the contact interference; the apparatus can measure constant, alternating magnetic field and components of a magnetic field in different direction. We can also change the position of probe to acquire a distribution of human magnetic field in three-dimensional space. Hence, with the help of computer analyzing, the distribution of bioelectric current sources that exert the magnetic fields in organisms can be obtained.

Nowadays, the human body magnetic diagrams being used include magnetocardiogram, magnetoencephalogram and magnetopneumogram. Among them, magnetocardiogram is a curve of magnetic field produced by the cardiac current varying with time. It is a new diagnosing technology in the field of cardiac function's non-damaging examination. Compared with the electrocardiogram, it can diagnose some diseases such as myocardial ischemia and coronary heart disease more sensitively and more accurately. The magnetocardiogram can give some information that cannot be obtained from ECG. For example, it has got the application in surveying the cardiac function of the fetus, for the reason that the signal from the fetus heart is so weak that it is often covered up by the signals from the maternal body. Even though the signal is hardly detected by ECG, but the heart rate of the fetus can displayed by the magnetocardiogram. Likewise, compared with the electroencephalogram, the magnetoencephalogram has many advantages. Nowadays, as the development of technology, the magneto-myogram, the magneto-hepatogram and the magneto-oculogram are also improved a lot. All in all, the magnetic diagnosis technique has got its increasingly wide application in medicine.

Another important application of magnetism in medicine is the nuclear magnetic resonance tomography (or NMR CT). It is a technology to display the distribution of nuclei of some chemical element, i.e. the distribution of the concentration of this element on a cross section in human body or in the organism of some creatures by means of the principle of the nuclear magnetic resonance and the computer processing technology. The nuclear magnetic resonance tomography for the nuclei of hydrogen element is the common application at present. This technology has more advantages than the computerized tomography of X-ray (or X-ray CT). The correlative details will be introduced in the latter chapters.

2. Magnetic Therapy Techniques

The method to make use of magnetic field acting on some particular parts of the body for treating diseases is known as magnetic therapy. The corresponding techniques can be divided into following categories.

(1) **Magnetostatic therapy**. Magnetostatic therapy is the application of the static magnetic fields produced by magnetic sheets, or DC electromagnet onto some acupoints or nidus locations to implement the therapy. The materials and equipments include magnetic sheets, magnetic needles, electromagnetic therapy devices, magnetic chairs, and magnetic beds, etc.

(2) **Motional magnetic field therapy.** It is the application of the alternating magnetic field with low frequency, pulsed magnetic field, rotating magnetic field produced by rotating magnetic sheets, and so on in the treatment of diseases.

(3) **Magnetized water therapy**. After flowing through the water magnetizer, normal water will turn into magnetized water immediately. Experiments show that the water been processed by magnetic field doesn't have any magnetism, but its oxygen content, PH value, osmotic pressure, and surface tension become different from ordinary water. The magnetized water is effective in the treatment of diseases like calculosis, hypertension and so on.

(4) **Magneto-fluid therapy.** Magneto-fluid is also called magnetic liquid, which has both magnetism and fluidity. Its main ingredients are magnetized powder, surface active agents and basic liquid. For example, by mixing the anticancer drug with magneto-fluid, and guiding the drug to the place where tumor located with an intense magnetic field outside the body, this method can improve the effect of the drug and reduce side effect.

Clinical applications of magnetic therapy have effects in the aspects of pain relieving, inflammation diminishing, detumescence, decompression, blood fat reducing, and so on. It has the advantages of economic, simple and convenient, painless, noninvasive, and has few side effects. Nowadays, the researches and applications of magnetic therapy are carried on in many countries. For example, Americans are curing tumors and cancers with heating method of superconductive magnetic field and high frequency magnetic field, etc.

A Brief Summarization of This Chapter

(1) Gauss' law in magnetism: $\oiint_S \boldsymbol{B}\cdot \mathrm{d}\boldsymbol{S}=0$

(2) Ampère's circuital law: $\oint_L \boldsymbol{B}\cdot \mathrm{d}\boldsymbol{l}=\mu_0\sum_{i=1}^{n} I_i=\mu_0\sum_{(\text{in})} I_i$

(3) Lorentz force and the motion of charged particles in the magnetic field.

1) Lorentz force: $\boldsymbol{f}=q\,\boldsymbol{v}\times\boldsymbol{B}$

2) The radius of gyration: $R=\dfrac{mv}{qB}$; the period of gyration: $T=\dfrac{2\pi m}{qB}$; the screw pitch: $h=v_{//}T=\dfrac{2\pi m v_{//}}{qB}$

(4) Ampère force: $\mathrm{d}\boldsymbol{F}=I\mathrm{d}\boldsymbol{l}\times\boldsymbol{B}$

(5) The torque on a current carrying coil in the magnetic field: $\boldsymbol{M}=\boldsymbol{m}\times\boldsymbol{B}$; $\boldsymbol{m}=INS\,\boldsymbol{n}_0$ is the magnetic moment of the current carrying coil.

(6) Faraday's law of induction: $\varepsilon_{\mathrm{i}}=-\dfrac{\mathrm{d}\Phi}{\mathrm{d}t}$

(7) The motional emf: $\varepsilon_i=\int_L(\boldsymbol{v}\times\boldsymbol{B})\cdot\mathrm{d}\boldsymbol{l}$

(8) The induced emf: $\varepsilon_{\mathrm{i}}=\oint_L(\boldsymbol{E}_{\mathrm{r}}+\boldsymbol{E}_{\mathrm{p}})\cdot\mathrm{d}\boldsymbol{l}=\oint_L\boldsymbol{E}\cdot\mathrm{d}\boldsymbol{l}$

(9) The self induced emf: $\varepsilon_{\mathrm{i}}=-\dfrac{\mathrm{d}\Phi}{\mathrm{d}t}=-L\dfrac{\mathrm{d}I}{\mathrm{d}t}$

Exercises 7

7-1. Try to illustrate with examples whether the magnetic inductions at any points on a magnetic line are constant vectors or not.

7-2. Inside the electronic devices, we usually twist two current-carrying wires with the current intensities of same magnitude and opposite directions together to reduce their magnetic fields in the distance. Try to explain the reason.

7-3. As shown in Figure for Exercise 7-3, three current carrying wires penetrate through the surface encircled by a closed path L. Find out whether the line integral along the path $\oint_L \boldsymbol{B}\cdot\mathrm{d}\boldsymbol{l}$ and magnetic field induction at each point on the path will change or not in the following cases:

(1) The direction of one of these currents is changed;

(2) The intensities of the currents are kept unchanged, the angle between one wire and the surface penetrated through, is changed;

(3) The positions of the wires and the distances among the three wires are changed within the range of the closed path L;

(4) One of the wires is taken out of the closed path L of the line integral.

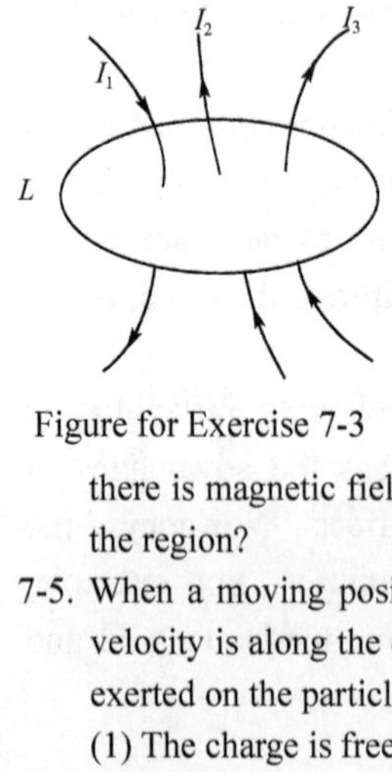

Figure for Exercise 7-3

7-4. In the case that the gravitational force is negligible, if a charged particle is passing across a particular region in the space but is not deflected, can you make sure whether there is magnetic field or not in this region? If the particle is deflected, whether there must be magnetic field in the region?

7-5. When a moving positive charge passes by point A in a magnetic field, shown as Figure for Exercise 7-5, its velocity is along the direction of axis x. Determine the direction of the magnetic induction, if the magnetic force exerted on the particle is in the following cases:

(1) The charge is free from any force;

(2) The direction of the force is along z axis, and the magnitude of the force is the maximum;

(3) The direction of the force is opposite to z axis, and the magnitude of the force is half of the maximum.

7-6. An electron gun shoots two electrons at the same time as shown in Figure for Exercise 7-6, the direction of their initial velocities are both perpendicular to the uniform magnetic field and the magnitudes of their velocities are respectively v and $2v$. After experienced the deflection by the magnetic field, which electron can be back to the starting point earlier? Find the ratio of the radius to the velocity for each charge.

7-7. Assume that the angle between the uniform magnetic field $\boldsymbol{B}$ and the normal direction of the rectangles current carrying wire frame is ϕ, as shown in Figure for Exercise 7-7. Find whether there is any relationship between the angle ϕ and the magnitude of the force acting on each of the four sides, whether there is any relationship between the angle ϕ and the resultant force acting on the frame, and whether there is any relationship between the angle ϕ and the resultant torque acting on the frame.

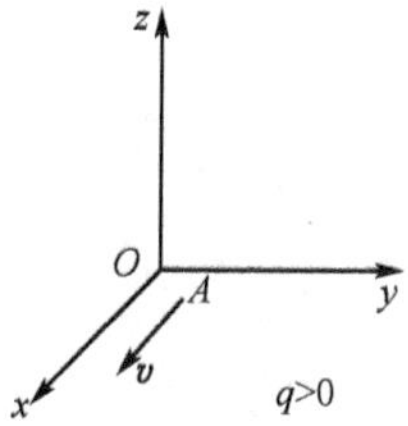

Figure for Exercise 7-5

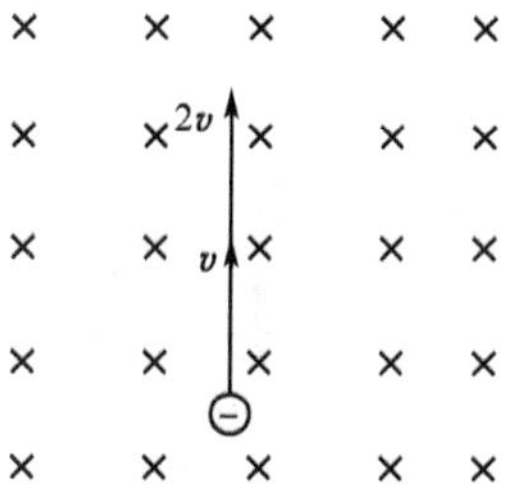

Figure for Exercise 7-6

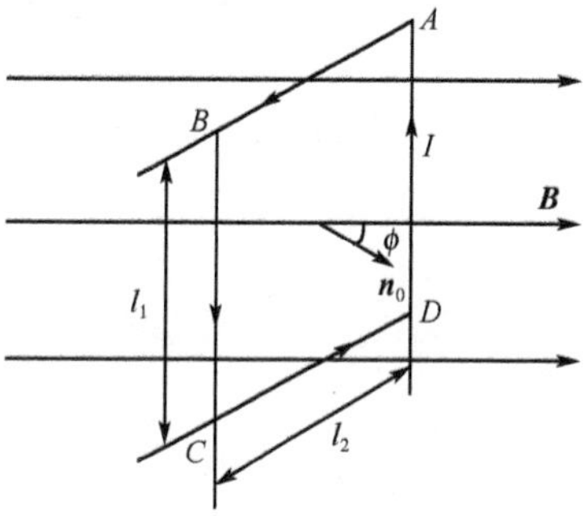

Figure for Exercise 7-7

7-8. Put a solid prism-like box $ABCDFE$ (see Figure for Exercise 7-8 for the sizes) in the magnetic field with a magnitude B=2.0 T following with the direction of x axis. Determine the magnetic fluxes through the surface of $ABCD$ and through the whole enclosed surface.

7-9. There is a square with the side length of b which is put beside an infinite long straight current carrying wire with the current intensity of I. The distance between them is a (see Figure for Exercise 7-9 for the direction of the current). Determine the magnetic flux through the square.

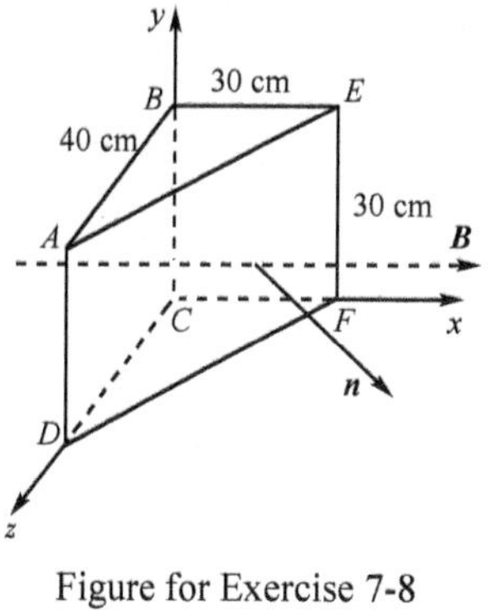

Figure for Exercise 7-8

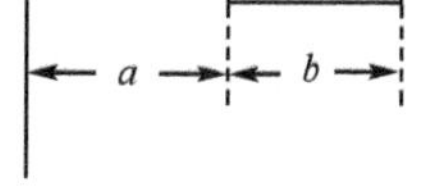

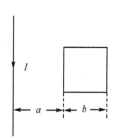

Figure for Exercise 7-9

7-10. There is an electric current flowing along the side wall of a long straight thin hollow metal tube. Try to find the distributions of magnetic inductions inside and outside the tube.

7-11. There is an infinite long column of conductor with the radius of R_1 coated by a cylinder. The inner and outer radiuses of the cylinder are respectively R_2 and R_3. A steady current I flows into the column and out of the cylinder, as shown in Figure for Exercise 7-11. Try to find the distribution of the magnetic induction in the space.

7-12. Two parallel straight long wires carry with currents intensities I and $4I$ respectively. The distance between them is d. Find the zero point of the magnetic induction, when the two currents are flowing in the same direction.

7-13. An infinite long straight current carrying wire and another straight current carrying wire AB are placed perpendicularly, as shown in Figure for Exercise 7-13. The currents are respectively I_1 and I_2, and the length of AB is l, the distance between the end A and the infinite long wire is a. Find the force acting on the wire AB.

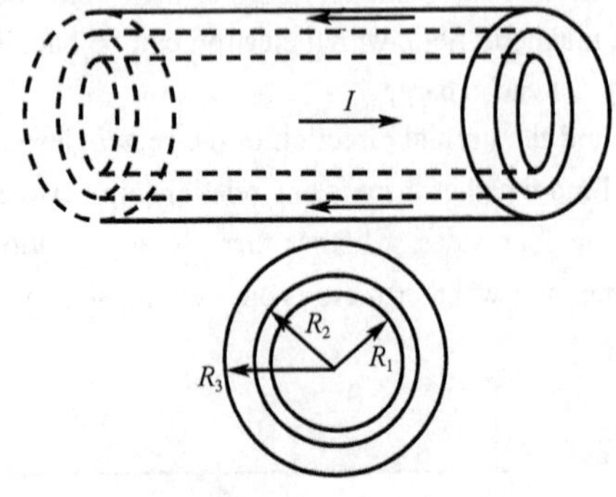

Figure for Exercise 7-11

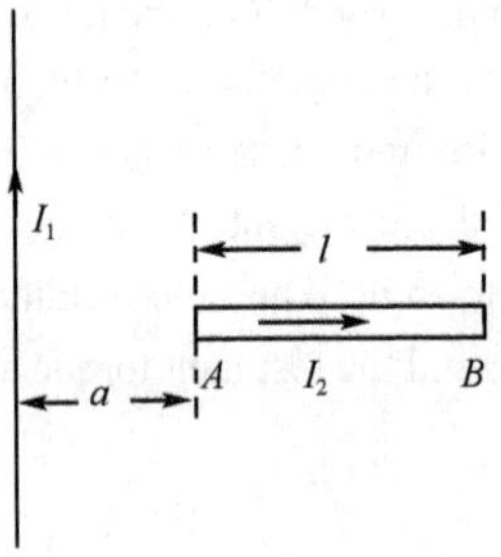

Figure for Exercise 7-13

Chapter 8 Mechanical Oscillations and Mechanical Waves

A **mechanical oscillation** (or **mechanical vibration**) refers to the motion of an object that moves back and forth about a fixed position. The phenomena of mechanical oscillations exist widely in many fields of the science and technology and also in daily life. There are so many mechanical oscillations, such as the reciprocating motion of the cylinder's piston, the heartbeat, the vibrations of the vocal cords, the strings' vibrations of some musical instrument, the tiny quiver at each part of a machine during its running etc.

There are many other phenomena in nature also belonging to the generalized oscillatory phenomena, such as alternating current, alternating electromagnetic field, and so on. In those cases, the motions are not essentially the mechanical motions, but in mathematical descriptions, the regularity of those motions is similar to mechanical oscillations.

The simplest periodic linear oscillation is the simple harmonic motion. Any complex oscillation can be considered as a composition of several or many simple harmonic motions, therefore, the simple harmonic motion is the most essential content of oscillatory theories.

A wave motion is the propagation process of an oscillation. The systems exciting the waves are called **wave sources**. Generally speaking, there are two kinds of waves. **Mechanical waves** are the disturbance and propagation of mechanical oscillations through the media. The ripples in the water due to a dropped pebble and a sound wave are examples of mechanical waves. **Electromagnetic waves** refer to the propagations of varying electric fields and varying magnetic fields. The radio waves, light waves, and the X-rays are examples of electromagnetic waves. They are a special class of waves that do not require media for propagating. These two kinds of waves are essentially different, but they have common characteristics and regularity of waves. For examples, they have certain propagation speeds, and can display the phenomena of reflection, refraction, diffraction and interference as well. We know that, the oscillations' propagations are accompanied by the energy transmissions, so waves are the propagating processes of energy transmission and crucial forms of motions of substances as well. So problems about waves can be encountered when we study in many physical phenomena.

In this chapter, we shall mainly discuss the essential nature and motion regularity of the simple harmonic motions and the simple harmonic waves; we then reveal some physical properties of sound waves and ultrasonic waves and introduce some applications of ultrasonic waves in medicinal field.

8.1 Simple Harmonic Motion

8.1.1 Simple Harmonic Motions and the Resonance Equation

In the case of periodic linear oscillations, the most basic and the most important instances are the **simple harmonic motions**.

Let's take the vibration of a spring oscillator as an example to discuss the basic regularity of a simple harmonic motion.

As shown in Figure 8-1, the left end of a light spring is fixed, and the right end is attached to an object with the mass of m, then place it on a smooth and horizontal plane. If the object is displaced a bit, it will oscillate back and forth by the action of the spring's elastic force. The whole system is called the **spring oscillator**.

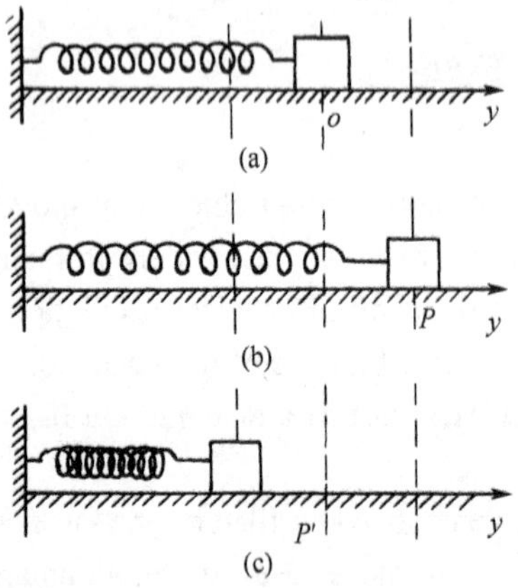

Figure 8-1 A system of spring oscillator

When the object is at the position of O, the spring has the original length, i.e., it is neither extended nor shortened, as shown in Figure 8-1 (a). There isn't any force in the horizontal direction acting on the object; and in the vertical direction, the gravity and the supporting force keep balanced with each other. In this way, if the object at the position of O, the resultant force acting on it is zero, then the position of O is called the equilibrium position.

Let's take the equilibrium position as the original position of the coordinate, the direction of object's vibration as y axis, and the direction from the equilibrium position to the right as the forward direction of y axis. When the object displaces from the equilibrium position during the oscillation, the resultant force acting on it is the elastic force of the spring along the y direction given by Hooke's law. If the displacement from the equilibrium position is y, the elastic force is directly proportional to the extension (or the compression) of the spring y, as shown in Figure 8-1 (b) and Figure(c), i.e.

$$F = -ky \tag{8-1}$$

where k is a positive constant called the coefficient of stiffness of the spring; and the negative sign in the equation signifies that the force exerted by the spring is always directed opposite to the displacement from the equilibrium position. We call the force in Equation (8-1) a linear restoring force. According to Newton's second law, the equation of motion of the object is

$$m\frac{\mathrm{d}^2 y}{\mathrm{d}t^2} = -ky \tag{8-2}$$

which is a homogeneous linear second-order differential equation. Equation (8-2) describes that the acceleration is proportional to the displacement of the object on the equilibrium position and is in the opposite direction of it. The oscillatory motion with this characteristic is called **simple harmonic motion**, or **harmonic motion**. Thus, we know that the motions of objects only under the actions of the elastic forces are harmonic motions. That is to say, if an object is only under the action of a linear restoring force (the word linear refers to the force is proportional to the displacement), its motion is a harmonic motion.

If we denote the ratio of k/m with the quantity ω^2, then Equation (8-2) can be rewritten as

$$\frac{\mathrm{d}^2 y}{\mathrm{d}t^2} + \omega^2 y = 0$$

The solution to it is the following cosine function

$$y = A\cos(\omega t + \phi) \tag{8-3}$$

or

$$y = A\sin(\omega t + \phi + \frac{\pi}{2})$$

where A and ϕ are constants. Thus, the displacement y of the object (or a particle) undergoing a simple harmonic motion is the cosine (or sine) function of time t. Equation (8-3) is called the **equation of simple harmonic motion**, also known as the **resonance equation**.

8.1.2 Three Elements of a Simple Harmonic Motion

1. Amplitude

By analyzing Equation (8-3) we know that, as time goes by, the displacement y of the object m is varying or reciprocating periodically between the values $+A$ and $-A$. Here A is the absolute value of the maximum displacement from the equilibrium position of the vibrating object. So A is called the amplitude of the simple harmonic motion.

2. Period and Frequency

The time required to complete a full oscillation (one round trip) for an oscillating particle is called the **period** of the harmonic motion, denoted by T. The unit of it is s. The reciprocal of the period is called the **frequency**, which represents the number of oscillations that the particle performs per unit time, denoted by ν. The unit of it is Hz. The quantity ω in Equation (8-3) is called the **angular frequency** or the **circular frequency** of the oscillation, it represents the oscillatory times of the oscillating particle in a time interval of 2π seconds, whose unit is rad/s, that is

$$T = \frac{1}{\nu} = \frac{2\pi}{\omega} \tag{8-4}$$

For a spring oscillator, because $\omega^2 = \frac{k}{m}$, its period should be

$$T = 2\pi\sqrt{\frac{m}{k}} \tag{8-5}$$

3. Phase

The quantity $(\omega t + \phi)$ in Equation (8-3) is called the **phase of the harmonic motion**, or the **phase**. The phase is a very important physical quantity. It can determine the motion state of an oscillating particle. Because the motion state of an oscillating particle is constantly changing during a period of oscillation, this varying physical quantity, phase $(\omega t + \phi)$, is chosen for describing the oscillating particle's motion state. For example, in the state of $(\omega t + \phi) = \frac{\pi}{2}$ and the state $(\omega t + \phi) = \frac{3\pi}{2}$, the particle is the same as the equilibrium position. But the motion states are not the same, because the corresponding velocities are different, i.e., the velocities' directions of the former and the latter are just opposite.

The constant angle ϕ is the phase when $t = 0$, called the **initial phase** (or the phase constant). Initial phase determines the displacement when $t = 0$. When two harmonic oscillations are compared to detect whether they are consistent in phase or not, and what the superposition result of them is, the factor playing the decisive role is the phase difference. If two harmonic motions have the same frequency, the corresponding simple harmonic motion equations for both of them can be written respectively as

$$y_1 = A_1 \cos(\omega t + \phi_1)$$

$$y_2 = A_2 \cos(\omega t + \phi_2)$$

Represented as $\Delta\phi$, the phase difference between them is

$$\Delta\phi = (\omega t + \phi_2) - (\omega t + \phi_1) = \phi_2 - \phi_1$$

We can describe the motion state of any simple harmonic motion system at any time with these three physical quantities, the amplitude, the frequency (or the period) and the phase, so these three physical quantities are called the " three elements" of a simple harmonic motion.

8.1.3 Velocity and Acceleration of a Simple Harmonic Motion

By the resonance equation $y = A\cos(\omega t + \phi)$ we see the functional relationship between the displacement of a particle undergoing simple harmonic motion y and the time t. Thus, we can obtain the velocity υ and the acceleration a of the particle from the equation:
The velocity is

$$\upsilon = \frac{\mathrm{d}y}{\mathrm{d}t} = -A\omega\sin(\omega t + \phi) \tag{8-6}$$

The acceleration is

$$a = \frac{\mathrm{d}\upsilon}{\mathrm{d}t} = \frac{\mathrm{d}}{\mathrm{d}t}[-A\omega\sin(\omega t + \phi)]$$

That is

$$a = -\omega^2 A\cos(\omega t + \phi) \tag{8-7}$$

In this equation, $A\cos(\omega t + \phi) = y$. Because the acceleration can be also expressed as $a = \frac{\mathrm{d}^2 y}{\mathrm{d}t^2}$, so Equation (8-7) can be written as

$$\frac{\mathrm{d}^2 y}{\mathrm{d}t^2} = -\omega^2 y$$

After being deformed, Equation (8-2) can be rewritten as

$$\frac{\mathrm{d}^2 y}{\mathrm{d}t^2} = -\frac{k}{m}y$$

For the ratio $\frac{k}{m} = \omega^2$, the two equations have just the same form. This indicates that $y = A\cos(\omega t + \phi)$ is indeed the solution of the differential Equation (8-2).

Example 8-1 A spring oscillator has the relationship between its displacement y and time t: $y = 5\cos(10\pi t + 0.5\pi)$ cm. Try to determine the amplitude, the frequency, the period and the initial phase of the oscillation; then find the displacement, the velocity and the acceleration at $t_1 = 1$ s.

Solution: By comparing the equation $y = 5\cos(10\pi t + 0.5\pi)$ cm with the general equation for simple harmonic motion Equation(8-3), we get,
the amplitude

$$A = 5 \text{ cm},$$

the angular frequency

$$\omega = 10\pi \text{ s}^{-1}$$

by using Equation (8-4), we have the period of the oscillation

$$T = \frac{2\pi}{\omega} = 0.2 \text{ s}$$

the frequency the oscillation

$$\nu = \frac{1}{T} = 5 \text{ Hz}$$

and the initial phase of the oscillation

$$\phi = 0.5\pi$$

By substituting $t_1 = 1$ s in the displacement expression, we have the displacement

$$y|_{t=1} = 5\cos(10\pi + 0.5\pi) = 0 \text{ cm}$$

the velocity

$$v = \frac{dy}{dt} = -5\times 10\pi \sin(10\pi t + 0.5\pi)$$

$$v|_{t=1} = -50\pi \sin 0.5\pi = -50\pi \text{ cm/s}$$

and the acceleration

$$a = \frac{dv}{dt} = -5\times(10\pi)^2 \cos(10\pi t + 0.5\pi)$$

$$a|_{t=1} = 0 \text{ cm/s}^2$$

8.1.4 Energy of a Simple Harmonic Oscillator

Taking the system of the spring oscillator shown in Figure 8-1 as the example, we shall discuss the energy of a simple harmonic motion.

Supposing an oscillating particle with the mass of m acted by the elastic force of a massless spring is undergoing a simple harmonic motion. Because the particle has the velocity, it should also have the kinetic energy. The corresponding kinetic energy is

$$E_k = \frac{1}{2}mv^2 \tag{8-8a}$$

In addition, the system has the elastic potential energy, too. The elastic potential energy is the work done by the external force to overcome the elastic force. If the equilibrium position of the particle is zero point of the potential energy, the elastic potential energy will be

$$E_p = \frac{1}{2}ky^2 \tag{8-9a}$$

Combining Equation (8-6) with Equation (8-8a) and Equation (8-3) with Equation (8-9a), we have

$$E_k = \frac{1}{2}m\omega^2 A^2 \sin^2(\omega t + \phi) \tag{8-8b}$$

$$E_p = \frac{1}{2}kA^2 \cos^2(\omega t + \phi) \tag{8-9b}$$

For a simple harmonic oscillating particle, both its velocity and displacement vary periodically with time, so its kinetic energy and potential energy will also vary periodically with time. When the particle gains the maximum displacement, the system's potential energy reaches the maximum value, but the kinetic energy is zero; well, if the displacement is zero, the potential energy is zero, but the kinetic energy reaches the maximum value. For a spring oscillator, its total energy (denoted by E) is the sum of its kinetic energy and potential energy, i.e.,

$$E = E_k + E_p = \frac{1}{2}m\omega^2 A^2 \sin^2(\omega t + \phi) + \frac{1}{2}kA^2 \cos^2(\omega t + \phi)$$

For a spring oscillator $m\omega^2 = k$, the formula can be written as

$$E = \frac{1}{2}kA^2 \tag{8-10}$$

or

$$E = \frac{1}{2}m\omega^2 A^2 \tag{8-11}$$

By the discussion above we know that, the kinetic and potential energy of a spring oscillator varies periodically with time. But its total energy (mechanical energy) does not change with time. That is to say, even the kinetic energy and the potential energy transform to each other during the oscillation. The mechanical energy of an isolated simple harmonic oscillator system is a constant during the motion and proportional to the square of the amplitude.

8.1.5 Superposition of Two Simple Harmonic Motions in the Same Direction and with the Same Frequency

Now let's suppose that there is an object undergoing two simple harmonic motions in the same direction along one straight line and with the same frequency. If we take this straight line as y axis and the equilibrium position of the particle as the origin point O of the y axis, then the two oscillations can respectively be expressed by the corresponding equations at any time t.

$$y_1 = A_1 \cos(\omega t + \phi_1)$$

$$y_2 = A_2 \cos(\omega t + \phi_2)$$

In the equations above, A_1, A_2 and ϕ_1, ϕ_2 represent respectively the amplitudes and initial phases of the two oscillations. According to the conditions set up, y_1 and y_2 are the displacements from the same equilibrium position and in the same direction of the straight line. According to the principle of superposition of motion, the resultant displacement of the object must be along the same straight line (y axis) and be the algebra sum of the displacements of the two oscillations, i.e.,

$$y = y_1 + y_2 = A_1 \cos(\omega t + \phi_1) + A_2 \cos(\omega t + \phi_2)$$

By using the trigonometric function formulae, we can get the simplification of it

$$y = A \cos(\omega t + \phi)$$

where A and ϕ have the values respectively

$$A = \sqrt{A_1^2 + A_2^2 + 2A_1 A_2 \cos(\phi_2 - \phi_1)} \tag{8-12}$$

$$\tan\phi = \frac{A_1 \sin\phi_1 + A_2 \sin\phi_2}{A_1 \cos\phi_1 + A_2 \cos\phi_2} \tag{8-13}$$

A and ϕ represent respectively the amplitude and initial phase of the resultant oscillation. It can be seen from the above results that the resultant motion of two simple harmonic motions, which is in the same direction and with the same frequency, is still a simple harmonic motion. And the direction and the frequency of the resultant motion are exactly the same as the two component oscillations'. The resultant oscillation's amplitude and initial phase can be determined by the amplitudes of and initial phases of those two oscillations.

By analyzing Equation (8-12) we can see that the resultant amplitude A is dependent not only on the component amplitudes A_1 and A_2 but also on the phase difference of the two component oscillations $\Delta\phi = (\phi_2 - \phi_1)$. Here, let's discuss two special cases.

1. Two Component Oscillations Are Cophase (or In-phase)

When $\Delta\phi = (\phi_2 - \phi_1) = \pm 2k\pi$ ($k = 0, 1, 2,\cdots$), the phase difference of two oscillations is an integer multiple of 2π, $\cos(\phi_2 - \phi_1) = 1$ and

$$A = \sqrt{A_1^2 + A_2^2 + 2A_1 A_2} = A_1 + A_2$$

Now, the resultant amplitude reaches the maximum value and the effect of the superposition of the two component oscillations is to make the amplitude of the vibration be strengthened. Just as shown in

Figure 8-2 (a): The two thin lines represent the motion curves of the two component vibrations and the thick line represents the motion curve of the resultant oscillation.

2. Two Component Oscillations Are Having the Reversed Phases (or Anti-phases)

When $\Delta\phi = (\phi_2 - \phi_1) = \pm(2k+1)\pi$ $(k = 0, 1, 2, \cdots)$, the two oscillations' phase difference $\Delta\phi$ is an odd multiple of π, $\cos(\phi_2 - \phi_1) = -1$ and

$$A = \sqrt{A_1^2 + A_2^2 - 2A_1 A_2} = |A_1 - A_2|$$

Now, the resultant amplitude (because the amplitude is always positive, the right side of the formula takes an absolute value) has the minimum value and the effect of the superposition of the two component oscillations decreases the amplitude of the vibration. The situation is shown in Figure 8-2 (b) .

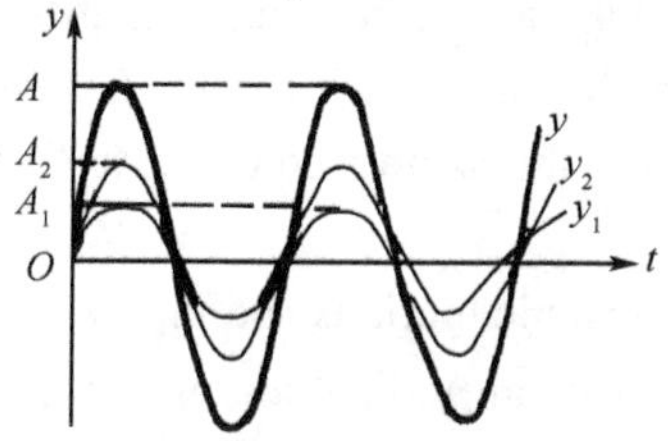

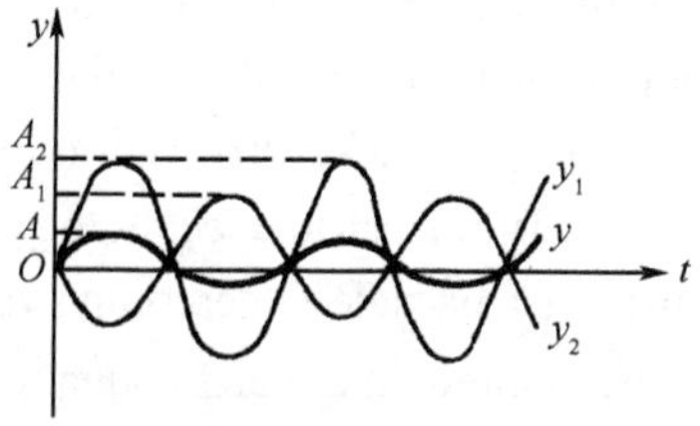

Figure 8-2 The situations of resultant amplitude

If $A_1 = A_2$, the result of the superposition will make the object be at rest ($A = 0$).

3. A General Situation (the Two Component Vibrations Are Neither Inphase Nor Antiphase)

When $\Delta\phi = (\phi_2 - \phi_1)$ is not the integer times of π, the amplitude of the resultant oscillation A has a value between $(A_1 + A_2)$ and $|A_1 - A_2|$.

Example 8-2 A particle is undergoing two simple harmonic motions along the same straight line: $y_1 = 4\cos(2t + \frac{\pi}{6})$ and $y_2 = 3\cos(2t - \frac{5\pi}{6})$, try to determine the amplitude, the initial phase and the equation of the resultant oscillation (where y is in cm and t is in s).

Solution: This is the problem about the superposition of two simple harmonic motions with the same frequency and in the same direction. By the motion equations given, we see that, the amplitudes $A_1 = 4$ cm, $A_2 = 3$ cm and the initial phases $\phi_1 = \frac{\pi}{6}$, $\phi_2 = -\frac{5\pi}{6}$, therefore, we know that the phase difference

$$\Delta\phi = \phi_2 - \phi_1 = -\frac{5\pi}{6} - \frac{\pi}{6} = -\pi$$

Using Equation (8-12) and Equation(8-13) we can evaluate the amplitude and the initial phase of the resultant oscillation and then get its equation of motion:

(1) The amplitude

$$A = \sqrt{A_1^2 + A_2^2 + 2A_1 A_2 \cos(\phi_2 - \phi_1)} = \sqrt{4^2 + 3^2 + 2\times4\times3\cos(-\pi)} = 1 \text{ cm}$$

$$\tan\phi = \frac{A_1\sin\phi_1 + A_2\sin\phi_2}{A_1\cos\phi_1 + A_2\cos\phi_2} = \frac{4\times\frac{1}{2} + 3\times(-\frac{1}{2})}{4\times\frac{\sqrt{3}}{2} + 3\times(-\frac{\sqrt{3}}{2})} = \frac{\sqrt{3}}{3}$$

(2) The initial phase

$$\phi = \frac{\pi}{6}$$

(3) The equation of the resultant motion is $y = \cos(2t + \frac{\pi}{6})$.

8.1.6 Superposition of Two Simple Harmonic Motions with the Same Frequency and in the Directions Perpendicular to Each Other

In the preceding discussion we dealt with some problems about the superposition of two harmonic motions with the same oscillatory direction. Moreover, there are also problems about the superposition of two harmonic motions with the oscillatory directions perpendicular to each other. The researches for this kind of problems, especially when the two oscillations have the same frequency, have their important meanings in applications in electrical technology and optics.

Supposing there is a particle undergoing two simple harmonic motions and the two motions have the same frequency (the common angular frequency is ω), the oscillatory direction of one is along the x axis and the other one is along the y axis, i.e., they are perpendicular to each other.

The equations for the two component simple harmonic motions are respectively:

$$x = A_1 \cos(\omega t + \phi_1)$$

and

$$y = A_2 \cos(\omega t + \phi_2)$$

At any moment t, the particle is at the position of (x, y). When t changes, the position of (x, y) also changes, so we can say that, the two equations above are the parameter equations of the particle's motion orbit by the parameter t. If the parameter t is eliminated, then we obtain the corresponding equation of the orbit in the right-angled coordinate system.

$$\frac{x^2}{A_1^2} + \frac{y^2}{A_2^2} - 2\frac{xy}{A_1 A_2}\cos(\phi_2 - \phi_1) = \sin^2(\phi_2 - \phi_1) \tag{8-14}$$

Equation (8-14) is an elliptic equation. For some special values of the phase difference $\Delta\phi = \phi_2 - \phi_1$ there will be some corresponding special cases.

(1) Two Component Oscillations Are In-phase

When $\Delta\phi = \phi_2 - \phi_1 = 0$, phase difference of two oscillations is 0 or they have the same phase. Equation (8-14) is simplified as

$$\left(\frac{x}{A_1} - \frac{y}{A_2}\right)^2 = 0$$

i.e.

$$\frac{x}{A_1} = \frac{y}{A_2} \quad \text{or} \quad y = \frac{A_2}{A_1}x \tag{8-15}$$

Now, the particle's moving trace is a straight line. The line is in the 1st and 3rd quadrants and passes through the original point of the coordinate, its slope is the ratio of the two oscillations' amplitudes $\frac{A_2}{A_1}$, as shown in Figure 8-3 (a).

With the change of time t, the particle's displacement from equilibrium position is

$$s = \sqrt{x^2 + y^2} = \sqrt{A_1^2 + A_2^2}\cos(\omega t + \phi)$$

From the equation above we know that, the resultant oscillation is a simple harmonic motion oscillating along that line. Its frequency is the same with the two oscillations' frequency and the amplitude is $\sqrt{A_1^2 + A_2^2}$.

(2) Two Component Oscillations are Anti-phase

When $\Delta\phi = \phi_2 - \phi_1 = \pi$, the two oscillations have conversed phases. Equation (8-14) is simplified as

$$\frac{x^2}{A_1^2}+\frac{y^2}{A_2^2}+2\frac{xy}{A_1 A_2}=0,\quad \left(\frac{x}{A_1}+\frac{y}{A_2}\right)^2=0$$

or

$$y=-\frac{A_2}{A_1}x \tag{8-16}$$

That is, the particle oscillates along another straight line $y=-\frac{A_2}{A_1}x$. The line is in the 2nd and 4th quadrants and passes through the original point of the coordinate. As shown in Figure 8-3 (b), the oscillation is similar to the above case.

(3) When $\Delta\phi = \phi_2 - \phi_1 = \frac{\pi}{2}$

In this case, Equation (8-14) is simplified as

$$\frac{x^2}{A_1^2}+\frac{y^2}{A_2^2}=1$$

As shown in Figure 8-3 (c), the motion orbit of the particle is an ellipse taking the coordinate axis x as its main axis. The arrow on the ellipse indicates the direction of motion of the particle.

(4) When $\Delta\phi = \phi_2 - \phi_1 = -\frac{\pi}{2}$

The simplified form of Equation (8-14) is still

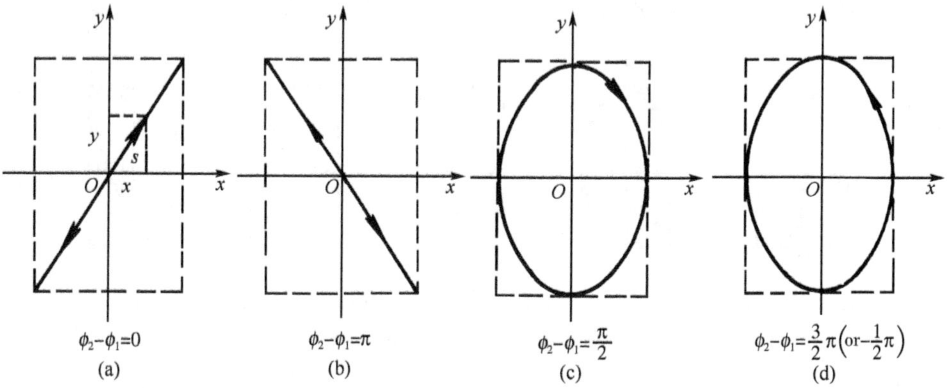

Figure 8-3 The composition of two simple harmonic motions with the same period and perpendicular oscillating directions

$$\frac{x^2}{A_1^2}+\frac{y^2}{A_2^2}=1$$

Then the motion orbit of the particle is the ellipse similar to the ellipse of the case (3), as shown in Figure 8-3 (d), but the direction of motion of the particle is just opposite to the direction of Figure 8-3(c)'s.

When the phase difference $\Delta\phi = \phi_2 - \phi_1 = \pm\frac{\pi}{2}$, if the amplitude of two vibrations is equal i.e. $A_1 = A_2$, the ellipse will become a circle, as shown in Figure 8-4.

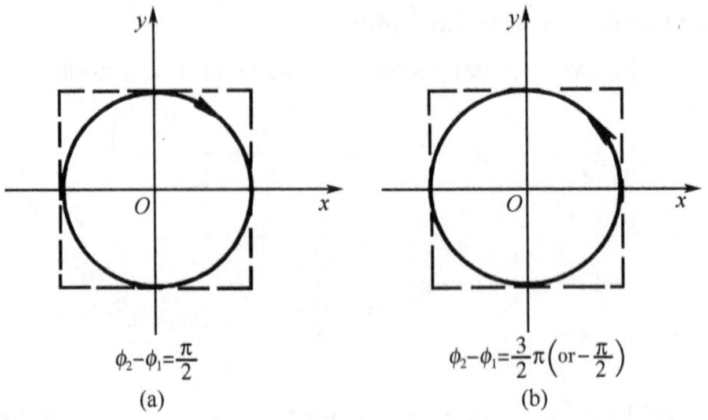

Figure 8-4 The composition of two simple harmonic motions with the same amplitude, a difference of phase $\Delta\phi = \pm\frac{\pi}{2}$ and perpendicular oscillating directions

In short, in the situation of the superposition of two harmonic motions with the same period and oscillating in mutually perpendicular directions, the motion orbit is an ellipse. The characters of the ellipse are defined by the phase difference of the two oscillations $\Delta\phi$. Figure 8-5 shows the diagrams of the superposition of two simple harmonic motions with the same frequency and in mutually perpendicular oscillating directions, in situations of several phase differences and different amplitudes.

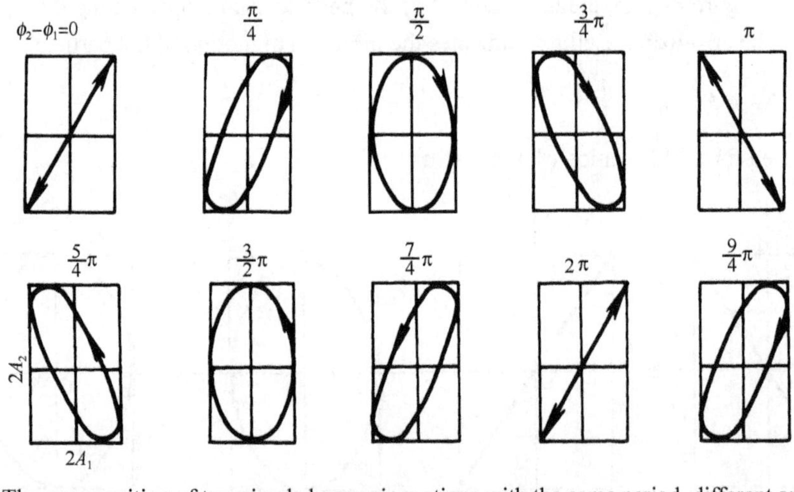

Figure 8-5 The superposition of two simple harmonic motions with the same period, different amplitudes and perpendicular oscillating directions

The above discussion also shows that: Any of a linear harmonic motion, an elliptical motion or a circular motion with a uniform speed can be represented by two simple harmonic motions in mutually perpendicular oscillatory directions.

For any two simple harmonic motions, if the ratio of frequencies of the oscillations is an integer, the traces of the resultant motion will be regular stable closed curves. Table 8-1 shows the diagrams of the resultant motions with the frequency ratios of 1:2 and 2:3, this kind of diagrams are known as the Lissajou's figures.

Table 8-1 Lissajou's figures

Phase difference / Rate of frequency	$\varphi_y - \varphi_z = 0$	$\varphi_y - \varphi_z = \pi/4$	$\varphi_y - \varphi_z = \pi/2$	$\varphi_y - \varphi_z = 3/4\pi$	$\varphi_y - \varphi_z = \pi$
$\omega_x : \omega_y = 1:2$	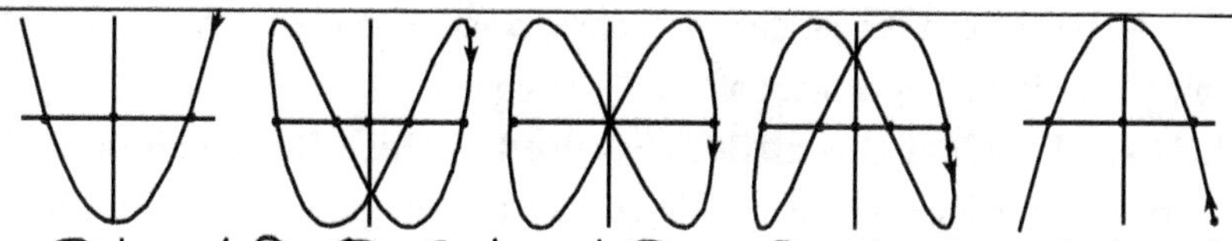				
$\omega_x : \omega_y = 2:3$	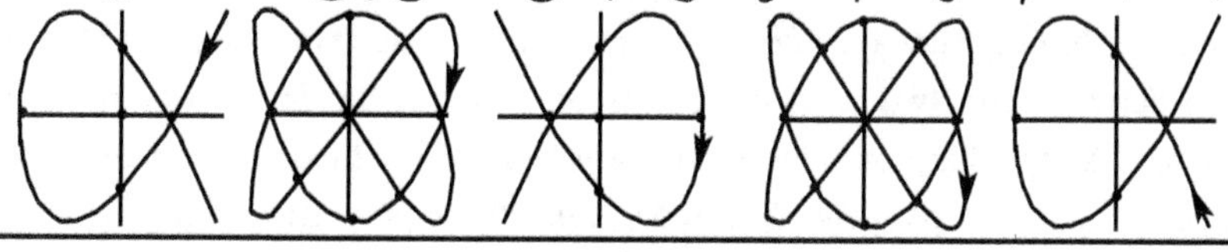				

8.2 Fundamental Theories of Wave Motions

8.2.1 Overview

The propagation of an oscillation in the medium forms a **wave motion**. Wave motions are a special kind of motions of substances. Sound waves, waves on the surface of water, the wave through a rope generated by the jitter of one end of it, pulse waves, seismic waves, light and electromagnetic waves, etc. are all wave motions. Different kinds of waves have different natures, and each has its particular properties and follows special rules. But in the expression, they possess many common characteristics and expressive rules, i.e., all of them have certain velocities and the energy transmission accompanied by, they can generate the phenomena of reflection, refracting, interference and diffraction, and they have similar mathematical expressions as well.

In this chapter, we shall mainly discuss the characteristics and the regularity of mechanical waves, or more concretely, of the most basic waves—sinusoidal harmonic waves. We shall also introduce the special forms of waves—sound waves and ultrasonic waves, which have many applications in medical studies.

If all the particles in the space of a medium are contacted each other by the elastic force, this medium is called the **elastic medium**. In the elastic medium, because of the connection of the elastic force, the oscillation of any particle will cause oscillations of neighboring particles. Oscillations of neighboring particles will cause more oscillations of other neighboring particles, in this way, the oscillations will propagate at a certain speed and spread out from the near to the distant in all directions. The processes of propagations of mechanical oscillations in the elastic media are called **mechanical waves**.

1. Two Conditions for Constituting a Mechanical Wave

(1) A **source of disturbance** (or a **wave source**), i.e., an object creating mechanical oscillation.

(2) The **medium** (elastic medium), i.e., the medium substance which is capable of propagating mechanical oscillations, such as air, water and so on.

2. Two Common Types of Mechanical Waves

The two basic types of mechanical waves are transverse waves (or shear waves) and longitudinal waves. We have known that, the mechanical waves are propagations of mechanical oscillations in the media. As a wave travels, if the particles of the medium undergo displacements parallel to the direction of propagation, the wave is called a **longitudinal wave**; and if the particles of the disturbed medium move perpendicularly to the direction of propagation, the wave is called a **transverse wave**. Generally speaking, the oscillatory situations of particles in the medium are very complex, so the wave motions resulted from the oscillations are also very complex. But these complex wave motions can be considered as superpositions of transverse waves and longitudinal waves. These two kinds of waves are all simple harmonic waves—the propagations of simple harmonic motions in elastic media—the topic of simple harmonic waves is the key content of our discussion.

3. Three Physical Quantities Required to Describe Mechanical Waves

There are three important commonly used physical quantities for describing mechanical waves, they are wavelength, frequency (or period as a substitution), and wave speed. One wavelength is the minimum distance between any two identical points on a wave; the frequency of the wave is the same as the frequency of simple harmonic motion of a particle of the medium; the wave speed is the velocity of the propagation of oscillatory state, it only depends on the properties of the medium through which the wave travels. These three physical quantities are denoted respectively by λ, ν (or T) and c; and the relationship among them is:

$$c = \frac{\lambda}{T} \quad \text{or} \quad c = \lambda\nu$$

8.2.2 Simple Harmonic Waves

If a wave source is performing a simple harmonic motion, it will cause a series of oscillations of the particles around it in the medium. The oscillations of the adjacent particles are all simple harmonic motions with the same frequency of the wave source. So the propagation of the simple harmonic motion of the source in elastic medium forms a **simple harmonic wave**. This kind of waves is the most essential and the simplest form of wave, so it has special significance to study the regularity of simple harmonic waves. As shown in Figure 8-6, a planar cosine harmonic wave is propagating along the direction of x axis. The source of it is just set at the origin of coordinate O, the wave speed is c; the x axis can represent the equilibrium position of each particle; the quantity y represents the displacement (or the distance from the equilibrium point) of each particle in the oscillatory direction. The initial phase of the wave source is supposed to be 0, the amplitude to be A, and the angular frequency to be ω. So the equation for the simple harmonic motion at the wave source is

$$y = A\cos\omega t \tag{8-17}$$

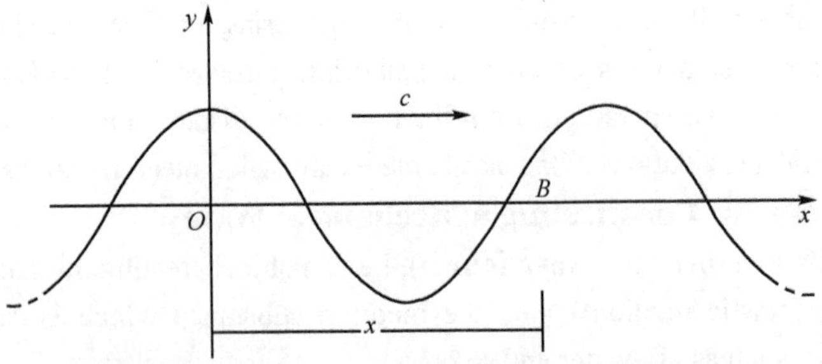

Figure 8-6 The graph for deriving the equation of wave

Suppose there is a particle at point B with a distance of x from the source in the direction of the wave propagation. The oscillation of the particle at point B is disturbed by the wave transmitted from point O. So the oscillation of point B is behind the oscillation of point O by a time interval $\frac{x}{c}$, it is just the time required for the wave traveling from point O to pont B. That means, the oscillating displacement of particle at point B at the moment t is equal to the displacement of particle at point O at the moment $(t-\frac{x}{c})$. Hence, the equation for the simple harmonic motion at point B can be written as

$$y = A\cos\omega(t-\frac{x}{c}) \tag{8-18}$$

Point B is selected at random, so Equation (8-18) represents the displacement at any point along the direction of wave transmission and at any time. We call this equation the **equation of a simple harmonic planar wave**, or the **wave equation** for short.

Because

$$\omega = \frac{2\pi}{T} = 2\pi\nu$$

and $cT = \lambda$, therefore, Equation (8-18) can be rewritten as

$$y = A\cos 2\pi(\nu t-\frac{x}{\lambda}) \tag{8-19}$$

or be rewritten as

$$y = A\cos 2\pi(\frac{t}{T}-\frac{x}{\lambda}) \tag{8-20}$$

Now let's discuss the physical significance of the wave equation. The wave equation contains two variables x and t. Here, three cases are discussed respectively as follows.

(1) If x is fixed (i.e., to consider the particle of the medium at this point "x"), then y is only a function of t. That is, the wave equation expresses the oscillating displacement of the particle at a fixed point with a distance of x from the origin O (or wave source) varying with the time t, it also expresses the motion state of the simple harmonic motion of the particle, or, it is the equation of the simple harmonic motion at point "x".

(2) If t is fixed (i.e., a general view of all particles on the wave curve at a given moment of "t"), then the displacement of y will only be the function of position x. The wave equation expresses the distribution of the displacements of particles on the wave curve at a given moment, it describes a waveform at a given moment "t".

(3) If x and t are both variables, then the wave equation expresses the displacements of different particles at different positions of the wave curve during an advancing time t, or more vividly, the wave equation, includes waveforms at different moments, which reflect the wave propagation, as shown in Figure 8-7.

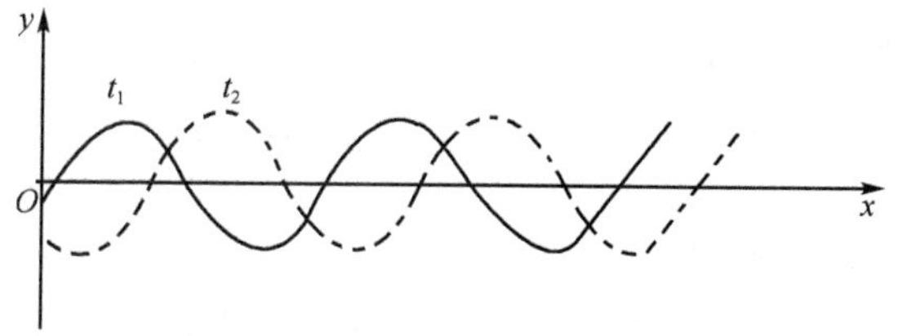

Figure 8-7 The graphs for showing the propagation of a transverse wave

Example 8-3 A simple harmonic wave has the wavelength $\lambda = 1.0$ m, the amplitude of $A = 0.4$ m, and the period of $T = 2.0$ s. (1) Try to write out the corresponding wave equation; (2) determine the equation for the simple harmonic motion of the particle at the point with a distance of $\frac{\lambda}{2}$ from the wave source.

Solution: (1) By substituting the numerical values of the wavelength $\lambda = 1.0$ m, the amplitude $A = 0.4$ m, and the period $T = 2.0$ s in the general wave equation $y = A\cos 2\pi(\frac{t}{T} - \frac{x}{\lambda})$ we have

$$y = 0.4\cos 2\pi(\frac{t}{2} - x)\ (\text{m})$$

(2) By using the equation above, with $x = \frac{\lambda}{2}$, we have the equation of harmonic motion at this point

$$y = 0.4\cos \pi(t-1)\ (\text{m})$$

8.2.3 Energy of Waves

When a wave propagates to somewhere in medium, the originally steady particles begin to oscillate, thus they begin to have kinetic energy. At the same time, the medium will have a deformation, and thus it will have the potential energy. For the wave propagation, the units of the medium oscillate from the near to the distant and one layer after another. Therefore, the energy is gradually transported out. This is one of the most important characteristics of wave motions, too.

The following study is on a planar simple harmonic wave. Supposing a wave is propagating in a medium with the density of ρ. For a volume element $\mathrm{d}V$ in the medium its mass will be $\mathrm{d}m = \rho \cdot \mathrm{d}V$. When the wave travels to it, the volume element obtains a kinetic energy of $\mathrm{d}E_{\mathrm{k}}$. Due to the deformation of the medium the element has the elastic potential energy of $\mathrm{d}E_{\mathrm{p}}$ simultaneously.

The oscillatory kinetic energy of this element is

$$\mathrm{d}E_{\mathrm{k}} = \frac{1}{2}v^2\mathrm{d}m = \frac{1}{2}\rho v^2\mathrm{d}V$$

The velocity v can be obtained from the equation of oscillation (8-18)

$$v = \frac{\partial y}{\partial t} = -A\omega\sin\omega(t - \frac{x}{c}) \tag{8-21}$$

If we substitute Equation (8-21) for the velocity in the expression of the kinetic energy, the kinetic energy of this element can then be expressed as

$$\mathrm{d}E_{\mathrm{k}} = \frac{1}{2}\rho A^2\omega^2\sin^2\omega(t - \frac{x}{c})\mathrm{d}V$$

Here we bypass the proof of $\mathrm{d}E_{\mathrm{k}} = \mathrm{d}E_{\mathrm{p}}$ and use the conclusion of illation directly, we can obtain

$$\mathrm{d}E_{\mathrm{p}} = \frac{1}{2}\rho A^2\omega^2\sin^2\omega(t - \frac{x}{c})\mathrm{d}V$$

so the total energy of this element is

$$\mathrm{d}E = \mathrm{d}E_{\mathrm{k}} + \mathrm{d}E_{\mathrm{p}} = 2\mathrm{d}E_{\mathrm{k}} = \rho A^2\omega^2\sin^2\omega(t - \frac{x}{c})\mathrm{d}V \tag{8-22}$$

Equation (8-22) can be rewritten as

$$w = \frac{\mathrm{d}E}{\mathrm{d}V} = \rho A^2\omega^2\sin^2\omega(t - \frac{x}{c}) \tag{8-23}$$

We call w the **energy density of the wave**, it represents the energy in a unit volume of medium. From the hint in Equation (8-23) we can see that the energy density of a wave is always changing with time. So we usually use the average value over a period of time. Because the mean square value of a sinusoidal function over a period of time is $\frac{1}{2}$, the **average energy density** during a period of time is

$$\overline{w} = \frac{1}{2}\rho A^2 \omega^2 \tag{8-24}$$

This formula is applicable to all simple harmonic planar waves.

From Equation (8-24) we see that, the energy of a mechanical wave is proportional to the square of its frequency and the square of its amplitude, and proportional to the density of medium.

We have already known that, the energy of a wave is transported with the wave propagation in the medium. The energy transported through an area of the medium in a unit time interval is called the **energy flow** through the area. In the medium, assume to take a cross section with the area of S perpendicular to the direction of the wave's propagation (wave speed c), and consider the energy through the area of S in a unit time interval. This quantity must equals to the energy in the volume of cS, as shown in Figure 8-8. Because energy is periodically varying, we usually use the average energy flow, denoted by $\overline{P}$, and its unit is W.

$$\overline{P} = \overline{w}cS$$

where $\overline{w}$ is the average energy density.

The average energy flow transported through a unit area and perpendicular to the direction of wave propagation is called the **energy flux density** or the **intensity of wave** I

i.e.,

$$I = \overline{w}\,c = \frac{1}{2}\rho c A^2 \omega^2 \tag{8-25}$$

here, I is actually a vector, which indicates the direction of energy flux density is the same as the direction of wave speed. The magnitude of I can express the strength of a wave, or the wave's intensity, and its unit is W/m^2.

In acoustics, the intensity of a sound wave referred to **intensity of sound** is an example of the definition above.

In Equation (8-25), $\rho c = Z$ is called the **acoustic resistance of the medium**, it only depends on the properties of the medium. A and ω are respectively the amplitude and the angular frequency of the wave, they depend on the properties of wave source. Equation (8-25) integrates the two necessary and sufficient conditions of constituting a mechanical wave. Here, I is proportional to Z, A^2, and ω^2.

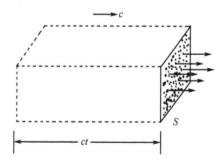

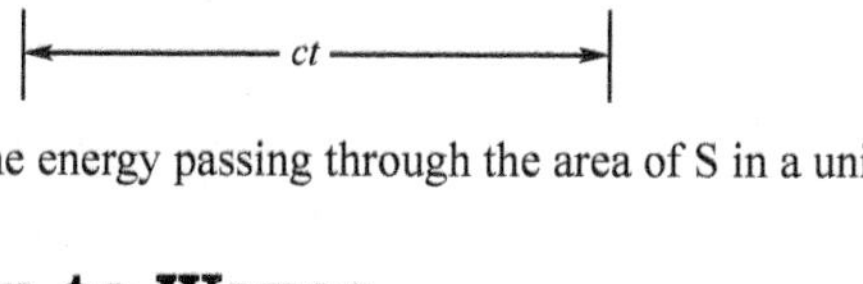

Figure 8-8 The energy passing through the area of S in a unit time interval

8.2.4 Absorption to Waves

In fact, as a planar harmonic wave propagating in a homogeneous medium, the medium will always absorb a portion of the energy. Hence, the intensity of the wave, the amplitude and the wave energy will gradually decrease. The energy absorbed will be converted into other forms of energy (such as the internal energy of the medium). This phenomenon is called the **absorption to the wave**. When the absorption happens, the regularity of attenuation of the planar wave's amplitude can be derived by the following method. Suppose there is a little attenuation of amplitude $-dA$ after the wave penetrates through a thin slice of medium with a thickness of dx. For the amplitude weakened, dA itself is a negative value. The decreased value of amplitude of $-dA$ is proportional to the amplitude of A (the corresponding value when the wave travels onto the thin slice) and also to the slice's thickness of dx, i.e.,

$$-dA = \alpha A dx$$

After the integral operation, we have

$$A = A_0 e^{-\alpha x}$$

where A and A_0 represent respectively the amplitudes at $x = 0$ and $x = x$, and α is a constant, and called the **absorption coefficient** of the medium. The above formula indicates the regularity of the attenuation of the planar waves' amplitudes.

Because the intensity of a wave I is proportional to the square of the amplitude A, we can also get the regularity of the attenuation of a planar wave's intensity, i.e.,

$$I = \frac{1}{2}\rho c A^2 \omega^2 = \frac{1}{2}\rho c A_0^2 e^{-2\alpha x}\omega^2 = I_0 e^{-2\alpha x} \tag{8-26}$$

In Equation (8-26), $I_0 = \frac{1}{2}\rho c A_0^2 \omega^2$ is the wave intensity at $x = 0$, and I is the wave intensity at $x = x$.

Example 8-4 The absorption coefficient of air to the sound wave is $\alpha_1 = 2\times10^{-11}\nu^2\ \mathrm{m}^{-1}$, the absorption coefficient of steel to the sound wave is $\alpha_2 = 4\times10^{-7}\nu\ \mathrm{m}^{-1}$. The quantity ν in the formulae represents the frequency of the sound wave. After penetrating respectively through air and steel, the intensity of an ultrasonic wave with frequency of 5 MHz will be both reduced to 1% of the original value. Determine the thickness of air x_1 and the thickness of steel x_2.

Solution: Using the formulae for the absorption coefficients given in the problem, with frequency ν= 5 MHz, we have the absorption coefficients of air and steel are respectively:

$$\alpha_1 = 2\times10^{-11}\times(5\times10^6)^2 = 500\,\mathrm{m}^{-1}$$

$$\alpha_2 = 4\times10^{-7}\times(5\times10^6) = 2\,\mathrm{m}^{-1}$$

By transforming the formula $I = I_0 e^{-2\alpha x}$, we get the expression of the thickness

$$x = \frac{1}{2\alpha}\ln\frac{I_0}{I}$$

By using the hint of $\frac{I_0}{I} = 100$ and substituting the values of α_1 and α_2 respectively into the expression of the thickness, we get the thickness of air is

$$x_1 = \frac{1}{1000}\ln 100 = 0.046\ \mathrm{m}$$

and the thickness of steel is

$$x_2 = \frac{1}{4}\ln 100 = 1.15\ \mathrm{m}$$

From the above solution we know the fact: For a high-frequency ultrasonic wave, it is hard to penetrate through gases, but easy to penetrate through solids.

8.2.5 Characteristics of Waves

Wave motions, either mechanical waves or electromagnetic waves, have the common characteristics of waves, i.e., they all have the propagation speed and the transportation of energy accompanied with. At the same time, they follow the regularity of the wave's propagation and can generate some phenomena such as reflection, refraction, diffraction, interference and so on.

1. Huygens' Principle

(1) The geometrical description of mechanical waves. The physical conceptions for describing the mechanical waves geometrically are wave rays, wave surfaces, and the wavefront. Figure 8-9 is the graph of showing the relative displacement of each particle from its respective equilibrium position, and showing the scene of each displacement's change with time. As for two-dimensional and three-dimensional waves, it is too difficult to dispaly them in this way. The usual method to describe a wave is to utilize the wave rays, the wave surfaces, and the wavefront. We connect all the homologous crest points together to form a surface and all the homologous trough points together to another surface; or more generally, if we connect all the points of some certain phase of oscillation to a surface, for different phases there will be some different surfaces corresponded in the medium, and these surfaces are called the **surfaces of wave**, shown in Figure 8-9 by the fine real lines. The leading wave surface in the front is called the **wavefront**, which is also called **the wave surfaces**, shown in Figure 8-9 by the outer thick real line. There are also some dotted lines in Figure 8-9, the tangential direction at any point on any dotted line represents the direction of propagation of the wave at this point; these dotted lines are called the **wave rays**, also known as the **wave lines**. The energy of wave is transported in the direction of the wave rays. In an isotropic medium, the wave rays are perpendicular to the wave surfaces.

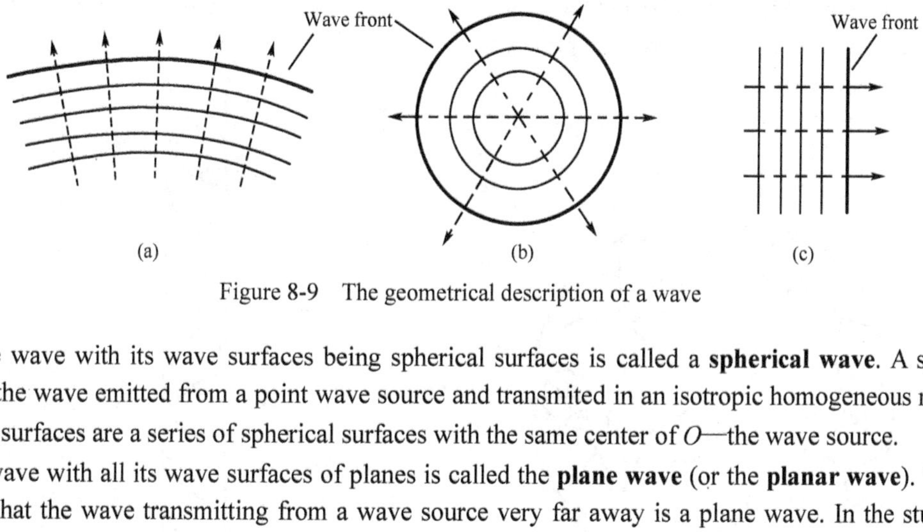

Figure 8-9 The geometrical description of a wave

The wave with its wave surfaces being spherical surfaces is called a **spherical wave**. A spherical wave is the wave emitted from a point wave source and transmited in an isotropic homogeneous medium, its wave surfaces are a series of spherical surfaces with the same center of O—the wave source.

A wave with all its wave surfaces of planes is called the **plane wave** (or the **planar wave**). We may assume that the wave transmitting from a wave source very far away is a plane wave. In the study of a plane wave, what we need is just to study the propagation along the direction of the wave rays. It is similar to the study of one-dimensional wave.

Wave surfaces, wave front and wave rays can lay out a picture of wave propagation vividly.

(2) Huygens' principle. Huygens' Principle tells us the regularity of the direction of the wave's propagation.

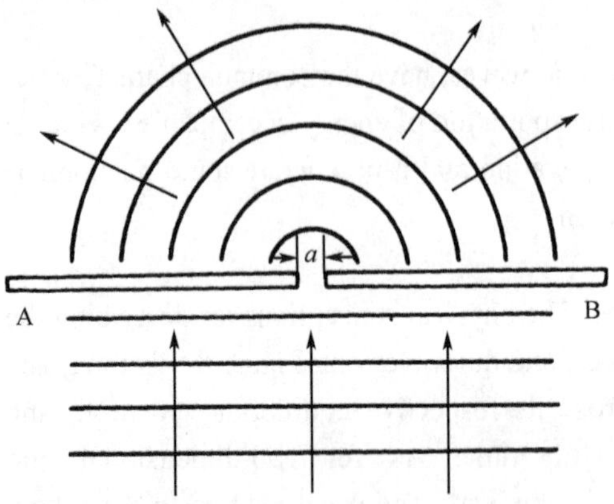

Figure 8-10 A wave passing through a small hole

By the previous discussion we have seen that, the wave is disturbed by the oscillation of the wave source, and the oscillation is spreaded out by the interactions of particles in the medium. In the continuously distributed medium, the oscillation of any particle will directly cause the oscillations of the particles near it. So, in the medium, any oscillating particle at any point can be seen as a new wave source. A wave of arbitrary shape propagating on the water surface is shown in Figure 8-10. If there is no obstacle encountered, the shape of the wavefront will keep on its original form during the wave's propagating process. If the wave encounters with an obstacle AB, which a small hole with the diameter of a is on it, as long as the hole's diameter is extremely small compared to the wavelength, no matter what the original wavefront's shape is, the new wavefront of the wave passed through the small hole will become the circular pattern taking the small hole as the center of it. This has nothing to do with the original waveform. This small hole can be considered as a new wave source, and this new wave source is called **wavelet**.

It was Huygens that summarized the above phenomenon and put forward the following principle in 1690. In the medium, any point that the wave arrives at can be regarded as a new wave source of transmitting the secondary wave (a wavelet). Thereafter, at any moment, the envelope (common tangent surface) of those wavelets "generated" from some certain wavefront is the new wavefront. This is **Huygens' principle**. Figure 8-11(a) and Figure 8-11(b) are respectively the examples of the application of Huygens' principle to spherical wave and plane wave.

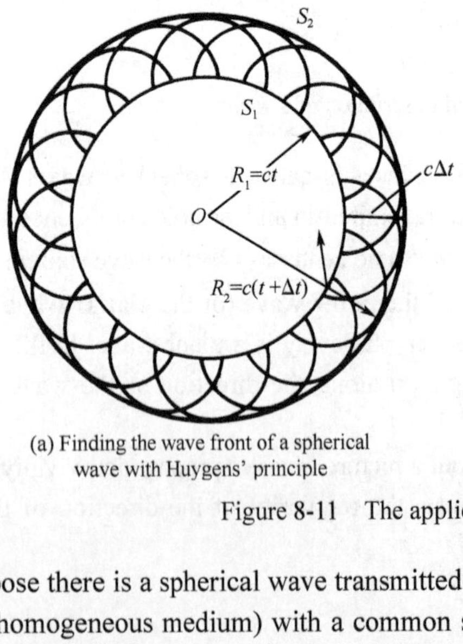

(a) Finding the wave front of a spherical wave with Huygens' principle

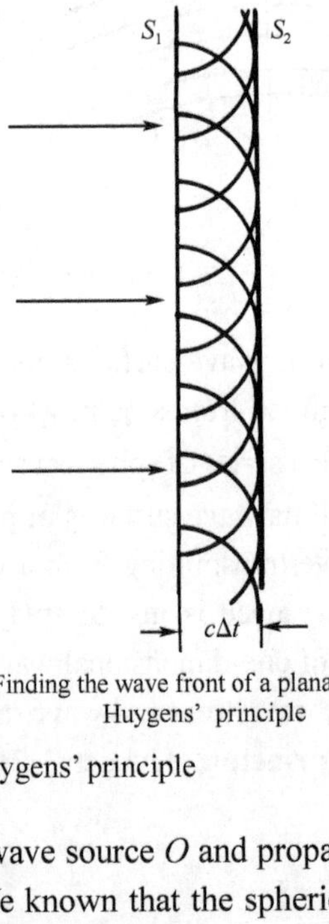

(b) Finding the wave front of a planar wave with Huygens' principle

Figure 8-11 The application of Huygens' principle

Suppose there is a spherical wave transmitted from the wave source O and propagated around (in an isotropic homogeneous medium) with a common speed c. We known that the spherical surface S_1 is the wavefront at the moment t, and its radius $R_1 = ct$, therefore, according to Huygens' principle the wavefront at moment $(t + \Delta t)$ can be determined. We acknowledge that, all the points on surface S_1 can be seen as the new wave sources of secondary wavelets. So we can draw a series of small hemispherical surfaces (as wavelets) with the common radius $r = c\Delta t$; the centers of them are corresponding points on the surface. The common tangent surface or the envelope of these wavelets S_2 is the new wavefront of the wave at the moment $(t + \Delta t)$, as shown in Figure 8-11 (a). The situation we discussed is in isotropic homogeneous medium, so it is clear that S_2 is also a spherical surface with the radius $R_2 = R_1 + c\Delta t$ and the same center O as S_1's. Similarly, if the wavefront of a plane wave is known as S_1 at a certain moment t, according to Huygens' principle, we can also obtain the new wavefront S_2 at a later moment $(t + \Delta t)$, as shown in Figure 8-11 (b).

Huygens' principle is applicable to any waves in propagating: Either the wave is a mechanical wave or electromagnetic wave; either the medium, which the wave transmits through, is uniform or non-uniform. As long as we know the wavefront at a certain moment t, according to this principle, we can determine the wavefront at the next moment $(t + \Delta t)$. By using this geometric method, we can also solve the problems of wave propagations in very broad ranges.

2. Interference of Waves

The phenomenon of interference of waves is one of special characteristics that sound wave possesses uniquely. Because only there is wave synthesis, the phenomenon of interference generates, which is not only significant to the optics and the acoustics, but also plays an important role in the development of the modern physics.

In daily life, we can identify the sound of each instrument when we are listening to a band playing, and also we are able to distinguish each voice if several people speak at the same time. This shows that : ① Each wave has the nature to maintain its original characteristics (frequency, wavelength, direction of vibration, etc.) unchanged, moreover, it keeps on transmitting forward in its original propagating direction and it will never be affected by other waves; ② in the area several waves encountered, the resultant displacement of each particle in the medium is the vector sum of the displacements caused by every wave separately at this point. This is so called **the principle of superposition of waves**. If two wave sources have the same frequency, the same oscillating direction and the same phase or have a fixed difference of initial phase, the two wave sources are called the **coherent wave sources**. The waves transmitted from two coherent wave sources are called **coherent waves**. When two coherent waves meet in space, according to the principle of superposition of waves, there will be some places where the oscillation is always strengthened, while, other places where the oscillation is always diminished or completely offset. This phenomenon is called the **phenomenon of the interference of waves**.

We will have a detailed discussion for the conditions of strengthening and diminishing of coherent waves with the example of lightwave, see Chapter 9 Wave Optics.

3. Diffraction of Wave

When a wave encounters an obstacle in the path it travels, it will change its direction of propagation and bypass the obstacle. This phenomenon is called **the diffraction of wave**. What shown in Figure 8-11 is a diffraction phenomenon, when a wave passes through a small hole. Due to the diameter $a \ll \lambda$, the small hole can be seen as a new wave source transmitting spherical wave, i.e., the wave will be transmitted outer along the radial direction of the spherical surface with the center of the small hole.

A person standing outside can still hear the speaking voice indoor, though there is the block of the wall. This is the result of diffraction of sound waves through the doors or windows. Theory and experiments show that the smaller the diameter or the longer the wavelength is, the more significant the diffraction phenomenon will be.

Wavelength of the sound waves are several meters, so the diffraction phenomenon of sound waves is obvious; the wave length of radio waves are several hundred meters, so the diffraction phenomenon of radio waves is more obvious. Even if there are mountains between the radio station and the receiver, the radio waves can also be received. Ultrasonic waves have very short wavelengths, hence, the diffraction phenomenon of ultrasonic waves is not obvious, and thus we can achieve directional transmissions of ultrasonic waves.

In wave optics, we shall discuss the diffraction phenomenon in more detail.

4. Doppler Effect

In everyday life, when a whistling ambulance is approaching to you, you will feel the higher tone or higher frequency; when the ambulance is passing by and moving away from you, you will feel the change in tone to lower, the frequency becomes lower. Actually, the tone of the ambulance siren does not change at all, but your ear really hears the change of the tone. The phenomenon, in which the received frequency is changed, takes place when the source or the observer moves relatively to the propagation medium. This phenomenon is called the **Doppler effect**.

The Doppler effect is a common feature of all kinds of waves in propagating. Here we only study this phenomenon in the example of sound waves. Generally, the waves can be divided into mechanical waves, electromagnetic waves and etc. The Doppler effect happens not only in the mechanical waves (for example, sound waves), but also in the electromagnetic waves (such as light waves). The formations of the Doppler effect in these two cases follow similar principles, but there are also essential differences existed between them, which lead to the fact that, we need two series of formulae to give descriptions respectively. We know the propagation of a mechanical wave is dependent on the elastic medium. In the discussion of the Doppler effect of a mechanical wave, for both the observer and the wave source, their motion velocities are relative to the medium. The two motions cause the different effects. However, in the discussion of a lightwave, for its propagation does not depend on the elastic medium, as long as there is a relative motion (relative speed v is known) between the light source and the observer, the relative formula of frequency variation caused by the Doppler effect can be determined. That is, we need not to distinguish which one is moving, the light source or the observer; what we need to know is the relative speed between them.

The Doppler effect has its important applications. For example, by the observation of the frequency variation of the electromagnetic wave emitted by a satellite, we can determine the operation situation of the satellite. This is one of the important applications of the Doppler effect in the modern science and technology. In addition, the Doppler effect can also be used to alarm, to inspect the speed of a vehicle. In daily life and scientific observations (for example, astronomical observations), we often encounter the phenomena that the wave source is moving or the observer is moving, or especially, they both moves relatively to the medium. Therefore, the study of the regularity of the Doppler effect and the research to its applications in practice are so significant. The following is the analysis of the phenomenon of the Doppler effect.

For simplicity, supposing the relative motion between the wave source S and the observer B is along the straight line connected them. The speed of the wave source relative to the medium is set to be v_S, the speed of the observer relative to the medium is set to be v_B, and c still represent the speed of the wave propagation in the medium. In addition, they are provided that: ① If the wave source approaches to the observer, v_S is positive; conversely, if the wave source leaves away from the observer, v_S is negative. ② If the observer approaches to the wave source, v_B is positive; contrarily, if the observer goes away from the wave source, v_B takes a negative value. ③ Wave speed c is constantly positive value. The following is our discussion.

(1) Both the wave source and the observer are static with respect to the the medium ($v_S = 0$, $v_B = 0$)

The number of completed oscillations of the wave source within a unit time (the frequency of oscillation) is the frequency of the wave disturbed by the wave source; while, the frequency felt by the observer is the number of the complete waveforms received within a unit time by the observer (by the instrument or by the human ear). Suppose, at a certain moment, the wavefront is just passing by the observer as shown in Figure 8-12 (a) I. After 1 s, this original wavefront will go forward a distance of the value of the wave speed c. Due to the wavelength is λ, so the number of the complete waveforms received by the observer within a unit time is

$$\nu' = \frac{c}{\lambda} = \frac{c}{cT} = \frac{1}{T} = \nu$$

That is, the frequency of the wave received by the observer is just the same as the oscillatory frequency of the wave source.

(2) The wave source is static and the observer is moving with the speed v_B with respect to the the medium ($v_S = 0$, $v_B \neq 0$)

a. The motion of the observer is toward the wave source: In this case $v_B > 0$, within a unit time, the original wavefront at the observer's place will advance a distance of the value of the speed c to the right; while, the observer own will go leftward a distance of the value of the speed v_B; which is equivalent to the fact that: Relatively, this wavefront leaves the observer and goes forward a total distance of $c + v_B$, as shown in Figure 8-12 (b) II. Within a unit time, the number of complete waveforms received by the observer is

$$\nu' = \frac{c+v_B}{\lambda} = \frac{c+v_B}{cT} = \left(\frac{c+v_B}{c}\right)\nu$$

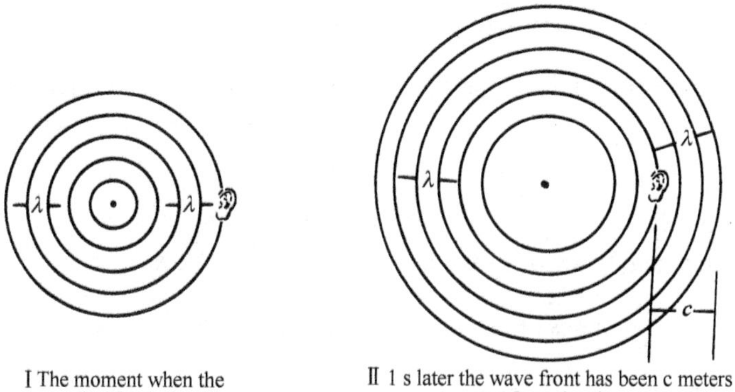

I The moment when the wave front just passes by the observes

II 1 s later the wave front has been c meters away from the observer

(a) Both the wave source and the observer are kept steady

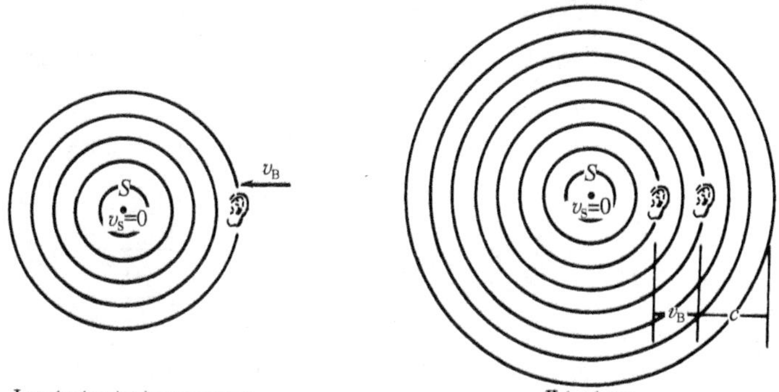

I at the beginning moment

II 1 s later

(b) The wave source is steady while the observer is moving

Figure 8-12 The Doppler effect

This indicates that, if the observer is moving toward the wave source the apparent frequency of the wave received (ν') will be $(\frac{c+\upsilon_B}{c})$ times of the real frequncy of the wave source (ν).

b. The motion of the observer is away from the wave source: In this case, the above formula can still be applied, but this time the speed υ_B is a negative value, thus the apparent frequency received by the observer is reduced. When $\upsilon_B = -c$, $\nu' = 0$. This corresponds to the situation that the observer is moving together with the original wavefront, and can certainly not receive the oscillation.

(3) The observer is static and the wave source is moving with the speed υ_S with respect to the the medium ($\upsilon_S \neq 0$, $\upsilon_B = 0$)

a. The wave source moves toward the observer: In this case, the speed $\upsilon_S > 0$, first, it is assumed that the speed $\upsilon_S < c$, the wave speed c depends only on the nature of the medium and is irrespective to the motion of the wave source, as shown in Figure 8-13. Suppose at some moment the wave source begins to emit a wave at point B. One period T later, the "head of the wave" will reach to the point C. If the wave source does not move, the waveform will be shown as the dotted curve. But in fact, after one period of time T, i.e., when the "wave end" is just emitted, the wave source itself advances to point B′, BB′ = $\upsilon_S \cdot T$. The whole wave is squeezed in the length B′C, as shown in real curve of the waveform. For the wave source is moving with a constant speed, the compression is uniform, the waveform has not distortion. The only thing happened is that the wavelength becomes shorter, and its value is

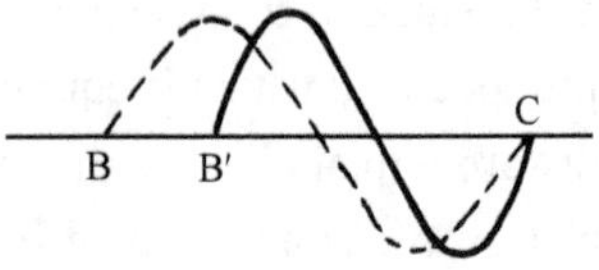

Figure 8-13 The Doppler effect for a moving wave source

$$\lambda' = \overline{B'C} = \lambda - \upsilon_S T = cT - \upsilon_S T = (c - \upsilon_S)\frac{1}{\nu}$$

According to the formula of the relationship among wave speed c, frequency ν and wavelength λ we can get

$$\nu' = \frac{c}{\lambda'} = \frac{c}{c - \upsilon_S}\nu \tag{8-27}$$

This indicates that, when the wave source is moving toward the observer, the apparent frequency felt by the observer is the $\frac{c}{c-\upsilon_S}$ times of the real frequency of the wave source.

b. The wave source moves away from the observer: In this situation the above formula can still be applied, but in the formula the value of υ_S will be a negative. Then $\nu' < \nu$, i.e., the observer feels that the apparent frequency becomes lower than the frequency of the wave source.

The conclusions of ② and ③ show that when either the wave source or the observer moves individually, even if $\upsilon_B = \upsilon_S$, the changed values of the frequency caused by the motions are different. When the wave source is moving relatively to the medium with speed υ_S, and the observer is at rest,

$$\nu' = \frac{c}{c-\upsilon_S}\nu = \frac{1}{1-\frac{\upsilon_S}{c}}\nu = \frac{1+\frac{\upsilon_S}{c}}{1-\frac{\upsilon_S^2}{c^2}}\nu = \frac{\frac{c+\upsilon_S}{c}\nu}{1-\frac{\upsilon_S^2}{c^2}}$$

If υ_S in the above formula is equal to υ_B, it is obviously that, ν' is never equal to the apparent frequency $\frac{c+\upsilon_S}{c}\nu$ felt by the moving observer with the speed $\upsilon_B = \upsilon_S$ while the wave source is at rest.

(4) Both the observer and the wave source move with respect to the medium ($v_S \neq 0$, $v_B \neq 0$)

Colligating the conclusions of ② and③, for the observer is moving with the speed v_B it corresponds to that the wave is moving with the speed of $c + v_B$ respect to the observer; meanwhile, because the motion of the wave source with the speed v_S, the wavelength is shortened with the ratio $\frac{c - v_S}{\nu}$. According to the basic relationship among the wave speed, the frequency and the wavelength, the apparent frequency felt by the observer is

$$\nu' = \frac{c + v_B}{\frac{c - v_S}{\nu}} = \frac{c + v_B}{c - v_S}\nu \tag{8-28}$$

Equation (8-29) includes all the situations discussed above. What we should pay close attention to is the signed provisions of v_B's and v_S's values when we use them. If v_B and v_S is not along the line connected the wave source and observer, the values of v_S and v_B in the above equation will be substituted by the component speeds in the direction of the connection line.

Example 8-5 A train whistles with the frequency of 2000 Hz and runs along the rail at a speed of 25 m/s. What will be the frequencies received by your ear, if (1) the train is moving toward you; (2) the train is moving away from you?

Solution: (1) When the train is moving toward you, $v_S = 25$ m / s, and the speed of sound is always $c = 340$ m/s. Substituting these values into $\nu' = \frac{c}{c - v_S}\nu$, we have

$$\nu' = \frac{340 \times 2000}{340 - 25} = 2159 \text{ Hz}$$

(2) When the train is moving away from you, $v_S = -25$ m/s, substituting it into $\nu' = \frac{c}{c - v_S}\nu$, we have

$$\nu' = \frac{340 \times 2000}{340 - (-25)} = 1863 \text{ Hz}$$

8.3 Sound Waves

8.3.1 Sound Waves

Sound waves (or acoustic waves) are mechanical waves. We have discussed the general regularity of mechanical waves in the previous section, and now we only discuss some of the special problems mentioned in acoustics.

When a propagating mechanical wave travels and comes into your ear, it will cause a corresponding forced oscillation of the eardrum, so as to stimulate the auditory nerve. Then it exerts the feeling of the sound. Thus, we call this kind of waves the **audible sound waves**, or the **sound waves** for short. In fact, only mechanical waves with the frequency band of about 20-20 000 Hz can cause the human's feeling of voice. Any frequency in this band is called the **audio frequency** (or **acoustic frequency**). The mechanical waves with frequencies higher than 20 000 Hz are called ultrasonic waves (or supersonic waves); the mechanical waves with frequencies lower than 20 Hz are called the infrasound waves (the frequency can be as low as 10^{-4} Hz). The waves caused by the earthquake and the tsunami are instances of infrasound waves. Oscillations within the audible frequency band are known as **acoustic oscillations**, the sound wave is the propagation of acoustic oscillations.

Considering the characteristics and functions of sound waves, 20 Hz and 20 000 Hz are not clear dividing lines. For example, high frequency audible sound waves will already have some of the characteristics and functions of the ultrasound waves. In the field of ultrasonic technology, the study of the characteristics and effects of the high frequency audible sound waves is often included, too.

The propagation of acoustic oscillations in the air is relatively important. Therefore, the speed of sound that we often talk about refers mainly to the propagation speed of sound in the air. The propagating speed of the sound waves depends on the nature of the medium and temperature, and is independent on the frequency of the sound waves. Under standard atmospheric pressure and at the temperature of 0℃, the speed of sound waves in the air is about 331 m/s. The higher the temperature is, the quicker the propagation of sound waves will be; while, the lower the temperature is, the slower the propagation of sound waves will be. At room temperature, the speed of sound is about 340 m/s. In the propagating process of sound, just as other waves, the sound waves have the features of the reflection, the refraction, the diffraction, and so on.

8.3.2 Sound Pressure, Sound Intensity and Sound Intensity Level

1. Sound Pressure and Sound Intensity

①**Sound pressure** Let's take the sound waves propagating in the air as an example to discuss the conception of the sound pressure. If there is not any sound wave passing through a range in the medium of air, the steady air pressure at any point is the atmospheric pressure P_0. When an acoustic wave is propagating, the pressures of all points in the air of this range will change, at some points the densities of the air become increased and at some other points the densities become decreased, i.e., in the denser places the pressure is bigger than P_0, while, in the thinner places the pressure will be lower than P_0. At a certain moment and at a certain point, the difference between the pressure of the steady medium and the pressure of the medium disturbed by the sound wave, or the changed amount of the pressure, is called the **instantaneous sound pressure** (or the sound pressure) at the point, denoted by P.

If the wave equation of the sound wave is

$$y = A\sin\omega(t-\frac{x}{c})$$

The sound pressure P at any point in the medium can be proved as

$$P = \rho c\omega A\cos\omega(t-\frac{x}{c}) \tag{8-29}$$

Equation (8-30) is called the equation of sound pressure. Where ρ is the density of the medium, c is the speed of sound; and ω is the angular frequency, A is the amplitude of the acoustic oscillation. If we define

$$P_{\text{m}} = \rho c\omega A \tag{8-30}$$

Then we can rewrite the expression of the sound pressure as

$$P = P_{\text{m}}\cos\omega(t-\frac{x}{c})$$

where P_{m} is called the **amplitude of sound pressure**, also called as the **acoustic amplitude** for short. The common-said sound pressure often refers to the effective sound pressure P_{e}. If the sound pressure varies with the cosine regularity, $P_{\text{e}} = P_{\text{m}}/\sqrt{2}$. The magnitude of the sound pressure corresponds to the strength of the sound waves.

② **Acoustic resistance** We have known that, in the transporting process of electricity in a circuit, there will be the existence of electric resistance, that is, there will be the existence of the energy loss. Similarly, in the propagating process of a sound wave, there will also be the acoustic resistance. We define the ratio of the sound pressure amplitude $P_m = \rho c A\omega$ and the amplitude of velocity $v_m = A\omega$ as the **acoustic resistance** (or the **acoustic impedance**), denoted by Z:

$$Z = \frac{P_m}{v_m} = \frac{\rho c \omega A}{\omega A} = \rho c \tag{8-31}$$

The unit of the acoustic resistance is kg/(m²·s). The acoustic resistance is a physical quantity to express the properties of the media. It affects the propagation of the sound waves severely. Table 8-2 lists several values of the acoustic resistances and the acoustic speeds in some media.

Table 8-2 **Values of the acoustic resistances and the acoustic speeds in several media**

Media	Speeds of sound c (m/s)	Densities ρ (kg/m³)	Acoustic impedances ρc [kg/(m²·s)]
Air	3.32×10^2 (0 ℃)	1.29	4.28×10^2
	3.44×10^2 (20 ℃)	1.21	4.16×10^2
Water	14.8×10^2	988.3	1.48×10^6
Fat	14.0×10^2	970	1.36×10^6
Brain tissue	15.3×10^2	1020	1.56×10^6
Muscle	15.7×10^2	1040	1.63×10^6
Denser bone	36.0×10^2	1700	6.12×10^6
Steel	50.0×10^2	7800	39.4×10^6

③ **Sound intensity** The sound intensity is the energy flux density or the intensity of a sound wave I, i.e., the average energy transported through a unit area perpendicular to the direction of the sound wave's propagation in a unit time interval. Equation (8-25) shows the sound intensity:

$$I = \frac{1}{2}\rho c A^2 \omega^2 \tag{8-32}$$

By Equation (8-30) and Equation (8-33), we can see that, if a sound wave has a higher frequency it will have the higher sound pressure and stronger sound intensity.

2. Sound Intensity Level

The audible sound waves have not only a certain range of frequency, but also have a certain range of the sound intensity. Both of the two ranges have the upper and lower extreme values. If the sound intensity is below the lower limit, it can not cause the sense of hearing; and if it is higher than the upper limit, it can only cause sense of pain.

It can be seen from the Figure 8-14 that if the sound frequency is 1000 Hz, the strongest sound intensity which can be heard by a normal person's sense of hearing is 1 W/m², and the minimum sound intensity can be heard is 10^{-12} W/m². Generally, this lowest sound intensity is defined as the standard of measurement of sound intensity, represented by I_0. Since there is a great disparity in the order of magnitude of the difference between the highest and the lowest sound intensities, a logarithmic scale is commonly used to describe the intensity extent of the sound waves. When the sound intensity of an sound wave is I, the common logarithm of the ratio of I to I_0 — the value of L— is a new scale to measure the intensity extent of the sound wave, i.e.,

$$L = \lg\frac{I}{I_0} \tag{8-33}$$

where L is called the **sound intensity level**, the unit of it is **bel**. In the practical application this unit bel is too large, so a conventional unit of 1/10 bel is usually used. This unit is known as **decibel** (dB). To take decibel as the unit, we should rewrite the above equation as

$$L = 10\lg\frac{I}{I_0} \quad \text{(dB)} \tag{8-34}$$

Table 8-3 lists the sound intensities and the sound intensity levels of several common sound waves.

Table 8-3 Sound intensities and sound intensity levels of several common sound waves

Types of sound	Sound intensities I (W/m^2)	Sound intensity levels (dB)
Sound of normal breath	10^{-11}	10
Sound of a clock	10^{-10}	20
Whispering	10^{-8}	40
Talking loudly	10^{-4}	80
Sound of a plane engine(5 m away)	10^{0}	120
Sound could result in deafness	10^{4}	160

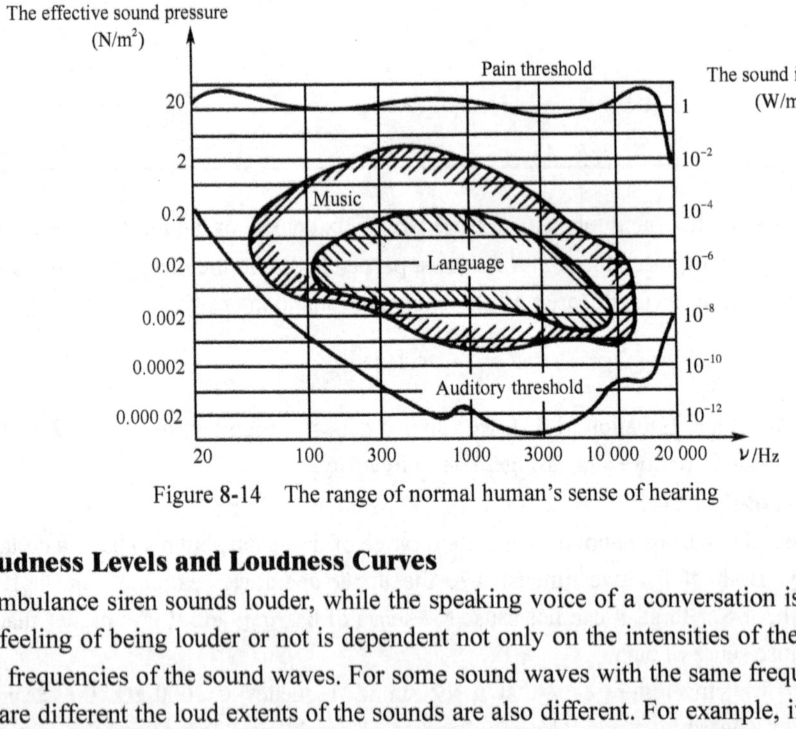

Figure 8-14 The range of normal human's sense of hearing

3. Loudness Levels and Loudness Curves

The ambulance siren sounds louder, while the speaking voice of a conversation is not so loud. This subjective feeling of being louder or not is dependent not only on the intensities of the sound waves, but also on the frequencies of the sound waves. For some sound waves with the same frequency, if the sound intensities are different the loud extents of the sounds are also different. For example, if two sound waves have the same frequency, the sound of 30 dB feels louder than the sound of 10 dB according to the feeling of the human ear. For some sound waves with the same sound intensity, if the frequencies of the sound waves are different, the sounds are felt different in the loud extent. For example, if two sound waves have the same sound intensity, the sound with the frequency of 1000 Hz feels louder than the sound with the frequency of 400 Hz according to the human ear hearing. The subjective loudness (the loud extent) of a sound is dependent not only on the sound intensity but also the frequency of the sound wave. In order to determine the degree of loudness of a sound, we shall compare this sound with a standard sound (usually, take the pure tone of 1000 Hz as the standard). To adjust the sound intensity level of the pure tone of 1000 Hz, till it feels as loud as the sound of being studied, here, this sound intensity level of the pure tone of 1000 Hz is defined as the **loudness level of the sound**. The unit of loudness level is phon. For example, a sound of 100 Hz and 49 dB feels as loud as the sound of 1000 Hz and 20 dB, so we can say that, the loudness level of the sound of 100 Hz and 49 dB is 20 phon.

By the defination of the loudness level, it is clear that, for the sound of 1000 Hz, its sound intensity level (in dB) is numerically the value of its loudness level (in phon); for a sound with the frequency of not 1000 Hz, its sound intensity level and its loudness level are numerically different. As shown in Figure 8-15, we can draw a series of curves each of them connects the points which correspond to the sounds with the same loudness level but the different sound frequencies, these curves are called the **loudness curves**.

For a sound with a certain frequency, it can not be heard by human ear until the sound intensity reaches to a specific value. So there will be a lowest value of the sound intensity level. If the sound intensity level is not lower than this value the sound can cause a sense of hearing. This weakest sound intensity is called the **threshold of hearing** to this frequency. The sounds with different frequencies have different thresholds of hearing. All thresholds of hearing in different frequencies correspond to the same loudness level of zero phon. The curve connecting the points of the loudness level of zero on different frequencies is called the zero loudness level curve or auditory threshold curve. In general, the sound with the loudness level below this curve can not be heard by human ear.

For a sound with a certain frequency, as the sound intensity becomes stronger, the loudness of the sound felt by human ear becomes bigger as well. If the sound intensity becomes strong enough, and reaches to a certain value, the sound will cause the sense of pain inside human ear. This value is called the **pain threshold**. The curve connecting the pain threshold points of different frequencies is called the **pain threshold curve**.

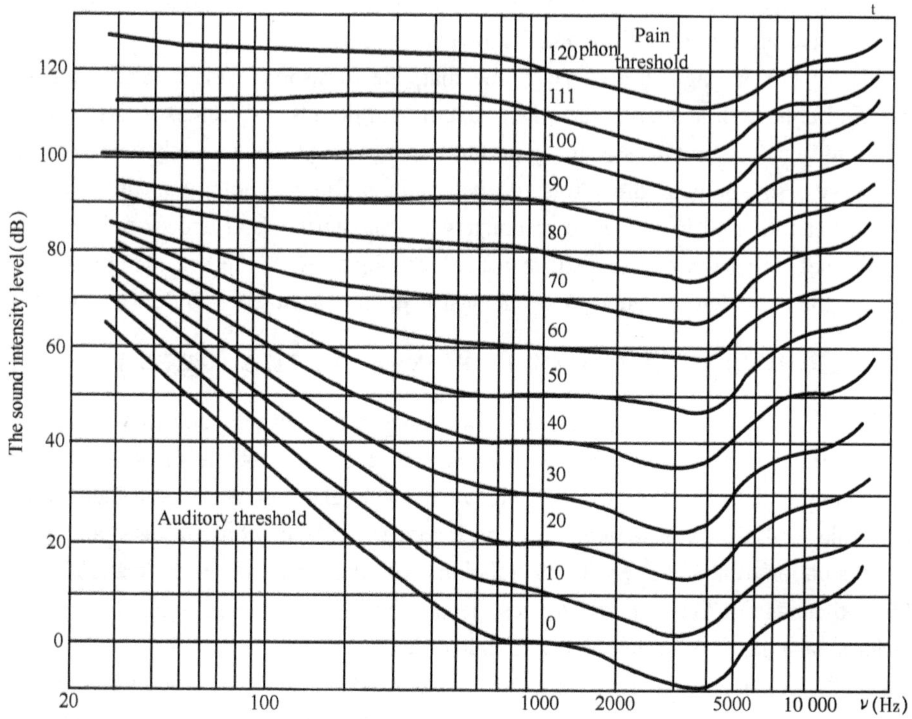

Figure 8-15 Loudness curves

Example 8-6 The noise generated by one running motor has the sound intensity of 10^{-7} W/m^2. Determine (1) the sound intensity level of the noise in decibels, when one motor is running; (2) the sound intensity level of the noise in decibels if two same motors are running simultaneously.

Solution: By applying Equation (8-35) $L = 10\lg\frac{I}{I_0}$ and $I_0 = 10^{-12}\,\text{W/m}^2$ we can get:

(1) $$L_1 = 10\lg\frac{I}{I_0} = 10\lg\frac{10^{-7}}{10^{-12}} = 50\ (\text{dB})$$

(2) $$L_2 = 10\lg\frac{2I}{I_0} = 10\lg 2 + 10\lg\frac{10^{-7}}{10^{-12}} = 53\ (\text{dB})$$

From the result of the above calculation, it can be seen that if the sound intensity increases twice, the increment of sound intensity level is only approximately the value of 3 dB.

8.4 Ultrasonic Waves and Infrasound Waves

8.4.1 Natures of Ultrasonic Waves

The mechanical waves with frequencies higher than 20000 Hz, which can not be heard by human ear, is called **ultrasonic waves** (or **supersonic waves**). For ultrasonic waves, besides the general natures of the mechanical waves, there are some particular properties.

(1) Good Directionality: Due to the shorter wave lengths, the diffraction phenomenon of ultrasonic waves is not significant, so their propagations are directive and along straight lines approximately. Like a beam of light, a beam of ultrasonic wave is easy-to-focus, and can be used as a directional transmission.

(2) Strong Intensity: Because the sound intensity is proportional to the square of the frequency, the ultrasonic waves have stronger intensities and the greater powers.

(3) Wonderful Penetrating Ability: We know that, the ultrasonic waves will be attenuated very greatly in the air, but have little attenuation when travelling in liquids and solids. So they can penetrate to certain depths within media, and have a strong penetrating ability, which is exactly contrary to the feature of the radio waves, so applying the ultrasonic waves in ocean technology is the most convenient. Ultrasonic waves can be used in oceans to reconnaissance submarines and underwater reefs, to measure the depth of the sea, to survey the seabed, to map the topography of the sea bottom, and to look for schools of fish in the ocean, etc. These have been constructed into a subject—underwater acoustics.

8.4.2 Effects of Ultrasonic Waves on the Matters

The propagating characteristics of an ultrasonic wave in a medium, such as velocity, attenuation, absorption, etc., are closely related with the macroscopic and non-acoustic physical quantities of the medium. For example, the velocities of ultrasonic waves have relations with the elastic modulus and the densities of media, and also with temperature, the ingredient compositions of gases and other relevant factors. The attenuation of sound intensity has relations with the void ratio of the material, viscosity and so on. Taking advantage of these characteristics, people have manufactured various kinds of ultrasonic instruments for measuring the correlative physics quantities.

In essence, the propagating characteristics of ultrasonic waves depend on the molecular properties of the media. Sound speed, absorption, the energy of the molecules, and molecular structures, etc., are closely related. It is convenient to measure ultrasonic waves, a lot of experimental data can be obtained, so in the productive practice and scientific research, many special effects of ultrasonic waves on materials have been found, and these special effects have got their wide applications.

The following is the introduction to three main characteristics of ultrasonic waves, i.e., mechanical effect, cavitation and thermal effect.

1. Mechanical Effect

When a beam of high-frequency ultrasonic wave propagates in a medium, the particles of the medium will undergo the forced oscillations with the same high frequency. If the power is strong enough, the mechanical structure of the medium will be damaged. This means the high-frequency ultrasonic waves have the ability of splitting, so they are often used for crushing, cutting, drilling, cleaning, and agglomerating.

2. Cavitation

When a beam of high-frequency ultrasonic wave with stronger power propagates in a liquid medium, it will cause the variation liquid denseness. In the areas with denser the medium is compressed; in the sparse areas the medium is extended. Since the liquid media have such weak anti-tensile ability, at some spots (especially where the liquid media containing impurities and bubbles) the liquid will be pulled off to form tiny cavities; well, the following positive sound pressure will generate the local high temperature, high pressure and discharging phenomenon at the moment of the cavities' closing. This effect is called cavitation. The cavitation effect of the ultrasonic wave is commonly used in cleaning, spraying, emulsifying, promoting chemical reactions, and so on. For example, if a chemical reaction can not occur under the situation of normal temperature and pressure, in the role of cavitation effect the reaction may often proceed. Another example is that: Mercury can be broken up into tiny particles, and can be evenly mixed together with water to form emulsion under the action of cavitation effect. In medicine, the cavitation effect can be used to mash drugs into various medicaments; the cavitation effect can also be used in food industry to produce various kinds of sauces. In the construction industry the cavitation effect can be used to process cement emulsion and other materials.

3. Thermal Effect

Thermal effect refers to the phenomenon that when a beam of ultrasonic wave acting on a material, its energy is partly absorbed by the material, so the material's temperature will become higher.

The absorption of ultrasonic wave can cause the rise of the medium's temperature. On the one hand, the higher of the frequency is, the more obvious of the effect will be; on the other hand, on the interface between two different media, especially on the interface between a fluid medium and a solid medium, or on the interface between a fluid medium and the suspended particles, a lot of ultrasonic waves energy will be converted into heat energy to cause the local higher temperature, and even to cause the ionization effect on the interface. Thermal effect has also many important applications.

The above three kinds of effects are the most basic functions of ultrasonic waves. In addition, ultrasonic waves have many other effects (such as the chemical effects, biological effects and so on).

8.4.3 Generation of Ultrasonic Waves

Ultrasonic frequencies (higher than 20000Hz) are much higher than the frequencies of normal sound (acoustic frequencies: 20–20 000Hz), so unlike the methods of generating audio vibrations, the methods to generate the ultrasonic waves are different. Even though there are many methods to generate ultrasonic waves, the current ultrasonic generators used in medical ultrasonic diagnostics, are mainly manufactured according to the principles of the piezoelectric effect. The piezoelectric effects include the positive piezoelectric effect and the inverse piezoelectric effect. The positive piezoelectric effect refers to the following phenomenon: If there is a compressing force applied in a certain direction of some crystals, as the compressed deformation occurs, there will be positive charges on the upper surface and negative charges on the undersurface, as shown in Figure 8-16 (a); if there is a stretching force in this direction, as the crystal's stretched deformation occurs, there will be negative charges on the upper surface and positive charges on the undersurface, as shown in Figure 8-16 (b). This means that if the compression and the stretch are applied in a certain direction of some crystal, the crystal's opposite surfaces will have converse charges. This phenomenon is known as the **piezoelectric effect** in physics. The crystal with the piezoelectric effect is called a **piezoelectric crystal**. If converse charges are put on the piezoelectric crystal's opposite surfaces (or an electric potential difference is acted on the direction), the crystal will have a compressed or stretched deformation in the corresponding direction. This phenomenon is called the **inverse piezoelectric effect**. If a high frequency (ultrasonic frequency) alternating voltage is put on a crystal with this character, the crystal will have a corresponding high-frequency mechanical oscillation and emit an ultrasonic wave.

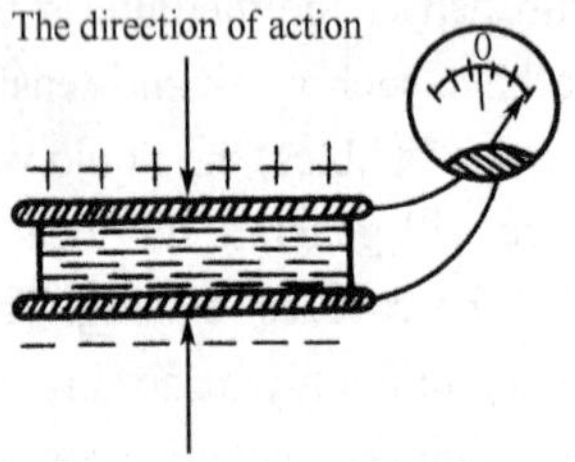

(a) When the crastal is compressed there are charges on the opposite surfaces

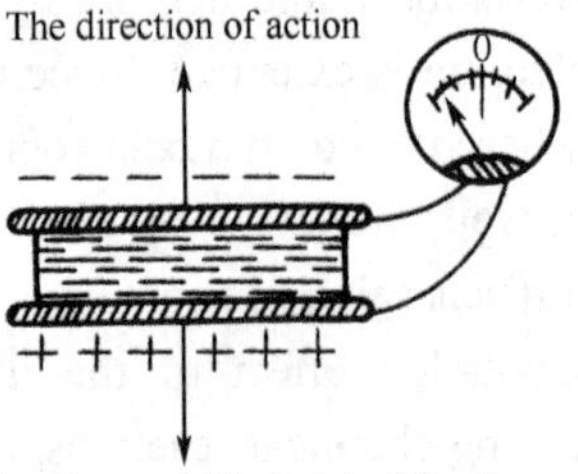

(b) When the crastal is stretched the charges on the corresponding surfaces are conversed

Figure 8-16 The principle of piezoelectric effect

In the probe of a common ultrasonic diagnostic apparatus, the main element is a piece of piezoelectric crystal. During operating, because of the inverse piezoelectric effect, the crystal piece is activated to generate ultrasonic oscillations, i.e., to convert electrical energy into mechanical energy. Due to the positive piezoelectric effect, the ultrasonic oscillation reflected back from the human body's organs will act on the crystal piece to generate a high-frequency alternating voltage on it, i.e., the mechanical energy is converted to electrical energy. Therefore, the ultrasonic probes are a kind of transducers. Nowadays, the commonly used crystal pieces in this kind of transducers are made of artificial or natural crystals such as lead zirconate, titanate barium, quartz, lithium sulfate, and so on.

8.4.4 Applications of Ultrasonic Waves in Medicine

There are fairly extensive applications of ultrasonic waves in medical treatment and diagnosis. In the recent years, there are reports of applications of ultrasonic waves in the treatments of diseases such as hemiplegia, facial paralysis, polio sequelae, mastitis, breast hyperplasia, and hematoma etc. Meanwhile, as a non-invasive and non-incursive diagnostic method, ultrasonic diagnostics is widely used in clinical examinations. In this section we shall only discuss the A-type, B-type, M-type, D-type ultrasonic diagnostic apparatus. These apparatus are designed upon the principles of reflection or on the physics laws. With various scanning methods, they can transmit ultrasonic waves into the human bodies and let ultrasonic waves spread within the organs. If there is a difference of acoustic resistance between normal tissue and pathological tissue, the ultrasonic wave will reflect and scatter from the corresponding interface, therefore, there will be echo signals received. Then, the echo signals will be treated and displayed as waveforms, curves or an image. According to the characteristics of different echoes, and combining with physiology, pathology, and anatomy knowledge in clinical analysis, doctors can make judgments to the locations and natures of patients' pathological changes.

1. A-type Ultrasonic Diagnostic Apparatus

Before examination a layer of acoustic coupling agent such as liquid paraffin should be applied between the probe and the skin to prevent the spacing, which will affect the intensity of ultrasonic wave transmitting into the body. For the acoustic resistances of different tissues and organs are different, so that, the different reflected waves are formed from the interfaces, and these waves are called echoes. Figure 8-17 is the working principle diagram of the A-type ultrasonic diagnostic apparatus. When the ultrasonic generator (U) is running there will be a beam of ultrasonic wave transmitting into the body, on any interface encountered a portion of ultrasonic wave will be reflected. The reflected waves can be received by the same probe (T), and transformed into electric signals then treated and displayed on the screen of the diagnostic apparatus as output echo pulses. On the displaying screen, the horizontal axis represents the distance (depth) of the different tissue interface away from the skin, and the vertical axis represents the intensity of corresponding echo pulse.

The diagram of echo pulses in Figure 8-17 (a) represents the normal tissue; the diagram in Figure 8-17 (b) represents the situation of a pathological tissue. Here, echo pulse "*i*" represents to the reflected wave when the ultrasonic wave reached the pathological tissue and echo pulse "*o*" represents to the reflected wave when the ultrasonic wave penetrated out the pathological tissue. By analyzing the waveform in Figure 8-17 (b), doctors can determine the location, size and nature of the pathological tissue or the foreign body appeared in the organ. Figure 8-18 (a) and Figure 8-18(b) are the echo diagrams of detecting a brain tumor with A-type diagnostic apparatus.

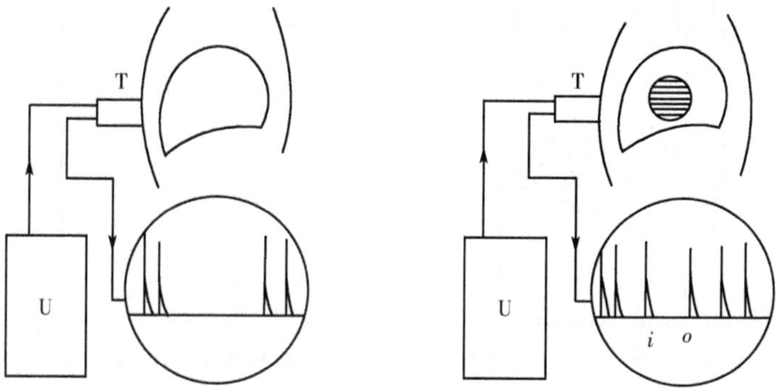

(a) (b)

Figure 8-17 The working principle of an A-type ultrasonic diagnostic apparatus

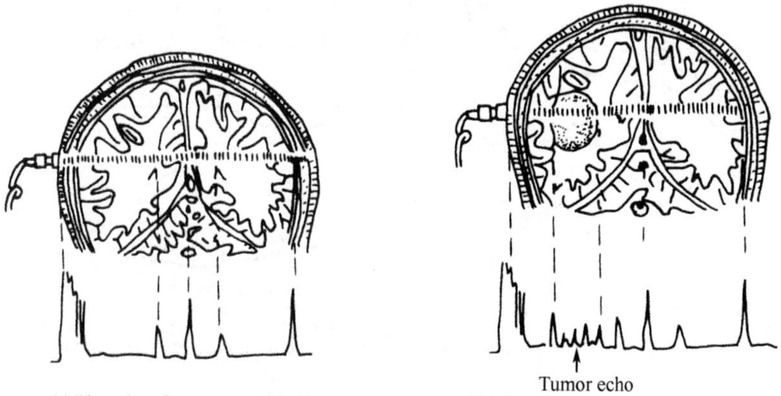

(a) The echos from a normal brain (b) The echos from a brain with a tumor

Figure 8-18 The echo pulses of brains

2. B-type Ultrasonic Diagnostic Apparatus

B-type ultrasonic diagnostic apparatus work on the principles similar to A-type ultrasonic apparatus'. The only main difference is that, in B-type ultrasonic diagnostic apparatus the display manner of amplitude modulation (used in A-type ultrasonic diagnostic apparatus) is improved as display of luminance modulation. That is, the stronger the echo is, the brighter the light element will be; and the weaker the echo, the dimmer the light element. If there isn't any echo the corresponding area will be fully dark. According to the characters of the echoes, doctors can observe the interfaces of various organs, tissues and the situations of the organs. The images displayed by B-type ultrasonic diagnostic apparatus are two-dimensional images of the site probed, they are more appropriate for examining the lesions in different parts of the body. Since B-type ultrasonic diagnostic apparatus can choose the site probed within a certain range, and have the function of displaying the continuously moving organs, so the echo images displayed by them are relatively close to the entity slice images seen visually. Therefore, it is easier for B-type ultrasonic diagnostic apparatus to be popularized than other types of ultrasonic diagnostic apparatus. Figure 8-19 is a diagram of B-type ultrasonic diagnostic apparatus. principle.

3. M-type Ultrasonic Diagnostic Apparatus (or Echocardiography Instrument)

M-type ultrasonic diagnostic apparatus are generally used for the diagnosis of cardiovascular diseases, so they are often called the echocardiographic instrument.

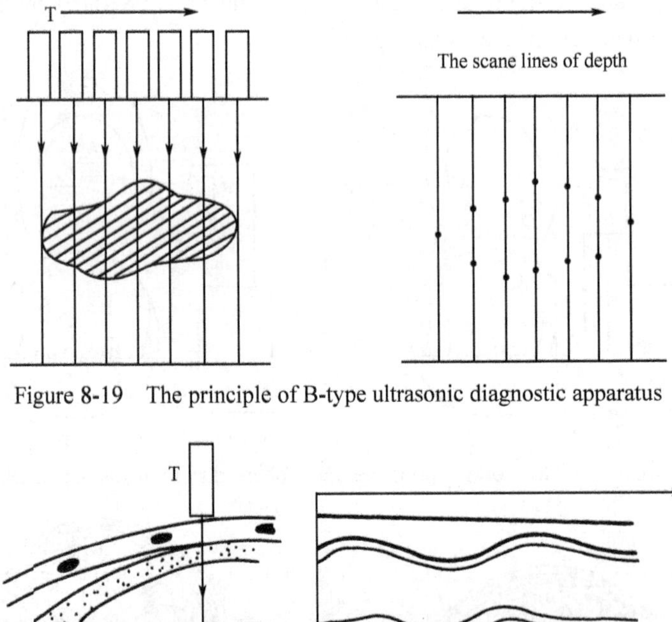

Figure 8-19 The principle of B-type ultrasonic diagnostic apparatus

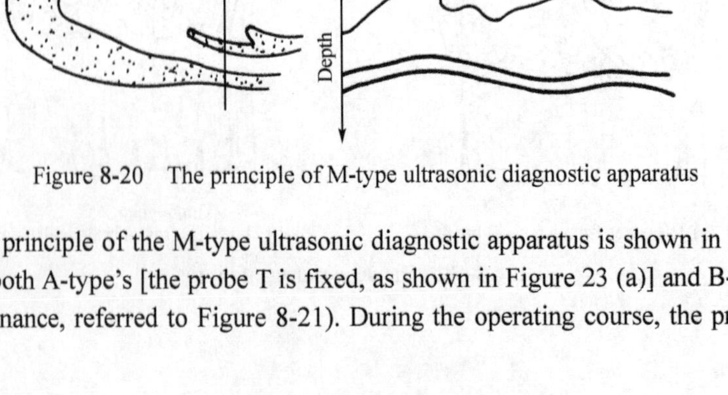

Figure 8-20 The principle of M-type ultrasonic diagnostic apparatus

The working principle of the M-type ultrasonic diagnostic apparatus is shown in Figure 8-20. It has the characters of both A-type's [the probe T is fixed, as shown in Figure 23 (a)] and B-type's (the echo is displayed by luminance, referred to Figure 8-21). During the operating course, the probe is at a certain position in front of the heart, as the heart beating regularly, a series of light elements moving up and down with the heart beat will be shown on the screen. As the scan line moving from left to right, these light elements are spreaded horizontally and an active state curve, which represents the structure of cardiac tissue layers during a beating period, will emerge. This is called echocardiography, and particularly suitable for the examination of heart function.

4. D-type Ultrasonic Diagnostic Apparatus (or Imaging Instrument)

The principle of the Doppler ultrasonic blood flow meter is based on Doppler Effect. This kind of instrument is widely used in clinical practice and mainly applied in the measurement of velocities of moving objects or fluids in vivo. Figure 8-21 shows the schematic principle of Doppler ultrasonic blood flow meter. It is a popular kind of D-type ultrasonic diagnostic apparatus.

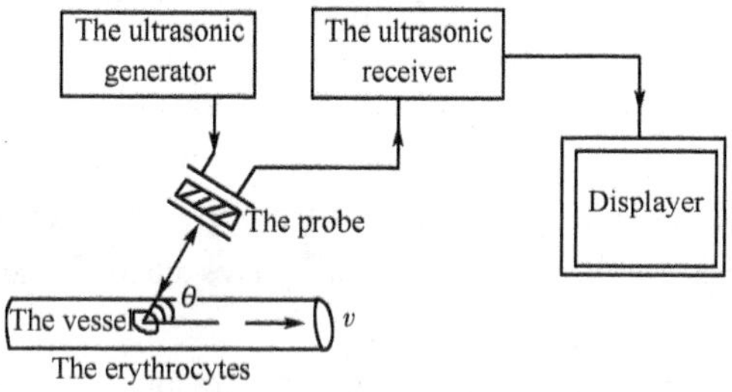

Figure 8-21 The principle of Doppler ultrasonic blood flow meter

When a beam of ultrasonic wave emitted by the probe meets the erythrocytes in the vessel it will be reflected. According to the Doppler effect, here, the ultrasonic generator is looked as the wave source, and the erythrocytes as observers moving with the speed υ, so the frequency received by the erythrocytes is different from the frequency of the ultrasonic generator ν. When this ultrasonic wave is reflected by the erythrocytes and received by the ultrasonic receiver (the probe), every erythrocyte is looked as a wave source in moving and the ultrasonic receiver as the observer keeping static. In this way, the frequency received by the ultrasonic receiver will change again. The calculation results show that the difference of the frequency received by the receiver and the frequency emitted from the ultrasonic generator $\Delta\nu$ and the blood flow speed υ have the following relationship

$$\upsilon = \frac{c}{2\nu\cos\theta}\Delta\nu \tag{8-35}$$

Where c is the propagation speed of the ultrasonic wave in the tissue, θ is the angle between the direction of the propagating wave and the direction of blood flow, and ν is the frequency of the ultrasonic wave emitted from ultrasonic generators.

Color Doppler flow imaging instrument is also called "color-ultrasonography". The principle of the instrument is by using of a high-speed phase-control array of scanning probes to get a plane scan. It belongs to a real-time two-dimensional blood flow imaging technology, which can show the anatomy configuration, size and the structure of the object and show the state of blood flow simultaneously. This provides an advanced kind of diagnostic apparatus for clinical application.

Ultrasonic waves can be applied not only for medical diagnosis but also for medical treatment. When the ultrasonic waves penetrate into the organismal tissue, the acoustic energy will convert to heat energy, i.e., the ultrasonic energy is absorbed by the tissue and results in the temperature of the tissue becoming higher. Meanwhile, the high frequency vibrations of ultrasonic waves will provide a special "massaging" function to the local tissue. Ultrasonic waves have a certain curative effect when they are applied to treat certain diseases such as arthritis, neuralgia, and so on.

8.4.5 Infrasound Waves

Infrasound waves, also known as sub-sonic waves, generally refer to the mechanical waves with the frequencies in the range of 10^{-4}-20 Hz. Volcanic eruptions, earthquakes, meteorites impinging against land, atmospheric turbulence, thunderstorms and other natural activities will accompany with infrasound waves. Because the frequencies of the infrasound waves are so low that the attenuation of the intensity is very limited. Comparing with the absorption to the sound waves, the absorbed energy of infrasound waves by the atmosphere is very little. For an infrasound wave, after having propagated in the atmosphere for millions meters, the absorption to it may be less than one thousandth of a decibel. For example, in 1883, the infrasound waves caused by a volcanic eruption located between Java and Sumatra traveled three circles around the earth, and lasted for 108 hours. The propagating speed of the infrasound waves is the same as the sound waves'.

With the development on various instruments to detect infrasound waves, the detection of infrasound waves has become a powerful tool to study the large-scale movement of the earth, the oceans, and the atmosphere. Researches on the generation, the transmission, the reception and application of infrasound waves and other aspects of researching on infrasound waves have founded a new branch of modern acoustics i.e., infrasonics.

Infrasound waves also affect on creatures. Intensive infrasound waves with some frequencies can cause fatigue and pain, and even result in blindness. It has been reported that intensive infrasound waves occured on the ocean may cause the seafarers suffering from the abnormally terrified feelings and disembarking hastily, and eventually, lead to the persons' disappearance. For these reasons, the institutions to forecast infrasound waves have been established in some countries.

A Brief Summarization of This Chapter

(1) The definition of a simple harmonic motion.

1) The motion of an object is under an elastic force or a quasi-elastic force i.e., to meet: $f=-ky$

2) Or to meet the differential equation of simple harmonic motion: $m\dfrac{\mathrm{d}^2 y}{\mathrm{d}t^2}=-ky$

3) Or to meet the the equation of simple harmonic motion: $y = A\cos(\omega t+\phi)$

(2) The three elements of the simple harmonic motion: Amplitude A, period T (frequency ν, angular frequency ω) and the phase $(\omega t+\phi)$;

1) The relationship between the angular frequency, frequency and period

$$\omega=\frac{2\pi}{T}=2\pi\nu$$

2) For a spring oscillator, its angular frequency

$$\omega=\sqrt{\frac{k}{m}}$$

3) The phase $(\omega t+\phi)$ determines the state of motion of an oscillating object at the moment t, the initial phase ϕ determines the state of motion of the vibration of the object at the initial moment $t = 0$.

(3) The total energy of a simple harmonic motion system is the sum of its kinetic energy and potential energy,

$$E=E_{\mathrm{k}}+E_{\mathrm{p}}=\frac{1}{2}kA^2$$

(4) The resultant motion of two simple harmonic motions in the same direction and with the same frequency is still a simple harmonic motion. The frequency of the resultant motion are exactly the same as the two component oscillations'. The resultant oscillation's amplitude and initial phase can be expressed respectively by:

$$A = \sqrt{A_1^2 + A_2^2 + 2A_1 A_2 \cos(\phi_2 - \phi_1)}$$

and

$$\phi = \arctan \frac{A_1 \sin \phi_1 + A_2 \sin \phi_2}{A_1 \cos \phi_1 + A_2 \cos \phi_2}$$

When the phase difference $\phi_2 - \phi_1 = 2k\pi,\ k = 0, \pm 1, \pm 2, \cdots$, the resultant oscillation's amplitude is the largest, $A_{max} = A_1 + A_2$;

When the phase difference $\phi_2 - \phi_1 = (2k+1)\pi,\ k = 0, \pm 1, \pm 2, \cdots$, the resultant oscillation's amplitude is the smallest, $A_{min} = |A_2 - A_1|$;

(5) Several physical quantities to describe a wave: The wavelength λ, the period T, the frequency ν, and the speed c of the wave, the relationship among them is

$$\lambda = cT = \frac{c}{\nu}$$

(6) The expression for a plane harmonic wave, i.e. the wave equation

$$y = A\cos\omega\left(t - \frac{x}{c}\right) \quad \text{or} \quad y = A\cos 2\pi\left(\nu t - \frac{x}{\lambda}\right) = A\cos 2\pi\left(\frac{t}{T} - \frac{x}{\lambda}\right)$$

where the displacement y is a dual function of the coordinates x and time t, this expression represents the displacement of the particle at any point x on the wave line and at any moment t, i.e., it means the propagation of the waveform.

(7) The average energy density of a wave is: $\overline{w} = \frac{1}{2}\rho\omega^2 A^2$

(8) The intensity of a wave or a sound wave is: $I = \frac{1}{2}\rho c\omega^2 A^2$

(9) Doppler Effect: When the wave source or the observer is moving with respect to the medium, the frequency received by the observer will change. This phenomenon is called Doppler Effect.

(10) The sound intensity level: $L = 10\lg\frac{I}{I_0}$ (dB), where $I_0 = 10^{-12}\ \text{W/m}^2$.

Exercises 8

8-1. There is a simple harmonic oscillation with the amplitude of A. Determine the distance that the oscillating particle traveled during a period of time.

8-2. An object is performing a simple harmonic motion, the equation of the motion is $y = 0.12\cos(\pi t - \frac{\pi}{3})$ (m).

Determine:

(1) The vibration amplitude, the frequency, the period and the initial phase;

(2) The position, the velocity and acceleration of the object when $t = 0.5$ s.

8-3. For a spring oscillator with the mass of $m = 0.64$ kg and the coefficient of stiffness $k = 100$ N/m, when $t = 0$, $y_0 = 0.10$ m, $\upsilon_0 = -1.25\sqrt{3}$ m/s. Try to determine:

(1) The angular frequency ω and period T;

(2) The amplitude A and the initial phase, and write the equation of this oscillation;

(3) The displacement, velocity, acceleration and the elastic force f acting on it when $t = \frac{6}{25}\pi$ s.

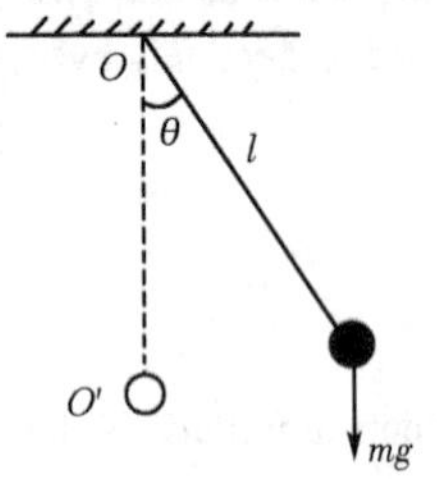

Figure for Exercise 8-5

8-4. An object is performing a simple harmonic motion along the y-axis as shown in Figure 8-1. The amplitude is 0.12 m and the period is 2s; when t = 0, the displacement of the object is 0.06 m, and it moves toward the positive direction of the y-axis. Determine the initial phase of this simple harmonic motion.

8-5. As shown in Figure 8-5, an even rod with the length of l and the mass of m is hanging on a horizontal axis O at one end, so that, the rod can swing freely in the in vertical plane. When the swing is very slight, try to prove that the motion of the rod is a simple harmonic motion, and find its period.

8-6. The equations of two simple harmonic motions in the same direction and with the same frequency are respectively $y_1 = 3.0\cos(\omega t + \pi)$ (cm) and $y_2 = 4.0\cos(\omega t + \frac{3\pi}{2})$ (cm) Determine the amplitude, the initial phase and the equation of the resultant oscillation.

8-7. The equation of a wave is $y = 0.05\cos\pi(5x - 100t)$ (m), Determine:

(1) The amplitude, the frequency, the period, the speed and the wavelength of the wave;

(2) The equation of oscillation and the initial phase of the oscillating particle at the point with a distance of x = 2 m from the wave source;

(3) The phase difference of the two oscillating particles respectively at point x_1 = 0.2 m and point x_2 = 0.35 m.

8-8. A plane harmonic wave with the frequency of ν = 12.5 kHz is propagating in a metal rod. The speed of propagation is $c = 5.0\times10^3$ m/s, and the amplitude at the wave source is A = 0.1 mm. Try to determine:

(1) The equation of oscillation at the wave source;

(2) The wave equation;

(3) The equation of oscillation of the particle at the point with a distance of 10 cm from the wave source;

(4) The phase difference of two oscillating particles respectively at the points with the distances of 20 cm and 30 cm from the wave source;

(5) The waveform equation when the wave source has oscillated for a time of 0.0021 s.

8-9. A large-amplitude ultrasonic wave with sound intensity of 120 kW/cm^2 can be generated in the liquid by the method of focusing the ultrasonic wave. If the frequency is 500 kHz, the density of the liquid is 1 g/cm^3, the sound speed is 1500 m/s, determine the amplitude of the oscillating liquid particles in this region of the liquid.

8-10. A car is traveling along a straight line. When it is passing by an observation station the observed frequency of the car's sound decreases from 1200 Hz to 1000 Hz, and we know that the sound speed in the air is 340 m/s. What is the speed of the car?

8-11. A train leaves a man and goes to the cave with the speed of 10 m/s. If the train whistles with the frequency of 2000 Hz,

(1) what is the frequency of the whistle heard directly by the man?

(2) what is the frequency of the whistle reflected from the mountain and then heard by the man (the speed of sound in the air is 340 m/s)?

8-12. A beam of ultrasonic wave with the frequency of 500 kHz, the sound intensity of 12×10^7 W/m^2, and the sound speed of 1500 m/s is travelling in the water (the density of water is 1000 kg/m^3). What is the amplitude of the sound pressure with the unit of the atmospheric pressure?

What is the amplitude of the displacement?

8-13. The range of sound intensity can be felt by human ears is from 10^{-12} to 100W/m^2. How to express this range with sound intensity level?

Chapter 9 Wave Optics

Generally, optics could be divided into geometrical optics and physical optics. The main study work of geometrical optics is the regularity of rectilinear propagation of light. The properties of rectilinear propagation of light only display in some special cases, and so far, the theories of rectilinear propagation is the basis for designing and manufacturing optical imaging instruments. The physical optics includes wave optics and quantum optics. In the theory of wave optics, the nature of light is the electromagnetic wave and the light is considered to travel in the form of wave. However, according to the theory of quantum optics, the particle property of light displays obviously. So, the features of light are including wave property and particle property.

In this chapter we'll research the wave optics, i.e., the study of the phenomena and the regularity of the propagating light and the applications. The wave optics mainly includes the interference, the diffraction, the polarization, and the absorption of light.

9.1 Light

9.1.1 Visible Light, Monochromatic Light, and White Light

Light is one kind of electromagnetic waves. The difference between light, radio wave, microwave, X-ray, γ-ray and other electromagnetic waves depends on their wavelengths.

The electromagnetic wave which could be sensed by human's eyes is the **visible light**. The wavelength range of the visible light is 350–770 nm. The color of visible light is related to the frequency (or the wavelength). The relationship between color, wavelength and frequency of the visible light is shown in Figure 9-1.

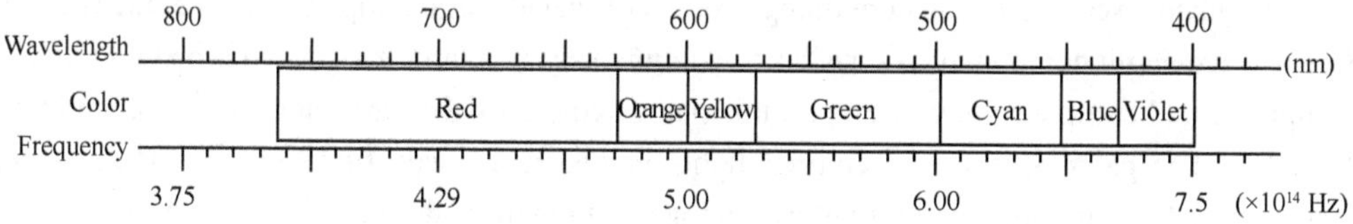

Figure 9-1 The color and the frequency of the visible light

The visual sensitivity of human eyes for different colors of light is different. The curve of relative sensitivity of human eyes for different colors of light is shown in Figure 9-2. The yellow-green light with the wavelength of 550 nm is the most sensitive one for human eyes; meanwhile, the red light and violet light have the lower sensitivities. There are not strict boundaries on both sides of the wavelength range of the visible light. For different people there are different boundaries and even for the same person the wavelength range will change with the intensity of light. The light with the wavelength longer than the longest wavelength limit of visible light is called the **infrared light**; and the light with the wavelength shorter than the shortest wavelength limit of visible light is called the **ultraviolet light**. The infrared light and the ultraviolet light are invisible for the human eyes.

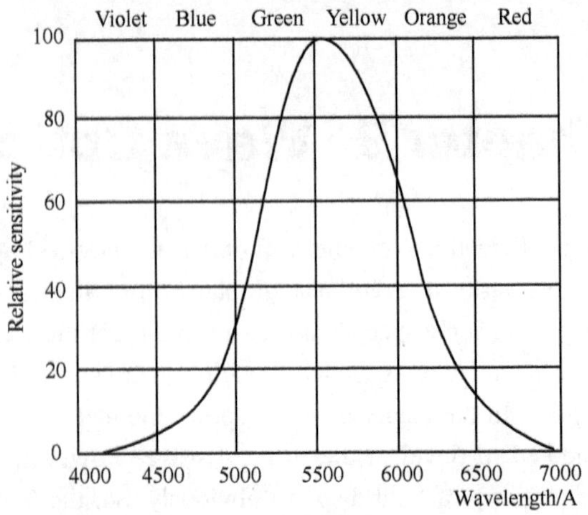

Figure 9-2 The relationship between relative sensitivity of human eyes and the wavelength of light

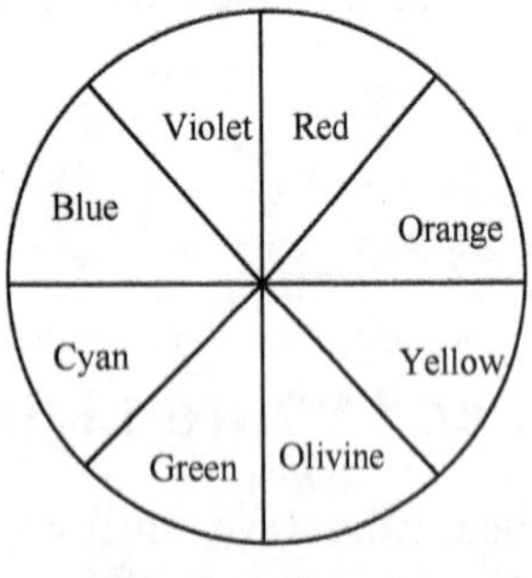

Figure 9-3 Complementary colors

The light containing only one wavelength is referred to as the **monochromatic light**. The strict monochromatic light does not exist in nature. In fact, the light from any light source contains a lot of different wavelengths. If the wavelength range of light is narrow enough, the light could be referred to as quasi-monochromatic light. The narrower the wavelength range is, the better the monochromatic property of the light will be. In practice, we can only get the quasi-monochromatic light. For example, the red light could be obtained from the white light by passing through the normal red glass, and the wavelength range is about several hundred angstroms. In laboratories, approximately monochromatic light could be obtained commonly from the laser source. For example, the yellow light with wavelength of 589.0 nm could be obtained by a sodium lamp.

The **white light** is the mixed light with various colors. The light from a common heat source (such as the sun or an incandescent lamp) is containing a series of wavelength components. The intensity of light of different wavelength component is distributed continuously in a large range. After being mixed, if two colored lights could compose the white light, this pair of colored lights are referred to as complementary colored lights. The pairs of opposite colored lights in Figure 9-3 constitute **complementary colored lights**, such as red and green, blue and yellow, orange and green, and so on. If a colored light is filtered out from the white light, the light remained will be the complementary colored light to the former one. For example, the green light could be obtained by filtering the red light from white light, and the yellow-green light could be obtained by filtering violet light from white light, and vice versa. Note that, both of the complementary colored lights are not monochromatic light.

9.1.2 Speed of Light in a Medium, and Wavelength

According to Maxwell's electromagnetic theory, the electromagnetic waves or light with different wavelengths have the same speed in vacuum. The speed measured with experiments is c = 299 792 458 m/s.

The speed of light in the medium is

$$\upsilon=\frac{1}{\sqrt{\varepsilon_0\varepsilon_r\mu_0\mu_r}} \tag{9-1}$$

where ε_0 and μ_0 are respectively the permittivity of vacuum and the permeability of vacuum; and ε_r and μ_r are the relative permittivity of the medium and the relative permeability of the medium. In the vacuum, $\varepsilon_r = 1$ and $\mu_r = 1$, so the speed of electromagnetic waves in the vacuum is

$$c=\frac{1}{\sqrt{\varepsilon_0\mu_0}} \tag{9-2}$$

If the known data was applied in the equation, the speed of electromagnetic waves is equal to the speed of light. This result suggests that there are some relationship between the electromagnetic phenomena and optical phenomena. Subsequently, the theory and practice shows that the light is one kind of electromagnetic waves, and the wavelength of light is much shorter than radio waves.

According to the Equation (9-1) and Equation (9-2), the speed of light wave in the medium is

$$\upsilon=\frac{c}{\sqrt{\varepsilon_r\mu_r}}$$

where $\varepsilon_r > 1$ and $\mu_r \approx 1$, their values are dependent on the properties of the medium. So, the speeds of light wave in different medium are different, and the speed of light wave in medium is lower than the speed of light wave in the vacuum.

The frequency of a light wave is dependent on its light source. So that, even spreading in different media the same light wave has the same frequency. According to the relationship between velocity, wavelength and frequency, i.e. $\lambda=\frac{\upsilon}{\nu}$, since the same light wave spreading in different media have different velocities, the same light wave spreading in different media would have different wavelengths, and the wavelength of light wave in a medium is shorter than the wavelength of light wave in the vacuum.

Example 9-1 The wavelength of a light wave in water is 440 nm, what is the wavelength of this light wave in air? Here the refractive index of water is $n = 1.33$, and $n=\frac{\lambda}{\lambda'}$ (λ' and λ represent respectively the wavelength of the light wave in medium and the wavelength of the light wave in the vacuum).

Solution: The refractive index of the air is about 1. So, the wavelength of light wave in air is equal to the wavelength of light wave in the vacuum approximately.

So the wavelength of the light wave in the air should be $\lambda = n\lambda'$.

$$\lambda = 1.33\times 440 = 588 \text{ nm}$$

9.2 Interference of Light

Light is one kind of electromagnetic wave, and the phenomenon of interference is one of the basic characteristics of the wave property of light.

When two special light waves on some conditions encounter, in the space where these two light waves met, there will be a stable distribution of the intensity of light or a stable distribution of bright and dark degree. This phenomenon is called the interference of light.

9.2.1 Coherent Lights

If two light waves have the same frequency, the common oscillation direction, and a constant phase difference, these two light waves are called **coherent lights** (these conditions are **conditions for coherence**), and there may be a corresponding phenomenon of interference.

The light wave from an ordinary light source (including heat light source or gas discharge light source) is the electromagnetic wave radiated out when the moving states of the atoms (or molecules) in the light source change. It corresponds to a series of random un-continuous spontaneous radiations. The duration for each radiation of an atom is rather short, only 10^{-10} - 10^{-8} s; and a wave with certain frequency and certain oscillating direction is radiated. It is called a **wave train**. The wave train irradiated in this case is very short (much less than a meter). The wave trains radiated by an atom at different moment or by different atoms in a normal light source are independent wave trains with random different oscillating directions and uncertain phase difference, and they are irrelative to each other. Therefore, when these un-continuous wave trains meet at a point P and superpose together, the phase differences and oscillating directions are haphazard, so the phenomenon of interference will not happen, since the conditions for the interference are unsatisfied.

Well, how to get the coherent lights?

The common method is that the light from one point on a normal light source is divided into two beams traveling in two different paths and then meeting together. The phenomenon of interference occurs when they meet because at this moment each original wave train after being divided on two paths has the same frequency, the common oscillation direction, and the constant phase difference. That is to say, these two beams that were derived by dividing from one point could satisfy the coherent conditions and play the roles of the coherent lights beams. The common methods to get coherent lights by divided light beams are usually the wave front segmentation method and the oscillation amplitude segmentation method. Both methods will be introduced later.

9.2.2 Optical Path, and Optical Path Difference

The optical path is different from the geometrical path. The geometrical path is the length of the path of light propagation, while the optical path depends not only on the geometrical path, but also on the refractive index of the medium n. Therefore, we call nr, the product of the refractive index and the geometrical path, the **optical path**, written as

$$\delta = nr \tag{9-3}$$

Generally speaking, the optical path is longer than the geometrical path. Only when the refractive index $n = 1$ (in the vacuum or in the air), the optical path will be equal to the geometrical path.

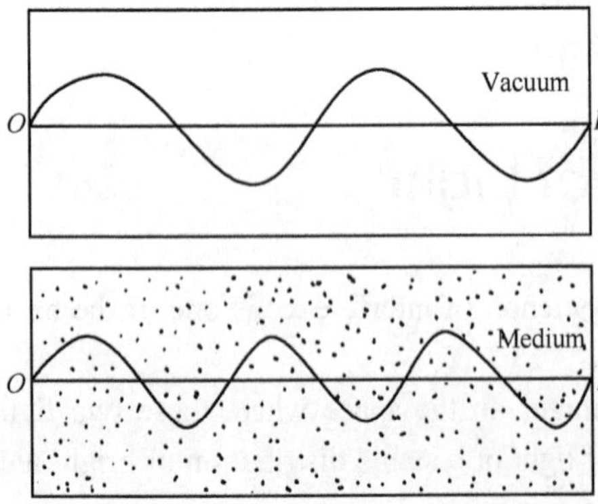

Figure 9-4 The schematic diagram of optical path

When a light propagates from the air to a medium, the wavelength of light in the medium $\lambda' = \dfrac{\lambda}{n}$ will be shortened i.e., in the same geometrical path r, the wave number will increase. As shown in Figure 9-4, compared with the case in the vacuum, the value of phase difference for the light arriving at the same position P through the medium will be changed. In this way, phase difference cannot be calculated based on the difference of geometrical path. For this reason, we introduce the concept of optical path, which is to say, for the same change of phase, the geometrical path r for light propagating in a medium is equal to the geometrical path *nr* of light propagating in the vacuum, and the change of phase is

$$\Delta\varphi = 2\pi \cdot \frac{r}{\lambda'} = 2\pi \cdot \frac{nr}{\lambda} \tag{9-4}$$

The relationship between the phase difference and the optical path difference is

$$\Delta\varphi = \frac{2\pi}{\lambda}\delta \tag{9-5}$$

With the concept of the optical path, we can correspond any propagation path of a monochromatic light in the different medium to the propagation path of this monochromatic light in the vacuum. And by this method, it becomes more convenient for the discussion of interference of light. For example, if two coherent light waves travel in the same medium (such as in the air) and the wavelength is constant, according to the relationship between the phase difference and the optical path difference, $\Delta\varphi = \frac{2\pi}{\lambda}\delta$, the phase difference could be determined by the geometrical path difference. Further more, in the case of the interference, the condition of bright and dark of light could also be determined.

9.2.3 Interference with the Division of Wave Front

We may generate two beams of coherent light by dividing a certain wave front of the monochromatic light emitted from a light source into two parts and superpose them at some place to exert the phenomenon of interference after reflection, refraction or diffraction with some optical devices. The methods of obtaining interferences in this way are called the methods of the **division of wave front**. If an interference phenomenon is obtained by the means of division of wave front, the interference is called the **interference with the division of wave front**.

1. Young's Double-slit Interference

In 1801, Thomas Young (1773-1829) obtained the interference phenomenon in the first place. Young's double-slit interference was achieved by superposing two coherent light beams got from a double-slit device, as shown in Figure 9-5. A monochromatic light beam irradiated out from a light source passes through the single slit S on the screen P_1 first; so that S can be looked as a slit light source. In front of S, two slits S_1, and S_2 are laid in a very close distance on the screen P_2, and the distance from S_1 to S is equal to the distance from S_2 to S. According to Huygens' principle, S_1 and S_2 can be looked as two secondary light sources; they can both produce light waves which satisfy the conditions for coherence. Therefore, S_1 and S_2 are called coherent light sources. In this way, the interference phenomenon will be produced when the light beams emitted by S_1 and S_2 respectively meet in the space. If a screen P_3 is place in front of S_1 and S_2, the steady interference fringes consisted of bright and dark bands will appear on it.

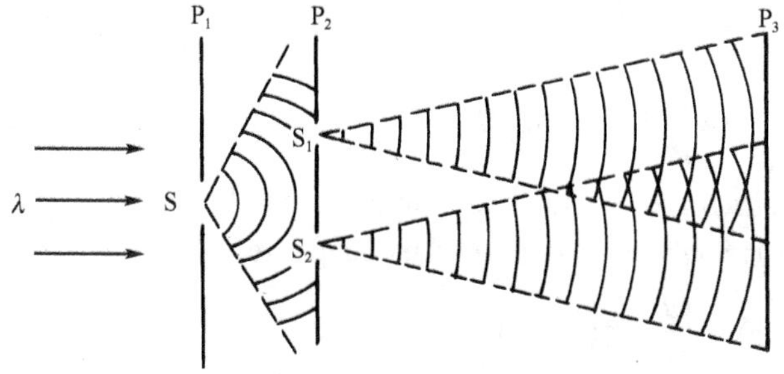

Figure 9-5 The experiment of Young's double-slit interference

The condition satisfied for producing the fringes consisted of bright and dark bands on the screen can be analyzed quantitatively below. As shown in Figure 9-6, the corresponding quantities are assumed as: The distance between S_1 and S_2 is d; the distance between the plane P_2 on which the double slits and the screen P_3 is D. To select a discretionary point P on the screen, and the distance from it to S_1 and S_2 are respectively r_1 and r_2. Therefore, the optical path difference between the lights emitted from S_1 and S_2 respectively to point P on the screen is $\delta = r_2 - r_1$.

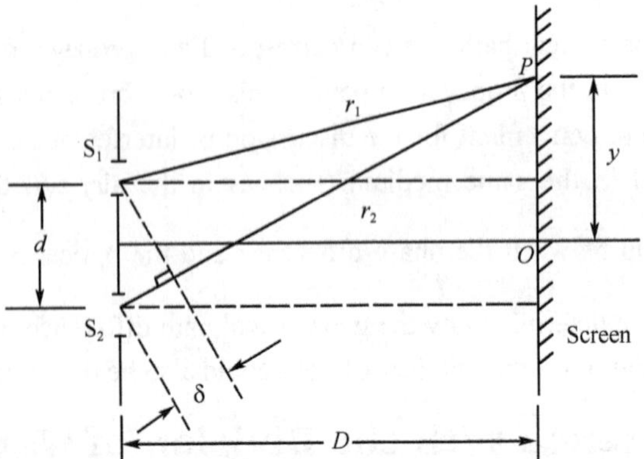

Figure 9-6 The schematics of Young's double-slit interference

According to the Pythagorean Theorem, there are

$$r_1^2 = D^2 + \left(y - \frac{d}{2}\right)^2$$

$$r_2^2 = D^2 + \left(y + \frac{d}{2}\right)^2$$

The subtraction result of two equations is

$$r_2^2 - r_1^2 = (r_2 - r_1)(r_2 + r_1) = \delta(r_1 + r_2) = 2yd$$

Because $D \gg d$, $(r_1 + r_2) \approx 2D$, therefore,

$$\delta = \frac{yd}{D} \tag{9-6}$$

If the optical path difference δ is an integer multiple of the wavelength λ of incident light, there will be a bright band appeared at point P. So the conditions for bright bands are

$$\left.\begin{aligned} &\delta = \frac{yd}{D} = \pm k\lambda \\ \text{or} \quad & \\ &y = \pm k\frac{D}{d}\lambda, \quad k = 0, 1, 2, \cdots \end{aligned}\right\} \text{bright bands} \tag{9-7}$$

If the optical path difference δ is the odd multiple of the half-wavelength of incident light, a dark band will appear at point P. So the conditions for dark bands are

$$\left.\begin{aligned} &\delta = \frac{yd}{D} = \pm(2k+1)\frac{\lambda}{2} \\ \text{or} \quad & \\ &y = \pm(2k+1)\frac{D}{d}\cdot\frac{\lambda}{2}, \quad k = 0, 1, 2, \cdots \end{aligned}\right\} \text{dark bands} \tag{9-8}$$

For point P, if the optical path difference δ follows neither the conditions of the bright bands nor the conditions of the dark bands, then point P is neither the brightest nor the darkest.

Experimental results show that, the distributions of interference fringes are symmetrical about point O on both sides; and the distance between adjacent two bright bands or two dark bands can be calculated with

$$\Delta y = \frac{\lambda}{d} D \tag{9-9}$$

According to Equation (9-9), we can get:

(1) Δy, the distance between adjacent two bright bands is proportional directly to the wavelength of the incident light λ, the shorter the wavelength of the incident light λ is, the smaller the distance between adjacent bright bands will be. If the white light is used in this experiment, the colored fringes from violet to red will appear on both sides except the central bright (white color) band since the bright bands corresponding to different wavelengths appear at different positions.

(2) If the values of d and D are known, after measuring the value of y for the k order bright band, the wavelength of the monochromatic light λ can be calculated from the above equation.

(3) Due to the wavelength of the monochromatic light λ is very short, the distance d between S_1 and S_2 should be short enough, and the distance D between the plate on which the double slits are and the screen P should be long enough, only in this way, Δy the distance between adjacent two bright bands, could be observed directly by human's eyes.

2. Lloyd Mirror Experiment

Lloyd mirror experiment is a kind of interference experiment that uses a reflective equipment to achieve the division of wave front. The experiment equipment is as shown in Figure 9-7.

In Figure 9-7, MB is a reflective mirror. As wave front W is emitted from the light source S, one part of it shoots directly on the screen P, and the other part casts on the mirror MB and is reflected to the screen. We can regard the reflected light as being radiated by a dummy light source S′. Comparing with Young's double-slit interference experiment, S and S′ compose a couple of coherent light sources, and at this time, the fringes with bright and dark bands can also be seen on the screen. The analysis and discussion of Young's double-slit interference experiment could also be applicable to the Lloyd mirror experiment.

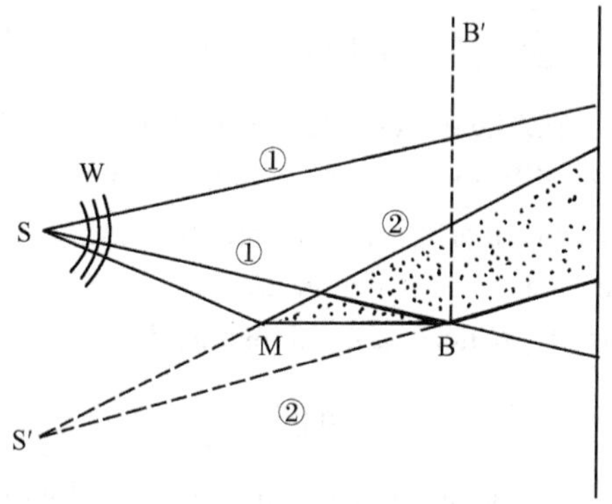

Figure 9-7 Lloyd mirror experiment

An important physical phenomenon can be observed in the Lloyd mirror experiment. If the screen is placed at the position B′B and touches the mirror, a dark band appears at the touching point. According to the analysis shown in Figure 9-7, the distances of light beams radiated by S and S′ and arrived respectively at point B are equal. It seems that the bright band should appear at point B. However, the fact of the experiment is that a dark band appears at the touching point, why does this phenomenon happen?

The study results show that when the incident light shoots from a medium with the smaller refractive index onto the surface of another with the bigger refractive index and is reflected, on the conditions of the incident angle $i \approx 0°$ or $\approx 90°$, the phase of reflected light has a phase transition of π comparing with that of the incident light. From the viewpoint of the optical path, it seems that there is an optical path difference of a half wavelength $\lambda/2$. This phenomenon is called the **half-wave loss**. In the Lloyd mirror experiment, the condition of the incident angle $i \approx 90°$ is followed and the light is incident from the optically thinner medium (air, the medium with smaller refractive index) onto the surface of the optically denser medium (mirror, the medium with bigger refractive index) and is reflected from it, so the phase of reflected light has a transition of π comparing with that of the incident light. Therefore, at the touching point B, the phase difference between reflected light and the light shoot directly on the screen P is π, and the result of the interference is a dark band.

9.2.4 Interference with the Division of Amplitude

When a beam of light is incident onto the interface of two transparent media, the energy of the light will be reflected partly and refracted partly. The method to divide a beam of light into two parts is called the method of the **division of amplitude**. The interference phenomenon generated by the method of the division of amplitude is called the **interference with the division of amplitude**. If the interference of the division of amplitude is realized with a thin film, the interference phenomenon is called the **film interference**. In daily life, the colorful fringes on soap films, on oil films floating on water by white light's shining are just the results of this kind of interference.

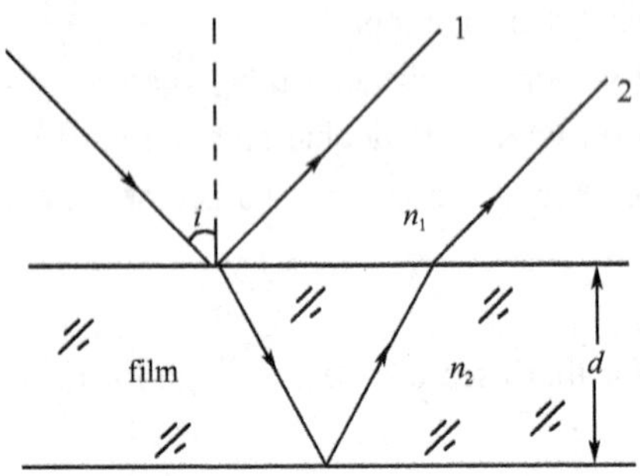

Figure 9-8 The film interference

Now, let's discuss the phenomenon of the film interference. As shown in Figure 9-8, there is a film with the refractive index of n_1 and the thickness of d. It is assumed that, a light beam emitted from a point at a monochromatic light source shoots onto the surface of the film with the incident angle of i. Then, part of the light beam is reflected by the surface of the film (light beam 1 as shown in the figure), and the other part of the light beam penetrates into the film and then is reflected by the bottom interface of the film, and refracted thereafter gets out from the upper surface of the film (light beam 2 as shown in the figure). The optical path of light beam 2 is longer than the optical path of light beam 1, and the optical path difference between light beam 2 and light beam 1 is $2nd$ (to assume that, the light beam is perpendicularly incident onto the film). Because the light is incident from the optically thinner medium onto the optically denser medium, the phase of reflected light 1 has a phase transition of π comparing with that of the incident light, than the half wave loss exerts. So the optical path difference between light beam 2 and light beam 1 should be $\delta \approx 2nd - \dfrac{\lambda}{2}$. According to the knowledge mentioned above, there are

1) The interference condition of bright bands

$$\delta = 2nd - \frac{\lambda}{2} = k\lambda \qquad (k = 0, 1, 2, \cdots) \tag{9-10}$$

2) The interference condition of dark bands

$$\delta = 2nd - \frac{\lambda}{2} = (2k-1)\frac{\lambda}{2} \qquad (k = 1, 2, 3, \cdots) \tag{9-11}$$

The discussion above is about the interference phenomenon of a monochromatic light. If the light source is polychromatic, the interference fringes should be multicolor, because there are lots of different wavelengths. For example, when the film of gasoline on the wet surface of road was shined by the sunlight, the multicolor fringes could be observed.

Example 9-2 As shown in Figure 9-9, a film of a transparent medium with the refractive index of n_t is covered on the surface of a glass base with the refractive index n. Now, a monochromatic light beam with the wavelength of λ is perpendicularly incident onto the film from air (with the refractive index of

n_0). If the lights reflected respectively from upper interface and bottom interface could just be canceled out each other, what is the thinnest thickness of the transparent medium (it is assumed that $n_0 < n_t < n$)?

Solution: As shown in Figure 9-9, the thickness of the film of the transparent medium is l, the condition of destructive interference is

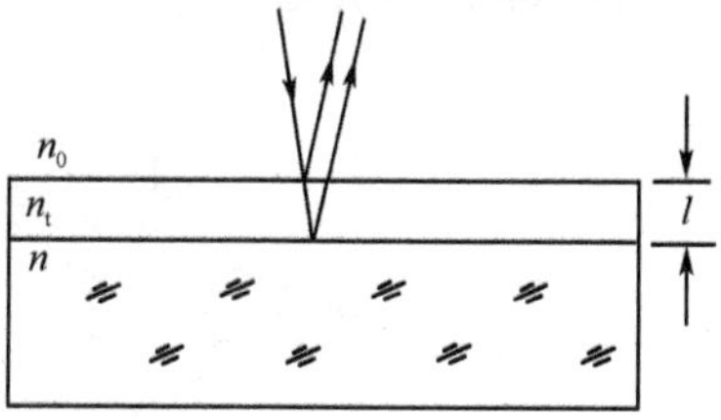

Figure 9-9 The antireflection film

$$2n_t l = (2k-1)\frac{\lambda}{2} \quad (k = 1, 2, 3, \cdots)$$

and the thinnest thickness of the film of the transparent medium should be ($k = 1$), and then

$$l = \frac{\lambda}{4n_t}$$

This kind of film of a transparent medium is called the **antireflection film**. An antireflection film plays the role of canceling the reflecting light and strengthening the penetrating light. The antireflection films are widely used in the optical instruments, such as the shots of microscope or camera lens, and lens of glasses. The commonly used material for antireflection films is magnesium fluoride (with the refractive index of $n = 1.38$). Oppositely, some other optical pieces require to be coated with films of transparent media for reducing the intensity the penetrating light and strengthening the reflecting light. This kind of film of transparent medium is called the **reflection increasing film**. For example, there are multilayer of films of high reflectivity for infrared on the surface of the astronaut helmets to preserve astronauts from the strong radiation of infrared from the universe.

9.3 Diffraction of Light

9.3.1 Diffraction Phenomenon of Light

Light as a king of wave, when it travels by a barrier in the transmission, it may bypass the barrier and spreads out to the shadowed regions of the barrier. This phenomenon is called the **diffraction of light**.

Diffraction phenomenon is another important feature of waves. Due to the wavelength of light is short and the size of the barrier is relatively larger, the diffraction phenomenon could not be observed generally. So, the obvious diffraction phenomenon could be observed when there is not much difference between the size of the barrier and the light wavelength, or thereabouts.

According to relevant distances between the light source and the diffraction slit (or barrier), and the screen, we can divide the diffraction phenomena into two kinds. The first one is what shown in Figure 9-10 (a) where the distances from the light source to the diffraction slit (or barrier) and to the screen are limited; this kind of diffraction is called **Fresnel diffraction**. In this kind of diffraction, due to the light rays from the light source S to the diffraction slit are not parallel, and the wave front is not a plane, the Fresnel diffraction could be observed conveniently, but the quantitative discussion of it is very complicated. The second one is what shown in Figure 9-10 (b) where the distances are “infinite” long, so the light rays of both the incident light and the diffracted light are respectively parallel; this kind of diffraction phenomenon is called **Fraunhofer diffraction.**

In fact, the diffraction phenomenon of the parallel light could be observed by two convergent lenses. As shown in Figure 9-10 (c), the light source S is placed on the focal point of lens L_1, and the screen P is placed on the focal plane of lens L_2, then the diffraction phenomenon of the parallel light could be obtained on the screen.

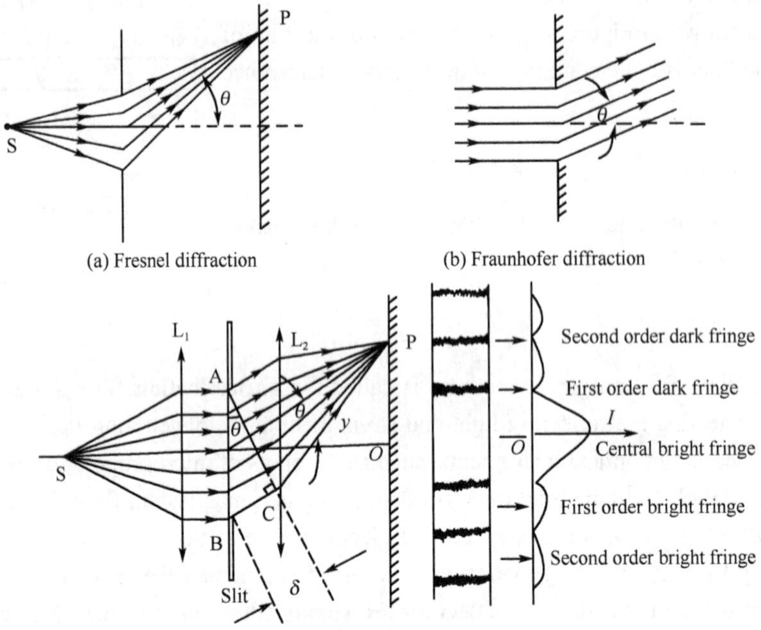

(a) Fresnel diffraction (b) Fraunhofer diffraction

(c) Using lens to satisfy the Fraunhofer diffraction

Figure 9-10 Different kinds of diffractions

9.3.2 Huygens-Fresnel Principle

According to the Huygens principle, every point on the wave front could be considered as the new wave source of the secondary spherical wavelet, and the enveloping surface of all the spherical wavelets constitute the new wave front at the next moment. However, Huygens principle could not explain the intensity distribution of the diffracted light, because the secondary spherical wavelets in Huygens principle do not involve the periodical characteristics of time and space of waves. So, the Huygens principle could not be used to study quantitatively the diffraction phenomenon. Fresnel, according to the principle of the wave superposition and interference, raised the concept of "the coherent superposition of wavelets", and this concept developed and extended Huygens principle. According to the Huygens-Fresnel principle, wavelets emitted from any points on the same wave front are coherent, as propagating and meeting at the certain point in the space, the result of the coherent superposition of all the wavelets determines the wave's amplitude at that place.

Huygens-Fresnel principle is the theoretical foundation of studying the diffraction phenomenon and it perfects the wave theory of light, too.

9.3.3 Single-slit Diffraction

The experimental apparatus of Fraunhofer single-slit diffraction is as shown in Figure 9-11. When a beam of parallel light is perpendicularly incident on the single slit, the diffraction light is focused by the lens L_2 on the screen placed at the focal plane, and the diffraction pattern is formed on it. The diffraction pattern is parallel to the slit, and appears as a group of fringes which are bright and dark bands distributed symmetrically on both sides of the central bright band as shown in Figure 9-11.

Figure 9-12 is the sectional sketch of Figure 9-11. In Figure 9-12, AB is the section of the single-slit with the width of a. In order to study conveniently, we enlarge the width of the single-slit. In fact, the width of the single-slit is much narrower than the diameter and the focal length of lens.

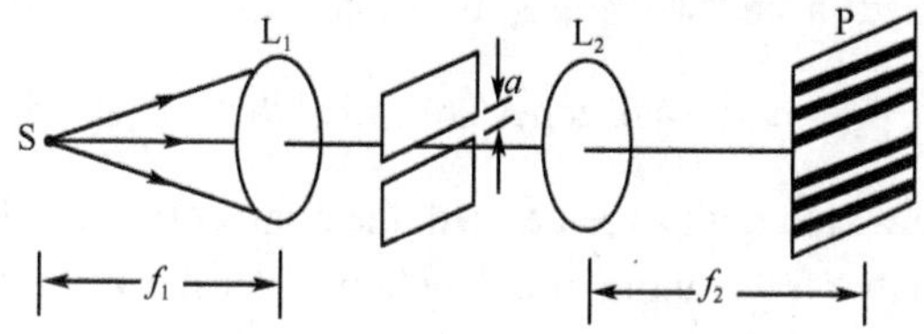

Figure 9-11 The scheme of Fraunhofer single-slit diffraction

A beam of monochromatic light is perpendicularly incident on the single-slit. According to the Huygens-Fresnel principle, every point on the wave front surface AB can be looked as a source of a coherent wavelet. As all the coherent wavelets only propagate forward, they will be focused by the lens L_2 and meet on the screen placed at the focal plane. The interference of these coherent wavelets occurs, so the diffraction pattern could be observed. The angle θ between the diffracted light and the normal direction of the slit is called the angle of diffraction. If the interference is enhanced or is weakened by the superposition of these coherent wavelets on any point on the screen should be determined by the optical path differences of all the diffracted lights arrived at this point.

Now, let's discuss this question by means of the simple and applicable method of Fresnel's half-wave zone.

As shown in Figure 9-12, point O is the intersection point of the screen and the perpendicular bisector of the single-slit AB. Due to the beam of parallel light is perpendicularly incident on the single slit, surface AB corresponds to a wave surface with the same phase, and the optical paths of all the rays are the same after being focused by the lens, so they keep the same phase as they arriving at point O; in this way, they will intensify to each others, and there will be a bright band at the central place O that is just faced to the center of the slit. This bright band is called the central band, which has its central angle of diffraction $\theta = 0$.

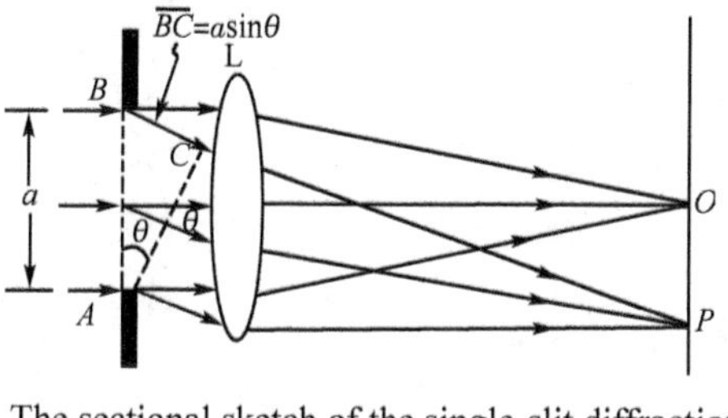

Figure 9-12 The sectional sketch of the single-slit diffraction experiment

To assume that, point P is a random point on the screen. As shown in Figure 9-12, a beam of parallel light is irradiated from AB and is focused by the lens L on the point P on the screen with the angle of diffraction θ. Here, it should notice that, the optical paths of the rays of the wavelets are not equal as they arrive at point P. It can be seen from Figure 9-12, the optical path difference between the rays of wavelets emitted respectively from point A and point B is

$$\delta = \overline{BC} = a\sin\theta \tag{9-12}$$

This is the biggest optical path difference between the rays of wavelets arriving at point P. It determines the intensity distribution at point P and the occurrence of bright bands or dark bands. The method of Fresnel's half-wave zone enables us to get the brief picture of the diffraction pattern distribution.

To draw a series of planes that are parallel to *BC* and let these planes cut the wave front *AB* into several pieces of wave zone with the equal area, as shown in Figure 9-13. If the optical path difference between the two rays emitted from two edges of some wave zone arriving at the focused point respectively is $\frac{\lambda}{2}$, then these pieces of wave zones are called the half-wave zones. On the conditions that the width of the slit a and the wavelength λ are defined, the number of the half-wave zones divided on the wave front *AB* is depended only on the angle of diffraction θ. As shown in Figure 9-12, according to the knowledge of plane geometry, if δ the optical path difference between *AB* and the focus point *P* equals m times of the half-wavelength, then the wave front *AB* could be divided into m pieces of half-wave zones. They will have the relationship of

$$a\sin\theta = \frac{\lambda}{2}\cdot m$$

The bigger of the angle θ, the more the half-wave zones could be divided into. Because the areas of all the pieces of half-wave zones are equal, the intensity of the optical vibrations on the focal point irradiated by the wavelets from the half-wave zones are equal too.

As shown in Figure 9-13 (a), if BC is just equal to even times of half of the wavelength, that is the wave front AB can just be divided into the even number of half-wave zones, therewith, for any two wavelets from two adjacent half-wave zones would interfere destructively in pair on the focal point of the screen, because the optical path difference is $\frac{\lambda}{2}$. And then, the dark band would appear on the corresponding place on the screen. According to the analysis above, when the diffraction angle θ meets the condition of a dark band would appear. Equation (9-13) is the equation for dark bands of single-slit diffraction. Where, k is the order of the dark band. The positive and negative symbols express that the dark bands are distributed symmetrically on both sides of the central bright band.

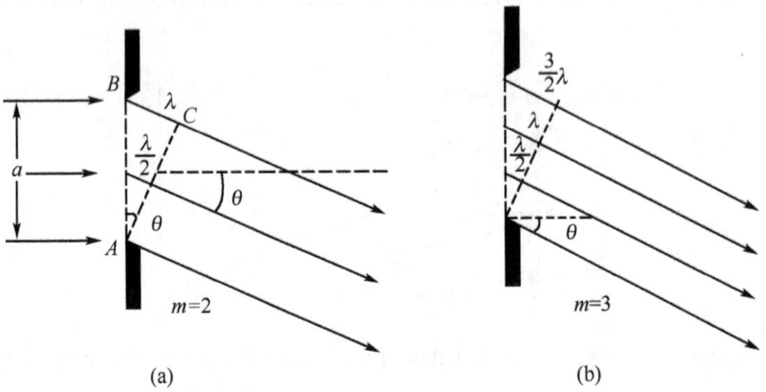

Figure 9-13 The division of Fresnel half-wave zones

$$a\sin\theta = \pm 2k\cdot\frac{\lambda}{2} = \pm k\lambda \qquad (k = 1, 2, \cdots) \tag{9-13}$$

As shown in Figure 9-13 (b), if BC is just equal to an odd number times of half of the wavelength, that is the wave front *AB* can just be divided into odd number of half-wave zones, at this time, the two wavelets corresponding to the adjacent two half-wave zones interfere destructively in pear, too; as the result, there must be an only one wavelet corresponding to the remain half-wave zone cannot be counteracted and it will arrive at point *P* after the lens' focusing. Therefore, there will be a bright band appeared at point *P*. According to the above analysis, when the diffraction angle θ meets the condition of a bright band would appear on the screen. Equation (9-14) is the equation for bright bands. Where, k is the order of the bright band, and the positive and negative symbols express that the bright bands distribute symmetrically by both sides of the central bright band.

$$a\sin\theta = \pm(2k+1)\cdot\frac{\lambda}{2} \qquad (k=0,1,2,\cdots) \tag{9-14}$$

To some angel θ, if neither the bright band condition nor the dark band condition could be satisfied, i.e., *AB* could not be divided into integer of half-wave zones, there will be some vibrations that could not be canceled out, and at the corresponding point on the screen there will be some light with the brightness between the bright and dark bands.

The distance between the two first order dark bands by both sides of the central bright band is its width. Normally, the diffraction angle is very small, so we have $\sin\theta \approx \theta$, and the distance x_1 from first order dark band to the center of central bright band is

$$x_1 = \theta f = \frac{\lambda}{a} f \tag{9-15}$$

where *f* is the focal length of the lens L. Therefore, the width of the central bright band is

$$\Delta x_0 = 2x_1 = 2\frac{\lambda}{a} f \tag{9-16}$$

The width of the *k*th order bright band is the distance between the centers of the *k*th order dark band and (*k*+1)th order dark band.

$$\Delta x = x_{k+1} - x_k$$

$$\Delta x = \frac{\lambda}{a} f \tag{9-17}$$

It is obvious that all other bright bands have the same width, and the width of central bright band is twice of the other bright bands'. If we know the Δx, *a* and *f*, we can determine the light wavelength of the light λ by Equation (9-17).

Example 9-3 A beam of parallel green light with the wavelength of 5460 Å irradiated from a mercury lamp is vertically incident on a single slit with the width of 0.437 mm. There is a lens with the focal length of 40 cm behind the single slit. What is the width of the central bright band on the focal plane?

Solution: According to Equation (9-16), we have

$$\Delta x_0 = 2\frac{\lambda}{a} f$$

$$\Delta x_0 = \frac{2\times 5.46\times 10^{-7}\times 0.40}{0.437\times 10^{-3}} = 1.0\times 10^{-3}\,\text{m} = 1.0\,\text{mm}$$

Example 9-4 On the conditions of Example 9-3, what is the distance between the second order dark band and the third order dark band ?

Solution: According to Equation (9-17), there is

$$\Delta x = \frac{\lambda}{a} f$$

and

$$\Delta x = \frac{\Delta x_0}{2} = \frac{\lambda}{a} f = 0.5\text{mm}$$

When the diffraction angle θ is very small, the width of the bright band by both sides of the central bright band is unrelated to the order of the band. The width is $\frac{\lambda}{a} f$, and it is depended only on λ, *a*, and *f*.

9.3.4 Hole Diffraction

If the slit from the experimental apparatus of single-slit diffraction is replaced with a small hole, there will be the diffraction phenomenon when the light beam travels through the small hole. As shown in Figure 9-14, it appears on the screen a diffraction pattern in which there is a round brightest spot at the center point surrounded by a series of the bright and dark rings with the decreasing brightness.

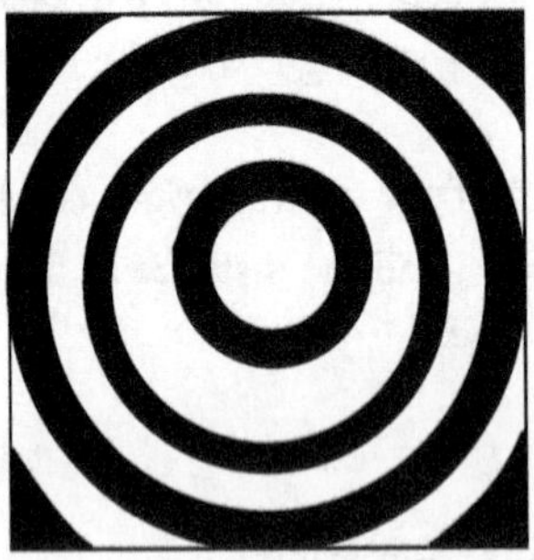

Figure 9-14 The pattern of hole diffraction

With the theoretical analysis we know that, the diffraction angle ϕ of the first order dark ring of the hole diffraction pattern meets

$$\sin\phi = 1.22\frac{\lambda}{D} \tag{9-18}$$

where λ is the wavelength of the monochromatic light, and D is the diameter of the small hole.

The studying of the hole diffraction has an important practical significance. Because the lenses and the diaphragms in most of the optical instruments can be looked as holes, the diffraction phenomenon will take place when the light beam penetrates through them. Therefore, the problem of the hole diffraction should be considered in the manufacture of optical instruments.

Usually, an optical instrument is an optical system constituted by some lenses. They could be replaced by a lens L, and equivalent to a small hole. When the image of an object is formed by an optical instrument, each point of object should have a corresponding point on its image. However, due to the diffraction of light, the point on the image is not a geometrical point, but an **Airy disk** with a certain size. Therefore, to two near points of object, two respectively corresponding Airy disks may overlap to each other, so that it may be impossible to get the resolvable images to the two object points. When two object points can just be resolved, the corresponding field angle to the lens light center to two object points is called the **minimum resolvable angle**. The reciprocal of the minimum resolvable angle is called the **resolution capability**.

9.3.5 Grating Diffraction

1. Grating Diffraction

The diffraction grating is composed of many parallel slits with equal separation distance and equal width. The grating is usually used to measure the wavelength, and to study the structure and intensities of spectral lines. The structure of the commonly used diffraction grating is the glass plate on which numerous parallel lines with equal separation distance and equal width are scratched. And the number of notches in every centimeter can reach to ten thousand or more. The scratched strips can be looked as strips of ground glass and scatter the light away. When a beam of light is irradiating on the grating, the light can only pass through the separation parts between scratched strips, and the separation parts are equivalent to single slits. To assume that the width of each slit is a, and the width of a scratched strip is b, then, $a+b$ is called the **grating constant** denoted by d; or $d = a+b$, as shown in Figure 9-15.

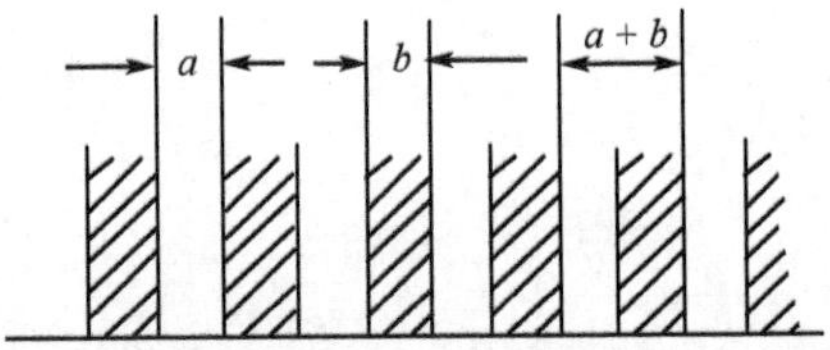

Figure 9-15 A grating

Generally, the grating constant of a normal grating is about the order of magnitude of 10^{-5}-10^{-6} m. There are two kinds of gratings. One is the transmission grating mentioned above, and the other is reflection grating.

Now let's study the regularities of the transmission gratings.

Figure 9-16 is the schematic of the transmission grating imaging. Here *MN* is the grating. When a beam of monochromatic light is irradiating on the grating, the wavelet through every slit produces the diffraction, and light waves through different slits will produce the interference. As the resultant effect of diffraction and the interference, there may be the fringes on the screen. It is assumed that the diffracting light waves irradiating along the direction of the diffraction angle θ from two adjacent slits are focused at point P on the screen by the lens L. If the corresponding optical path difference $d\sin\theta$ is just the integral times of the wavelength of incident light, these wavelets will interfere and enhance each others in pairs, so that a bright band will appear. Therefore, the general condition of the bright bands of the grating diffraction is that

$$\delta = d\sin\theta = \pm k\lambda \qquad (k = 0,1,2,\cdots) \tag{9-19}$$

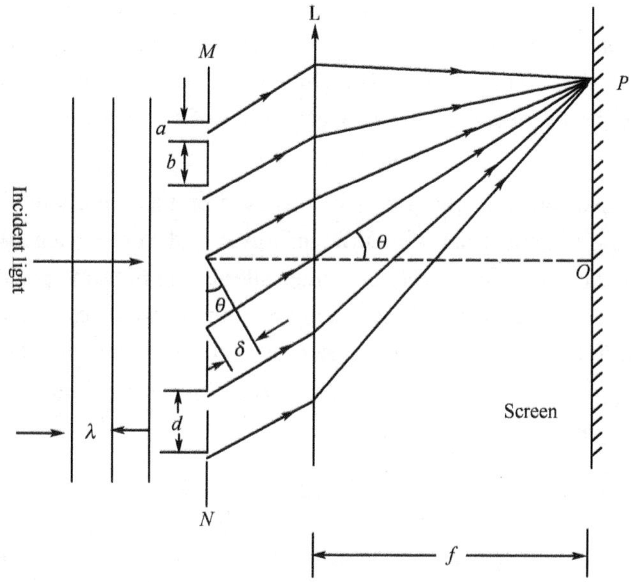

Figure 9-16 The schematic of the formation of grating diffraction

Equation (9-19) is called the **grating equation**. According to the grating equation above, the bright band corresponding to k is called the kth order bright band. It can be proved that the smaller the grating constant is, the bigger the diffraction angle θ will be, and the longer the distance between bright bands will be. When the grating constant d is fixed, the diffraction angle θ is proportional to the wavelength. Therefore, when a beam of polychromatic light is irradiating on the grating, a colored bright bands of the same order will spread out from violet to red without overlap together, except the central bright band. This phenomenon is called the **grating dispersion**. Sometimes in the direction of a certain diffraction angle θ, although the θ satisfies the condition of Equation (9-19), this θ happens to meet the condition of Equation (9-13) for dark band of single slit diffraction as well as, the result is that this bright band will not appear. It is called the **order shortage phenomenon**. On the condition that the above two equations are satisfied, the quantity $\sin\theta$ can be eliminated from the simultaneous Equation of (9-13) and Equation(9-19), i.e.,

$$a\sin\theta = \pm k'\lambda$$

$$(a+b)\sin\theta = \pm k\lambda \quad (9\text{-}20)$$

$$k = \frac{a+b}{a}k'$$

Therefore, when the formula of $\frac{a+b}{a}$ is an integer, the order shortage phenomenon will take place on the bright bands which k is integer.

According to the grating equation, it can be proved that when the wavelength of incident light is fixed, the smaller the grating constant is, the longer the distance between bright bands will be, and the brighter the bands will be. Therefore, the wavelength could be determined accurately by the grating equation.

Meanwhile, some spectrum bands in the spectrums of high orders may superpose with each other. In other words, the bright bands of different order corresponding to the lights with different wavelengths may appear at the same position on the screen. Therefore, the optical path difference corresponding to the same diffraction angle θ, should meet the enhancing conditions of both wavelengths, i.e.,

$$d\sin\theta = k_1\lambda_1 = k_2\lambda_2 \quad (9\text{-}21)$$

So, the superposing phenomenon could only be observed on the condition of different wavelengths with different orders. If in the same order with different wavelengths or the same wavelength in different orders, there will only be the change of density of fringe patterns, but not superposing phenomenon,

Example 9-5 A beam of light from a mercury lamp(λ=590nm) irradiates on a diffraction grating with the grating constant of 1/5000 cm. What is the biggest order of bright band could be observed?

Solution: According to the grating equation $d\sin\theta = k\lambda$, when the value of sinθ is the biggest, the order of bright fringe is the biggest too. So we have

$$k = \frac{d}{\lambda} = \frac{10^{-2}}{5000\times 590\times 10^{-9}} = 3.4$$

Due to k should only be an integer, the number of k = 3 will be adopt, so, the third order of bright band is the biggest order that could be observed.

2. Grating Diffraction Spectrum

It is known from the grating equation that, as the grating constant $a+b$ and the order of bright band are fixed, the value of diffraction angle θ is related only with the wavelength of incident light. When the diffraction angle is very small, θ seems to be proportional to the wavelength λ. Since the light with the short wavelength has the small diffraction angle and the light with the long wavelength has the big diffraction angle. Therefore, in a bright band of the same order, the diffraction angle of violet light is smaller than the diffraction angle of red light. To irradiate a beam of white light on a grating, we can find that all of the diffracting bright bands are colored spectral bands, except the central main bright band which is still white one with the mixed light of all colors. These spectral bands are called the **diffraction spectrums**. In each order of colored bright band arranged symmetrically by two sides of the central main bright band the colors are distributed separately from violet to red. The violet light is close to the central bright band, and the red light is away from the central bright band as shown in Figure 9-17 (a). Therefore, the grating could also be used in spectrophotometer. As shown in Figure 9-17, the width of spectrum band is increased with the increase of the order. A part of the second order spectral band and a part of the third order spectral band are superposed to each other. Therefore, in the grating diffraction spectrum, a part of spectral band with the longer wavelength will superpose with the other part of spectral band of the high order with the shorter wavelength, except in the first order spectral band. So, for getting a complete continuous grating spectrum the first order spectral band of the grating diffraction spectrum should be chosen.

There will be the dispersion for the white light when it is refracted by a prism. The corresponding colored spectral band is called **dispersion spectrum**. This is because the refraction index of the glass is related with the wavelength of light. And the deflection angle of the light passing through the prism is not proportional simply to the refraction index. The deflection angle of the red light passing through the prism is the least, and the deflection angle of the violet light is the biggest as shown in Figure 9-17 (b). The scatter range of the violet light is bigger than that of the red light in the spectral band.

The main differences between the diffraction spectrum and the dispersion spectrum of prism are mentioned as follow.

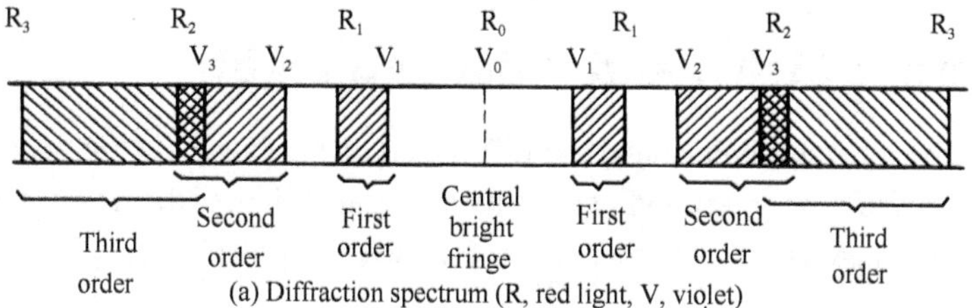

(a) Diffraction spectrum (R, red light, V, violet)

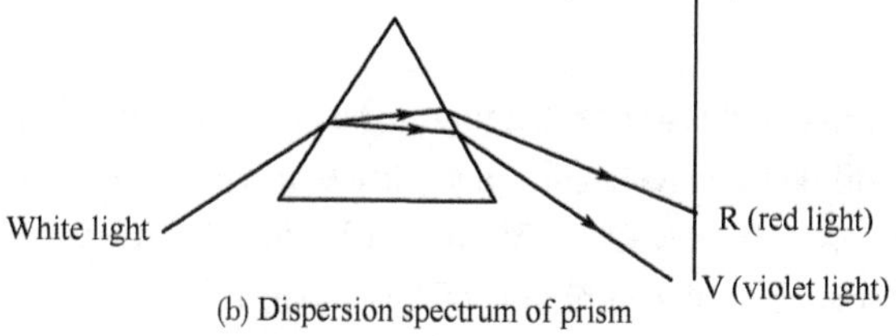

(b) Dispersion spectrum of prism

Figure 9-17 The diffraction spectrum and the dispersion spectrum of prism

(1) In the grating diffraction spectrum, the diffraction angles of the lights with different wavelengths are proportional to the wavelengths. The distances from different colored spectral lines to the centre on the screen are also proportional to the wavelengths. So the diffraction spectrums are arranged uniformly. However, in the dispersion spectrum of prism, the shorter the wavelength is, the bigger the deflection angle is and the more significant the phenomenon of dispersion will be. Therefore, the scatter range of the violet light is bigger than that of the red light in the spectral band. So, the dispersion spectrum is not uniformly arranged.

(2) In the grating diffraction spectrum, the distribution of the colored spectral lines in any spectral band are according to the increase of the diffraction angles from smaller to bigger corresponding to the colors from violet to red. Oppositely, in the dispersion spectrum of prism, the distribution of the colored spectral lines are according to the increase of the deflection angles from smaller to bigger corresponding to the colors from red to violet.

The grating diffraction spectrums formed by lights from different kinds of light sources are different. The spectrum of light emitted from a broiling object is a continuous spectral band, which is called the **continuous spectrum** and consists of every wavelength of the visible light. The spectrum formed by the light from the atoms emitting of the gas inside a discharging tube or of some material being heated in a flame is called the **bright line spectrum**, which consists of some individual bright lines corresponding to certain wavelengths. Every element has its characteristic spectral lines. This result suggests that the characteristic spectral lines emitted by atoms are related to the internal structures of the atoms. To heat an object till emitting light with continuous spectrum, and let the light pass through certain material then irradiate to a grating, we can obtain a spectrum with a series of dark lines appeared in it. This kind of spectrum is called **absorption spectrum**. For certain substances there are certain characteristic absorption spectrums. The wavelengths corresponding to the dark lines in the absorption spectrum are just the wavelengths corresponding to the bright lines in the bright line spectrum. According to the bright line spectrum or the absorption spectrum of some material, we can qualitatively analyze the elements and compounds contained in the material. We can also make the quantitative analysis for the elements contained in it with the intensities of the spectral lines. This method is called **spectrum analysis**, and it has been applied widely in the pharmacology researches.

9.4 Polarization of Light

9.4.1 Nature Light, and Polarized Light

The phenomena of the interference and the diffraction of light indicate the wave character of light. The phenomenon of the polarization of light confirms further that light is the transverse wave. The reason is that, it is only for transverse waves that could produce the polarization phenomenon, but not for longitudinal waves.

1. Natural Light

Light emitted by a normal light source (sunlight, the incandescent lamp) is the composition of the electromagnetic waves of different wavelengths and different vibrating directions radiated by numerous molecules and atoms. It involves light vectors ***E***s in all directions, and has no directional dominates. This means that in every possible direction, the amplitude of ***E*** is equal. This kind of light is called the **natural light**.

The representation of nature light is as shown in Figure 9-18. Figure 9-18 (a) shows that the amplitudes of light vectors ***E***s can be regarded as equal in every possible direction. Using decomposition method, we can decompose the natural light vectors ***E***s into two mutually perpendicular and independent components with the same amplitude [as shown in Figure 9-18 (b)]. Moreover, each component contains half of the natural light energy, and axis z represents the direction of the travel of light. For describing light travel more simply, we often use the vertical short lines with arrows to express the light waves vibrating in the direction of the paper plane, and the black spots to express that vibrating perpendicularly to the paper plane. For describing the natural light, the numbers of the short lines and the spots are uniformly distributed [Figure 9-18 (c) and Figure 9-18(d)].

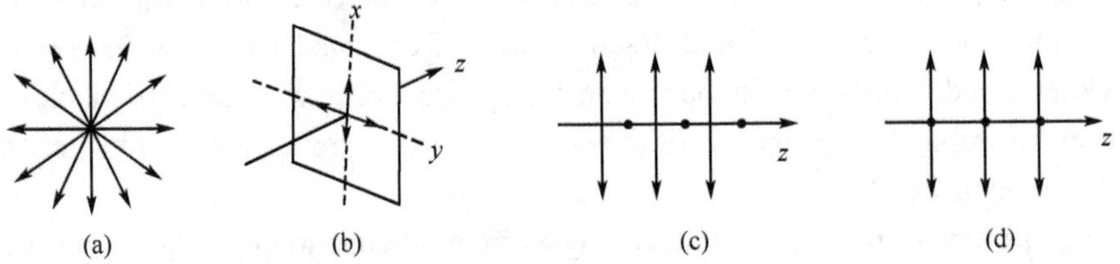

Figure 9-18 The representation of nature light

2. Polarized Light

Light with its vibration only in a certain direction, is called the **linear polarized light**. The plane consisted of the vibrating direction of the polarized light and its propagating direction is called the **vibration plane**. Because light vector ***E*** is always in this plane, the linear polarized light is also called the **planar polarized light**.

Figure 9-19 is the schematic diagram for linear polarized lights. Figure 9-19 (a) shows the linear polarized light with the vibrating direction in the paper plane, and Figure 9-19 (b) shows the linear polarized light with its vibrating direction perpendicular to the paper plane.

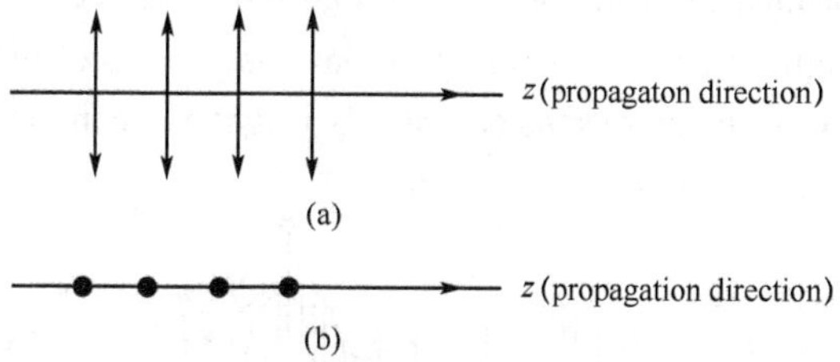

Figure 9-19 The schematic diagram of linear polarized lights

In optical experiment, a linear polarized light can be obtained by removing the vibration of certain direction from the natural light. For example, as we have known, the vector of the natural light $\boldsymbol{E}$ can be decomposed into two mutually perpendicular and independent components with the same amplitude. If one of the two mutually perpendicular vibrations can be partly removed, this kind of light is called the partial polarized light. And, if one of the two mutually perpendicular vibrations can be completely removed, this kind of light is called the complete polarized light, i.e., the linear polarized light. A polarized light can only be distinguished from the natural light with the help of instruments.

9.4.2 Polarizer, and Polarization Analyzer

1. Polarizer

The optical device to transform the natural light into the linear polarized light is called a **polarizer**.

There are many kinds of polarizer, but the function of them is to let the light vibrating in only one direction pass through. This specific direction is called polarization direction of the polarizer, also known as the transmission axis (the direction of PP′ as shown in Figure 9-20). The polarizer is the commonly used one of polaroids.

In practice, polaroids are produced with small crystals of dichroism arranged along some certain orientations on the thin films of polyvinyl alcohol.

2. Polarization Analyzer

The polaroids can be used not only for making the nature light be the polarized light, but also for checking if the light is the polarized light, and a polaroid played the latter role is called the **polarization analyzer** or the **analyzer**.

The division of the polarizer and the analyzer is according to their functions. Figure 9-20 shows the polaroid used as a polarizer in different orientations.

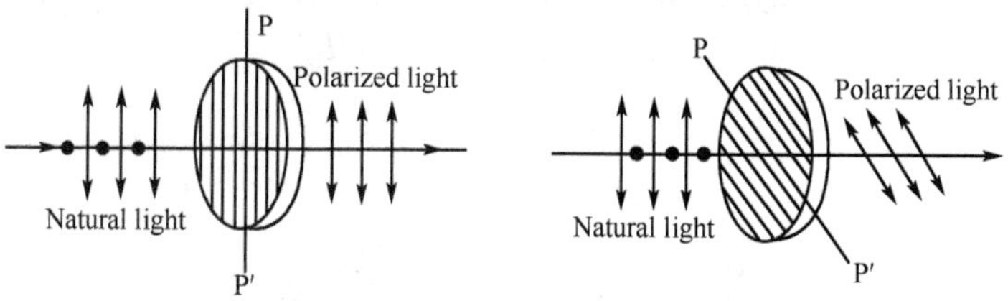

Figure 9-20 The polarizer

As shown in Figure 9-21, there are two polaroids PP′ and AA′, while, a beam of natural light shoots on and passes through them. If AA′ has the same polarization direction [the angle between PP′ and AA′ is 0°, as shown in Figure 9-21 (a)], the light passed through PP′ can pass totally through AA′; this results in a bright field with the strongest light intensity.

If the polarization directions of them are perpendicular to each other [as shown in Figure 9-21 (b)], the polarized light passed through PP′ can not pass through AA′, and the result is that the visual field is complete dark without any light intensity. Therefore, during the process of turning AA′ a round, the light passed through the two polaroids undergoes the completely bright and completely dark situations twice.

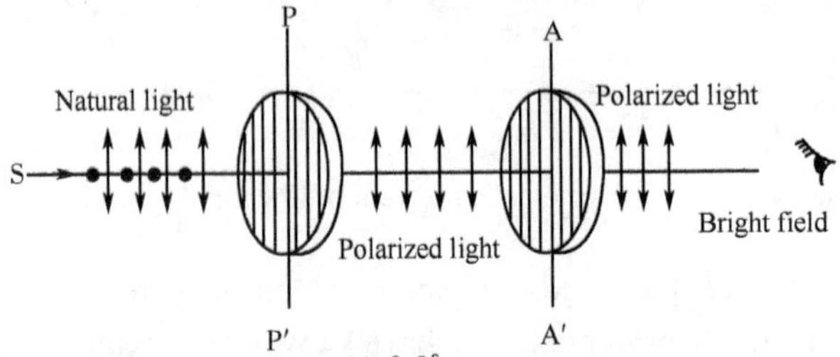

(a) θ=0°

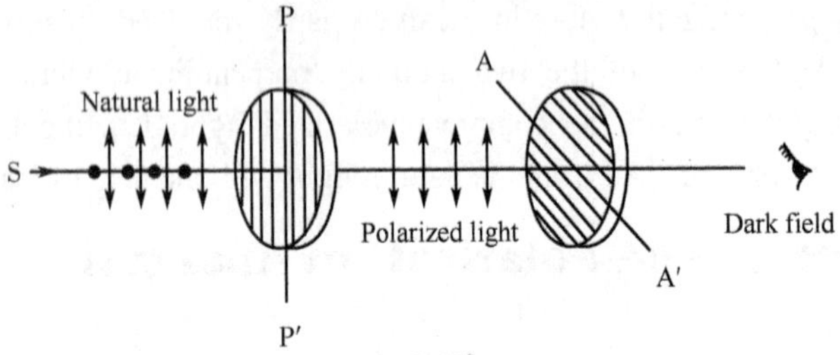

(b) θ=90°

Figure 9-21 Polarizer and polarization analyzer

The polarization analyzer can be used not only for distinguish the nature light from polarized light, but also for determining polarization direction.

9.4.3 Malus Law

In Figure 9-22, PP′ and AA′ represent a polarizer and an analyzer respectively, where θ is the angle between their polarization directions. Assume the intensity of polarized light passed through PP′ is I_0, and its amplitude is E_0. Here, E_0 is decomposed into two mutually perpendicular components (E_1 and E_2), and E_1 has the same direction with the polarization direction of AA′, so

$$E_1 = E_0 \cos\theta$$
$$E_2 = E_0 \sin\theta$$

For the function of the analyzer, it will just allow the component E_1 which is parallel to its polarization direction passing through and block the component E_2.

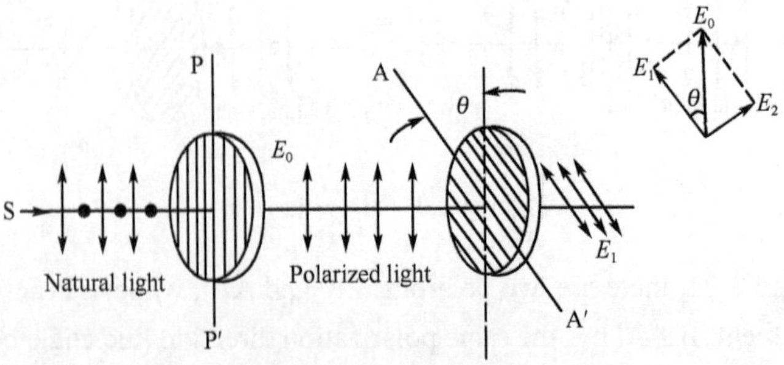

Figure 9-22 Malus law

Because the intensity of light is proportion directly to the amplitude, i.e., $E_1^2 = E_0^2 \cos^2\theta$, the intensity of light passing through the polarization analyzer AA′ should be

$$I = I_0 \cos^2\theta \tag{9-22}$$

Equation (9-22) is called Malus law. This law shows that: The intensity of the polarized light passed through the analyzer depends on the polarization direction of the analyzer. After passing through the analyzer, the polarized light with the original intensity of I_0 will change its intensity to $I_0 \cos^2\theta$.

Example 9-6 There are two light sources with the different intensities located at the same place. Now, they are observed with the same pair of polaroids (one is as polarizer, and the other is as the polarization analyzer). When the angle between their polarization directions is 30°, the ray of natural light from one source is allowed to pass through them; and when the angle between their polarization directions is 60°, the ray of natural light from the other source is allowed to pass through them. Moreover, the intensities of the two rays of light passed through the polaroids in these two cases are just the same. Determine the ratio of the intensities of the two rays of nature light from the two light sources.

Solution: Assume that the intensity of the first ray of natural light is I_1, and the intensity of the second ray of natural light is I_2. We know that the intensities should be reduced to half of the original values, which are $I_1/2$ and $I_2/2$ respectively, after they passed through the polarizer; and we also know that the intensities of the rays of light passed the polaroids $I_1' = I_2'$. According to Malus law, there are

$$I_1' = \frac{I_1}{2}\cos^2\theta_1 \qquad \theta_1 = 30^\circ$$

$$I_2' = \frac{I_2}{2}\cos^2\theta_2 \qquad \theta_2 = 60^\circ$$

So, the ratio of the intensities is

$$\frac{I_1}{I_2} = \frac{\cos^2 60^\circ}{\cos^2 30^\circ} = \frac{1}{3}$$

9.4.4 Optical Rotation

When a beam of polarized light passes through some special transparent materials, the vibration plane of this polarized light will rotate an angle as shown in Figure 9-23. This characteristic is called the **optical rotation** or the **optical activity** and the materials, such as quartz, turpentine, and the solutions of the saccharides, which have the strong activity of the optical rotation, are called **optically active materials**. The phenomenon that the vibration plane of a polarized light rotates an angle after penetrating through some material is called the **phenomenon of the optical rotation**, as shown in Figure 9-23.

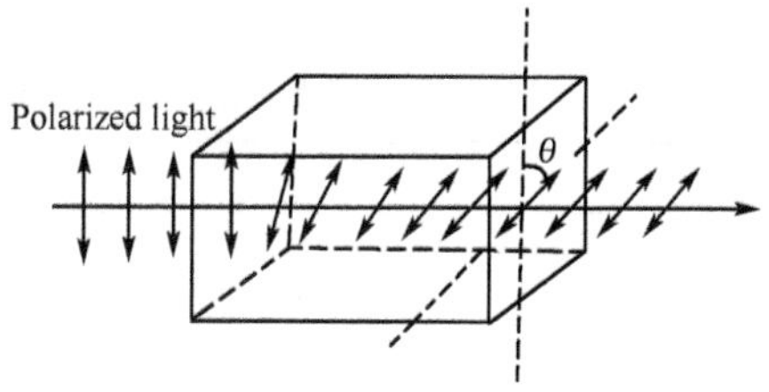

Figure 9-23 The phenomenon of the optical activity

The optical activity includes levo-rotation and dextro-rotation. Watching opposite to the ray of incident light, if its vibration plane is rotated clockwise, the corresponding optical activity is called **dextro-rotation**; and if its vibration plane is rotated counterclockwise, the corresponding optical activity is called **levo-rotation**. The crystals of quartz in nature and the solutions of different saccharides have the properties of the optical rotations of levo-rotation and dextro-rotation; glucose is dextrorotary, and fructose is levorotary.

According to the experiments, when a beam of monochromatic polarized light with certain wavelength penetrates through some optically active material, the rotation angle of its vibration plane is proportional directly to the thickness of the material. The corresponding formula is

$$\theta = \alpha l \tag{9-23}$$

This equation is called the optical activity law. Where the constant α is called the **specific rotation**, and different materials have different specific rotations. Moreover, the specific rotation is also related to the wavelength. Table 9-1 represents how the specific rotation is changed when the wavelength changes.

Table 9-1 The specific rotations of quartz for different wavelengths

λ (Å)	α (°/mm)
4046.56	48.945
4358.34	41.548
5085.82	29.728
5460.72	25.535
5892.90	21.724
6438.47	18.023
7281.35	13.924

In a solution, the rotation angle of vibration plane is also in proportional directly to the concentration of the solution C besides to its thickness l.

$$\theta = \alpha' C l \tag{9-24}$$

where α' is the **specific rotation of the solute** with the unit of (°)·cm^3/(dm·g), which is related to the wavelength of incident light and temperature of the solution. Based on Equation (9-24), the concentration of an optical rotary solution can be detected with the instrument called the polarimeter. Figure 9-24 is the basic principle diagram of the polarimeter. A beam of natural light emitted from the monochromatic light source (a sodium lamp) is transformed to a plane polarized light by the polarizer A, and then the rotation angle of vibration plane can be detected by the polarization analyzer B after the polarized light passes through the sample solution poured in the glass tube T. Generally, the units of θ, C, and l are respectively (°), g/cm^3, and dm. The specific rotations of some medicines are also called their specific rotary powers, the specific rotary powers of some medicines are listed in Table 9-2. In pharmacology analyses, we can measure the rotation angle of some solution with a polarimeter first, then find out the specific rotation of its solute. Finally, by applying Equation (9-24) we can detect the concentration of the solution reliably. So, this is a widely adopted method.

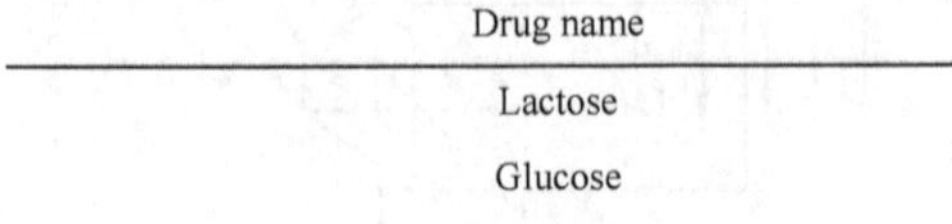

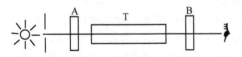

Figure 9-24 Principle diagram of the polarimeter

Table 9-2 The specific rotations of some medicines

Drug name	α' [(°)·cm^3/(dm·g)]
Lactose	+52.2-+52.6
Glucose	+52.2-+53
Cane sugar	+65.9
Cassia oil	−1-+1
Castor oil	+50 above
Menthol	−49-+50
Camphor (alcoholic solution)	+41-+43
Santonin (alcoholic solution)	−170-−175

9.4.5 Optical Rotation Saccharometer

A saccharometer is an optical measurement instrument designed base on the principle of optical rotation, its structural diagram is shown in Figure 9-25. Linear polarized light produced by polarizer P_1 passes through a solution of saccharides, and the rotation angle of vibration plane θ can be detected with the polarization analyzer P_2. Then, the concentration of the solution C can be determined by Equation (9-24). This method is not only reliable but also fast.

Example 9-7 There is a piece of quartz crystal of dextro-rotation placed perpendicularly with its surface to the optical axis. Its optical rotation can just offset the rotation of the vibration plane of the yellow sodium light with the wavelength of 5892.90 Å caused by a solution. This solution is the solution of levorotary fructose with the concentration of 10% and the length of 20 cm. What is the thickness of the quartz crystal piece? Here we known the specific rotation of this kind of fructose is 88.16 °·cm^3/(dm·g).

Solution: Assume that the thickness of the quartz crystal piece is l, based on Equation (9-23) and Equation (9-24), we have

$$\alpha l = \alpha' C l'$$

According to Table 9-1, we know that $\alpha = 21.724°/\text{mm}$, l' is the length of fructose solution. Hereby,

$$l = \frac{\alpha' C l'}{\alpha} = \frac{88.16 \times 0.10 \times 2.0}{21.724} = 0.81 \text{ mm}$$

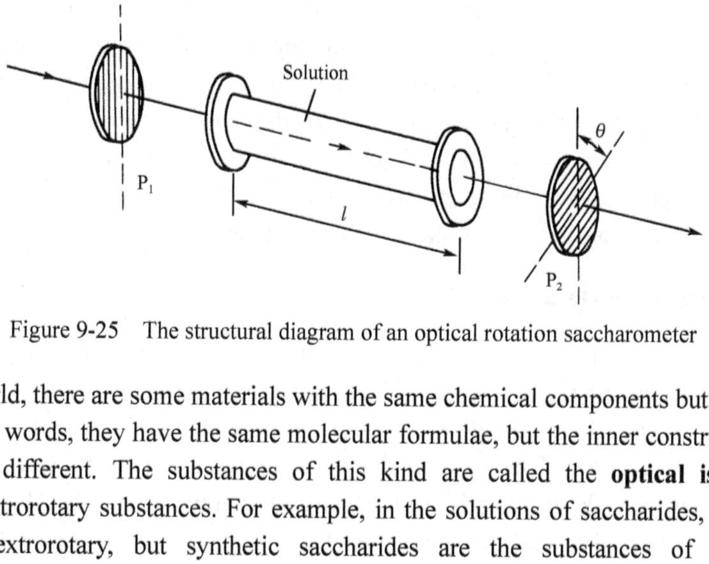

Figure 9-25 The structural diagram of an optical rotation saccharometer

In natural world, there are some materials with the same chemical components but different chemical structures. In other words, they have the same molecular formulae, but the inner constructional sequences of molecules are different. The substances of this kind are called the **optical isomers**, including levorotary and dextrorotary substances. For example, in the solutions of saccharides, the saccharides in nature are all dextrorotary, but synthetic saccharides are the substances of levo-rotation and dextro-rotation with half and half. Creatures prefer the dextro-rotary saccharides to the levo-rotary ones for digestive absorption. In addition, proteins are composed of over twenty kinds of amino acids, and the amino acids inside the creatures are all levorotary except the simplest glycine. This means the amino acids to construct any proteins of any kinds of creatures are all levorotary, no matter what kinds of creatures from which the proteins come. But the synthetic amino acids are equally the substances of levo-rotation and dextro-rotation.

Many organic medicines and alkaloid, all kinds of saccharides and amino acids inside creatures have the optical rotation; and they include levorotary and dextrorotary optical isomers. It is important to distinguish levo-rotation from dextro-rotation for understanding the structures of molecules and their properties. Although the levorotary and dextrorotary optical isomers of some medicine have the same molecular formula, the therapeutic effects of them may be completely different. For example, only the levorotary chloramphenicol has curative effect, the synthetic syntomycin is the mixture of levorotary chloramphenicol and dextrorotary chloramphenicol, so its therapeutic effect is only half of the pure levorotary syntomycin. In general, the optical rotation saccharometer is also used to study the levo-rotation and the dextro-rotation of substances.

9.5 Absorption of Light

9.5.1 Absorption of Light

When a light wave passes through some medium, its energy will be absorbed more or less, which results in its intensity reduces with the depth of penetration (It should be noted that the absorption discussed in this section does not include the reduction of the intensity caused by scattering).

The essence of the absorption of media to light is the interaction between light and molecules and atoms in media. A part of light energy is transformed to the energies of molecules and atoms, and this results in the reduction of the light energy or the absorption of light on the macroscopic viewpoint.

In general, the absorption is selective. In other words, for the lights with different wavelengths there will be different absorbing degrees. For example, the absorption of quartz to the visible light is extremely little, and that to the infrared light with the wavelength of 3.5-5.0 μm is very intense. The former is called the general absorption, which has the character of absorbing with little and being almost fixed in a given wavelength range. The latter is called the selective absorption, which has the character of absorbing with a lot and changing the degree of absorption remarkably for different wavelengths. The absorption of every substance to light consists of these two kinds. That is to say, a certain substance which is transparent to some wavelength ranges may be non-transparent to the other wavelength ranges. For quartz, it is transparent to the visible light and non-transparent to infrared light.

9.5.2 Absorption Laws

A ray of monochromatic light with the intensity of I_0 is perpendicularly incident onto a homogeneous substance with the thickness of l, as shown in Figure 9-26. It is assume that there is a film of the substance with the thickness of dx at the place with the distance of x from the surface. When the light arrives at the film its intensity is I_x; and there must be a differential intensity reduction of dI_x after the light passing through the film. It can be proved that this reduction of light intensity dI_x is proportional to both the intensity of the light when it arrives at the film I_x and the thickness of the film dx, i.e.,

$$-\mathrm{d}I_x = kI_x\mathrm{d}x$$

where k is called the **absorption coefficient**, which is related to the property of the substance and the wavelength of incident light. For dI_x is a negative quantity, the negative sign is put into the equation. The above equation can be also rewritten as

$$\frac{\mathrm{d}I_x}{I_x} = -k\mathrm{d}x$$

To perform the integral between 0-l, and assume the intensity of incident light is I_0, and the intensity of the light penetrated is I, we have

$$\int_{I_0}^{I} \frac{\mathrm{d}I_x}{I_x} = -k\int_0^l \mathrm{d}x$$

or

$$\ln I - \ln I_0 = -kl$$

i.e.,

$$I = I_0 e^{-kl} \tag{9-25}$$

Equation (9-25) is called **Lambert law**. By this equation we can find that the intensity of light decreases exponentially with the increase of the thickness of the substance, i.e., the absorption to light increases sharply with the increase of the thickness.

Experiments indicate that, when light is absorbed by the solute dissolved in some transparent solvent, the absorption coefficient k is proportional directly to the concentration of the solution C, i.e., $k = \chi C$, where χ is called **molar absorption coefficient**, which is only dependent on the molecular property of the solute rather than the concentration of the solution. In this way, Equation (9-25) can be expressed as

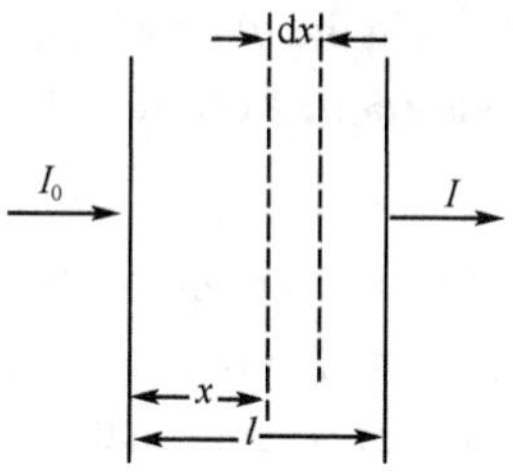

Figure 9-26 The absorption of light

$$I = I_0 e^{-\chi Cl} \tag{9-26}$$

The equation above is called **Lambert-Beer law**. It suggests that the light energy absorbed is proportional directly to the number of molecules in light path, and it is only correct when the absorption capacity of every molecule is not affected by the surrounding molecules. Therefore, this law is only applicable for the solutions with lower concentrations.

On the condition that the above law is tenable, the concentration of a solution can be determined by detecting the proportion of the light absorbed in the solution with Equation (9-26).

The important application of Lambert-Beer law is to detect the concentrations of solutions. Let a monochromatic light passes respectively through the congener solution with a standard concentration and the solution with unknown concentration of the same thickness. Because the concentrations are different, the absorptions to the light are different; and the intensities of the light penetrated will be different, too. Based on this, the concentration of the unknown solution can be determined. This method is called **colorimetric method**, which is a commonly applied method for pharmacology analysis.

In biology and chemistry, Equation (9-26) can be rewritten as

$$\frac{I}{I_0} = e^{-\chi Cl}$$

where I and I_0 are still the intensities of incident light and penetrated light respectively, and C and l are the concentration and the thickness of the solution respectively.

To assume

$$T = \frac{I}{I_0}$$

that is $T = e^{-\chi Cl}$, therefore we have

$$\lg T = -\chi Cl \lg e$$

If again to assume $A = -\lg T$ and $\varepsilon = \chi \lg e$, we have

$$A = \varepsilon Cl \tag{9-27}$$

where ε is called the **extinction constant**, which is related to the kind of the absorption substance. Its unit is m^2/mol. A is called the **absorbance**, which indicates the extent of the absorption to the light. The bigger the value of A is, the stronger the absorption to the light will be. In addition, $T=\frac{I}{I_0}$ is called the **transmissivity** or the **transmittance**.

Equation (9-27) indicates that the absorbance is proportional directly to the product of the concentration and the thickness of the solution.

Example 9-8 The absorption coefficients of the glass and the air are $k_1 = 10^{-4}\,\text{m}^{-1}$ and $k_2 = 10^{-7}\,\text{m}^{-1}$, respectively. Determine the thickness of the air through which the light absorbed is equal to the light absorbed in the glass with the thickness of 1 cm.

Solution: According to Lambert law, the intensity of light absorbed by some substance is

$$I_0 - I = I_0(1-\text{e}^{-kl})$$

When two beams of light with the same intensity penetrate respectively through the glass and the air, if the light absorbed in the glass with the thickness of l_1 and the light absorbed in the air with the thickness of l_2 are equal, there must be

$$1-\text{e}^{-k_1 l_1} = 1-\text{e}^{-k_2 l_2}$$

i.e.,

$$k_1 l_1 = k_2 l_2$$

$$l_2 = \frac{k_1 l_1}{k_2} = \frac{10^{-4}\times 10^{-2}}{10^{-7}}\,10\,\text{m}$$

That is to say, the light absorbed by the glass with the thickness of 1 cm is corresponding to the light absorbed by the air with the thickness of 10 m.

A Brief Summarization of This Chapter

(1)Interference of light:

1) The conditions of coherent light: Two light waves with the same frequency and the common oscillation direction, meanwhile, the phase difference between them is fixed.

2) The ways to get coherent light waves: The method of the division of wave front and method of the division of amplitude.

(2) Optical path: The product of the refractive index of some medium and the geometrical path of the light propagated in it, denoted as

$$\delta = nr$$

(3)The relationship between the phase difference and the optical path difference: $\Delta\varphi = \frac{2\pi}{\lambda}\delta$

(4)Young's double-slit interference:

1) The condition for bright bands: $\delta = \frac{yd}{D} = \pm k\lambda$ or $y = \pm k\frac{D}{d}\lambda$, $(k=0,1,2,\cdots)$

2) The condition for dark bands:

$$\delta = \frac{yd}{D} = \pm(2k+1)\frac{\lambda}{2} \quad \text{or} \quad y = \pm(2k+1)\frac{D}{d}\cdot\frac{\lambda}{2}, \quad (k=0,1,2,\cdots)$$

Where D is the distance between the double-slit and the screen, and d is the distance between the double slits.

(5) Film interference:

1) The condition of the interference with bright fringe: $\delta = 2nd - \frac{\lambda}{2} = k\lambda$ $\quad (k=0,1,2,\cdots)$

2) The condition of the interference with dark fringe: $\delta = 2nd - \frac{\lambda}{2} = (2k-1)\frac{\lambda}{2}$ $(k = 1, 2, 3, \cdots)$

(6) Single-slit diffraction:

1) When the diffraction angle meets the condition of $a\sin\theta = \pm 2k \cdot \frac{\lambda}{2} = \pm k\lambda$ the dark band would appear.

2) When the diffraction angle meets the condition of $a\sin\theta = \pm(2k+1)\cdot\frac{\lambda}{2}$ the bright band would appear.

(7) Grating diffraction:

1) Grating constant: $d = a + b$ (a is the width of the slit, and b is the width of the scratched strip)

2) Grating equation: $\delta = d\sin\theta = \pm k\lambda$ $(k = 0, 1, 2, \cdots)$, the bright band will appear when the grating equation is satisfied.

(8) Malus law: When a beam of polarized light with the intensity of I_0 passes through an analyzer, its intensity becomes $I_0 \cos^2\theta$ (where θ is the angle between the polarization directions of the polarizer and the analyzer).

(9) Lambert-Beer law: $I = I_0 e^{-\chi Cl}$.

Exercises 9

9-1. In the experiment of Young's double-slit interference, the distance between the double slits is 0.2 mm, and the distance between the double-slit and the screen is 80 cm. On the screen the distance between the first order bright band and the third order bright band is 5 mm. What is the wavelength of the monochromatic light used in this experiment?

9-2. In the experiment of Young's double-slit interference, the third order bright band with the wavelength of 500 nm is overlapping with a third dark band with the other light. What is the wavelength of the other light?

9-3. A beam of parallel light with the wavelength of 500 nm irradiates on a slit with the width of 0.1 mm. There is a lens with the focal length of 500 cm located behind the slit and a screen is placed at the focal plane of the lens. What are the width of the central bright band and the width of other order bright band?

9-4. A beam of monochromatic light irradiates perpendicularly on a grating which is made by scratching one thousand strips within 1 mm. The angle between the first order of bright band and the direction of incident light is 30°. What is the wavelength of the monochromatic light?

9-5. A beam of monochromatic light with the wavelength of 600 nm irradiates perpendicularly on a grating and the angle between the first order of bright band and the direction of incident light is 28.7°. How many strips are scratched within 1 mm?

9-6. A beam of monochromatic light with the wavelength of λ irradiates perpendicularly to a transparent film with the refractive index $n > 1$. If we want to enhance the intensity of the reflected light, what is the thinnest thickness of the transparent film?

9-7. A light source is observed with a pair of polaroids and the angle between their polarization directions is 45°; meanwhile, another light source is observed with a pair of polaroids and the angle between their polarization directions is 60°. The intensities of the two rays of light observed through these two pairs of polaroids are just the same. Determine the ratio of the intensities of the two rays of nature light from the two light sources.

9-8. When a ray of light penetrates through certain solution, the corresponding transmissivity is 1/2. If the thickness of the solution is fixed and its concentration is changed, the transmissivity is measured to be 1/8 then. What is the ratio of the two concentrations of the solution?

9-9. For certain solution of cane sugar, the specific rotation of it is 66.4° $cm^3/(dm \cdot g)$ to the sodium light at the temperature of 20 ℃. Now pour some of the solution fully into a polarization tube with length of 20 cm and detect its rotation angle as 8.3℃. Determine the concentration of this solution of cane sugar.

9-10. The absorption coefficient of the glass is $10^{-2}\,cm^{-1}$ and the absorption coefficient of the air is $10^{-5}\,cm^{-1}$. If the light absorbed by the glass with the thickness of 2 cm is just equal to that absorbed by a layer of the air with some thickness, determine the thickness of the air layer.

Chapter 10 Geometrical Optics

After a light ray passes by an obstacle whose size is much larger than the wavelength of the light ray, diffraction is not obviously visible. In this case, the wave nature of light is negligible and we can consider that light travels straight. In geometrical optics, the radial lines coming outward from the light source are called light rays. The transmitting regularities of light rays in transparent media and image formations of objects are discussed with geometrical methods in geometrical optics. The theoretical fundamentals of geometrical optics are the law of light traveling straight, the law of light traveling independently, the law of reflection and the law of refraction.

The theories of geometrical optics have been widely used in primary designs of optical instruments. This chapter mainly introduces the basic principles of geometrical optics and regularities of image formation. Based on these, the dioptrics of human eyes, image formations of optical microscopes and fiber optics will also be studied.

10.1 Refraction on a Spherical Surface

10.1.1 Refraction on a Spherical Surface

Refraction happens when a light ray strikes on the interface of two transparent materials. If the interface has the shape of a section from the surface of a sphere, the refractive phenomenon on it is called refraction on a spherical surface.

1. System of Refraction on a Spherical Surface

Figure 10-1 shows a system of refraction on a spherical surface. *MN* is the spherical refractive interface, the center of curvature is point *C* and the radius is *r*. The principal axis is a straight line drawn through point *C*. The spherical surface *MN* crosses the principal axis at point *P* that is called the vertex of the spherical surface. Assume the left medium has the refraction index of n_1 and the right medium has the refraction index of n_2 ($n_1<n_2$). Light rays that are near and parallel to the principal axis are from a light source, refracted from the left material into the right one, and cross the principal axis at the image point *I*. The distance from the object point *O* to the vertex *P* is the **object length** *u*. And the distance from the image point *I* to the vertex *P* is the **image length** v .

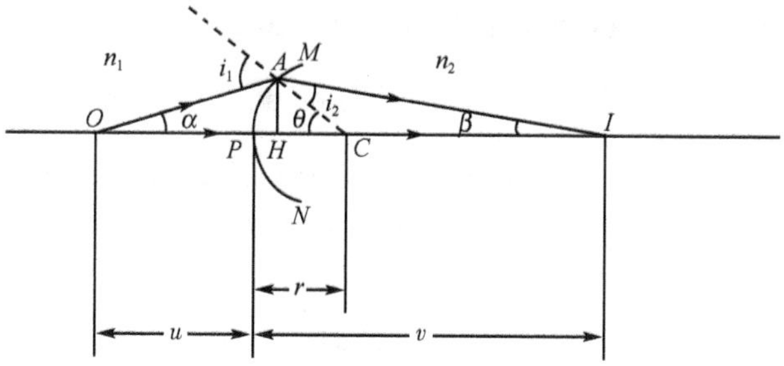

Figure 10-1 System of refraction on a spherical surface

2. Formula of Refraction on a Spherical Surface

First, let's discuss the regularity of image formation obeyed by paraxial rays from the object point *O*.

Assume two incident rays entering a spherical surface. Ray *OP* travels along the principal axis through the vertex and follows a radius of the spherical surface; as a result, the ray strikes the surface perpendicularly. Another paraxial ray *OA* travels along a line that passes in any arbitrary direction, and therefore passes through point *I* after refraction from the interface. The image of the object point *O* is point *I*. A normal line *AC* is drawn through point *A*, and the corresponding angle of incidence is i_1 and the corresponding angle of refraction is i_2.

According to the law of refraction, we obtain:

$$n_1 \sin i_1 = n_2 \sin i_2$$

Because the ray *OA* is near and parallel to the principal axis, angles i_1 and i_2 should be very small. So we have the approximate expressions of $\sin i_1 \approx i_1$ and $\sin i_2 \approx i_2$. As a result, the equation above can be rewritten as the approximate equation

$$n_1 i_1 = n_2 i_2$$

Consider the two triangles$\triangle OAC$ and $\triangle IAC$, $i_1 = \alpha + \theta$, $i_2 = \theta - \beta$. Substituting these values for i_1 and i_2 into the equation above and rearranging it, we have

$$n_1 \alpha + n_2 \beta = (n_2 - n_1)\theta$$

A vertical line passing through point *A* is drawn at point *H*. α, β, θ are small enough to follow the approximations for small angles, so their radians can be represented by their tangents $\tan\alpha \approx \alpha$, $\tan\beta \approx \beta$, $\tan\theta \approx \theta$, i.e.,

$$\alpha = \frac{\overline{AH}}{u}, \quad \beta = \frac{\overline{AH}}{v}, \quad \theta = \frac{\overline{AH}}{r}$$

Substituting these relations into the equation above, Equation (10-1) is gotten by eliminating $\overline{AH}$.

$$\frac{n_1}{u} + \frac{n_2}{v} = \frac{n_2 - n_1}{r} \tag{10-1}$$

Equation (10-1) is referred to the **law of refraction on a spherical surface.** It applies in concave or convex spherical imaging, when the light rays near and parallel to the principal axis.

We must agree on a sign convention in the application of Equation (10-1). It is object and image distances are both positive when the object and image are both real and both negative when virtual. The radius of curvature is positive when incident light ray strikes toward the convex surface and negative when incident light ray strikes toward the concave surface. Light ray travels initially from left to right toward the spherical surface. The order of n_1 and n_2 are dependent on the direction in which incident light ray travels through the spherical surface.

3. Refractive Power, Focal Point, and Focal Length

The right part of Equation (10-1) $\frac{n_2 - n_1}{r}$ depends on the refractive index of the two materials and the radius of curvature. For a given material and a spherical surface, it is a constant. The quantity is used to describe the extent to which a spherical surface refracts light and referred to the **refractive power** Φ of a spherical surface.

$$\Phi = \frac{n_2 - n_1}{r} \tag{10-2}$$

If the unit of the radius of curvature is m in SI units, refractive power of a spherical surface is measured in **diopter**, donated by D. From Equation (10-2), refractive power of a spherical surface is inversely proportional to the radius of curvature, and proportional to the difference of the refractive index of the two materials. The larger r is, the smaller Φ will be, while, the bigger the difference between n_1 and n_2, the stronger the refraction power is.

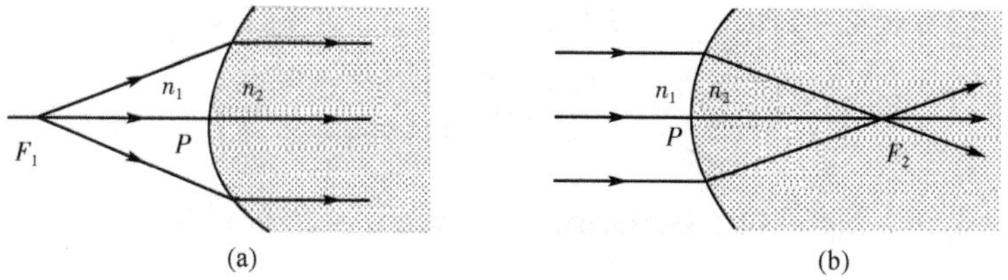

Figure 10-2 Focal point and focal length of a spherical surface

If the source of light lies at some point F_1 on the principal axis, the light rays from it will be changed into the parallel rays after being refracted by a spherical surface, as shown in Figure 10-2 (a). The point F_1 is referred to the first focal point of the refractive system. The distance from point F_1 to the vertex P is called the first focal length, denoted by f_1. Substituting $v=\infty$ into Equation (10-1), we obtain the first focal length as expressed by Equation (10-3)

$$f_1=\frac{n_1}{n_2-n_1}r \tag{10-3}$$

When the light rays traveling parallel with the principal axis are refracted on a spherical surface, the refracted rays will be focused at point F_2 on the axis, as shown in Figure 10-2 (b). This point is defined as the second focal point of the refractive system. The distance from point F_2 to the vertex P is called the second focal length, denoted by f_2. Substituting $u=\infty$ into Equation (10-1), we obtain the second focal length

$$f_2=\frac{n_2}{n_2-n_1}r \tag{10-4}$$

According to Equation (10-3) and Equation (10-4), the first focal length f_1 is usually not equal to the second focal length f_2 and the values of them could be positive or negative. The values of two focal lengths depend on the refractive indices of two materials and the radius of curvature. When f_1 and f_2 are positive, the points F_1 and F_2 are real focal points, because refractive system causes incident parallel rays to converge at the focal point. When f_1 and f_2 are negative, the points F_1 and F_2 are virtual focal points, which cause incident parallel rays to diverge after exiting the system.

Comparing Equation (10-3) with Equation (10-4), we find

$$\frac{f_1}{f_2}=\frac{n_1}{n_2} \tag{10-5}$$

The relation between two focal lengths and refractive power reduces to

$$\Phi=\frac{n_2-n_1}{r}=\frac{n_1}{f_1}=\frac{n_2}{f_2} \tag{10-6}$$

Using Equation (10-6), we have that the refractive power is equal although the two focal distances are not equal for a spherical surface.

Example 10-1 Converge light rays are propagating through a medium with the refractive index of n=1 and strike onto another medium with the refractive index of n'=1.5, as shown in Figure 10-3. The vertex of the light rays is at the point of 3 cm to the right side of the concave interface with the radius of 3 cm. Determine the location of the image.

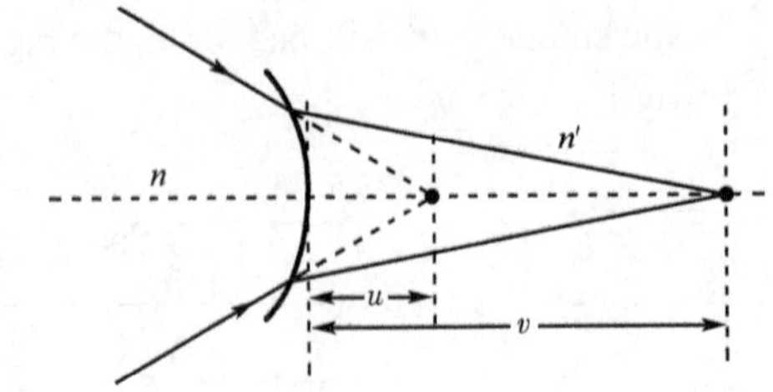

Figure 10-3 Refraction on a concave spherical surface

Solution: Using the equation for a spherical surface with n=1, n'=1.5 and u= –3cm, we have

$$\frac{1}{-3}+\frac{1.50}{\upsilon}=\frac{1.50-1}{-3}$$

The image distance is υ= 9 cm. The positive value of υ indicates that the image is a real image and is behind the concave interface as shown in Figure 10-3.

10.1.2 System of Coaxial Spherical Surfaces

When a system is consisted of two or more spherical surfaces, and the curvature centers and vertical points of these spherical surfaces are on the same straight line, this system is called the system of coaxial spherical surfaces. The straight line is called the principal axis of the system. For example, human eye can be considered as a system of coaxial spherical surfaces.

For the light rays near and parallel to the principal axis, the image of a system of coaxial spherical surfaces can be determined by the repeated applications of the simple equation to each of the spherical surfaces. The image produced by the first spherical surface serves as the object for the second one; then the image produced by the second one serves as the object for the third one to determine the image produced by the third one, and so on; until the image produced by the last one of the system is found.

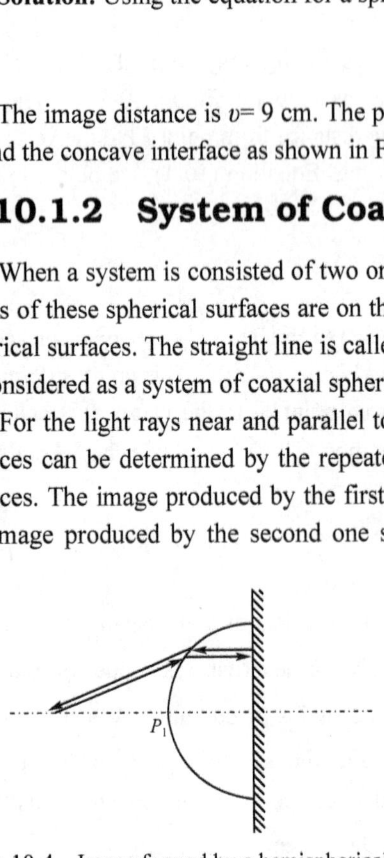

Figure 10-4 Image formed by a hemispherical glass

Example10-2 A glass hemisphere has the refractive index of 1.5 and the radius of 5 cm. The plane surface of the hemisphere is plated as a silver-gilt mirror, as shown in Figure 10-4. When a small object is placed in front of the vertex with the distance of 10 cm, determine the location of the final image of the object formed by this system with the repeated method mentioned above.

Solution: For the first spherical surface, using the spherical surface equation with n_1=1.0, n_2=1.5, u_1=10 cm, r= 5 cm, we have

$$\frac{1.0}{10}+\frac{1.5}{\upsilon_1}=\frac{1.5-1.0}{5}$$

and we can get $\upsilon_1=\infty$

After refracted on the first refractive surface, light rays travel parallel to the principal axis, are reflected in the silver-gilt mirror, and strike back on the spherical surface. Here, the spherical surface is considered as the second refractive surface. Therefore, light rays travel parallel to the principal axis from right to left toward the second refractive surface, $u_2=\infty$. Using the spherical surface equation

$$\frac{1.5}{\infty}+\frac{1.0}{v_2}=\frac{1.0-1.5}{-5}$$

we have

$$v_2=10\ \text{cm}$$

The final image lies 10 cm left to the vertex, as shown in Figure 10-4.

10.2 Lenses

A lens, made up of a transparent medium, is a system of coaxial spherical surfaces with only two refracting surfaces and one or both the surfaces being parts of the curved surfaces. The commonly used lenses are spherical lenses, which have one or both of the refracting surfaces being spherical surfaces. Other kinds of lenses are those which have one or both of the refracting surfaces shaped as cylindrical surfaces, elliptical surfaces or other forms. In this book or other textbooks, only thin spherical lenses are dealt with, unless there are special declarations.

If the central thickness of a lens is small compared with the distance from the object to the image and with the radiuses of curvature of its spherical surfaces, its thickness can be neglected in solving problems about image formation and it is called the **thin lens**. According to the structures, lenses can be classified into convex lenses and concave lenses. Lenses can also be divided into converging lenses and diverging lenses according to the optical properties.

10.2.1 Thin-lens Equation

A thin-lens with the index of refraction n is placed in a medium with the index of refraction n_0, as shown in Figure 10-5. Light rays from an object point O are refracted by the thin-lens and converge at point I. The drawing shows that the object distance, image distance and the radius of curvature of the first front surface of the lens are respectively u_1, v_1, and r_1. The drawing also shows that the object distance, image distance and the radius of curvature of the back surface of the lens are respectively u_2, v_2, and r_2. The object distance and image distance of the thin-lens are respectively u and v. Since the thickness of thin-lens is negligible, these parameters are measured from the optical center and the relationship between the parameters u_1, v_1, u_2, v_2 and u, v is given by $u_1=u$, $v_1=-u_2$, $v_2=v$. Substituting these quantities into the equation For the refraction of a spherical surface, i.e. Equation (10-1).

For the two refraction interfaces, we have

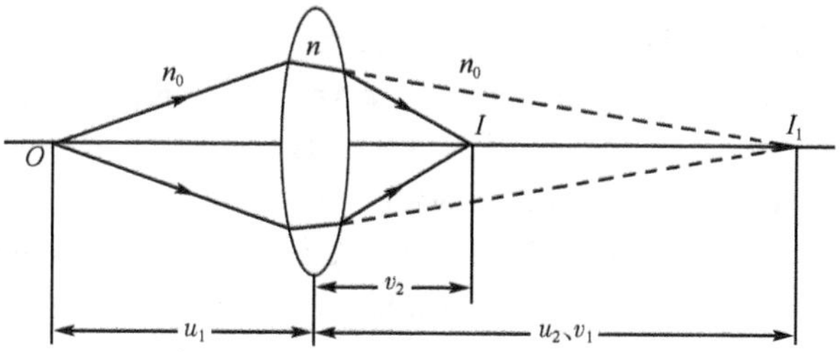

Figure 10-5 Image formed by a thin lens

$$\frac{n_0}{u}+\frac{n}{v_1}=\frac{n-n_0}{r_1},\quad \frac{n}{-v_1}+\frac{n_0}{v}=\frac{n_0-n}{r_2}$$

By combining the two equations above and rearranging terms, we have

$$\frac{1}{u}+\frac{1}{v}=\frac{n-n_0}{n_0}(\frac{1}{r_1}-\frac{1}{r_2}) \tag{10-7}$$

Because the air is the medium on both sides of the thin-lens, $n_0=1$, Equation (10-7) is simplified as

$$\frac{1}{u}+\frac{1}{v}=(n-1)(\frac{1}{r_1}-\frac{1}{r_2}) \tag{10-8}$$

Equation (10-7) and Equation (10-8) are important results known as the thin-lens equations. They are both applicable for both thin convex and thin concave lenses, and the signs of the quantities u, v, r_1 and r_2 in these expressions obey to the sign conventions used with the refraction of spherical surface.

There are two focal points for a thin lens. If the medium in front of the lens is the same as the medium at the back of the lens, these two focal distances can be proved to be equal i.e., $f_1=f_2=f$ by Equation (10-7) and the value is

$$f=[\frac{n-n_0}{n_0}(\frac{1}{r_1}-\frac{1}{r_2})]^{-1} \tag{10-9}$$

If the thin lens is placed in air, $n_0=1$, Equation (10-9) will be simplified as

$$f=[(n-1)(\frac{1}{r_1}-\frac{1}{r_2})]^{-1} \tag{10-10}$$

The focal distance of a thin lens depends on the material of the thin lens, the radiuses of curvature of its two spherical surfaces, and the medium where the thin lens is placed. Substituting Equation (10-10) into Equation (10-8), we find that

$$\frac{1}{u}+\frac{1}{v}=\frac{1}{f} \tag{10-11}$$

Equation (10-11) is an important result known as the **thin-lens Gauss formula**. It is applicable in the case of a thin lens which is in the same medium. The sign conventions are the same as previously mentioned. The shorter the focal length of a thin lens is, the larger refractive power of a thin lens is. Therefore, the reciprocal of the focal distance is used to describe the ability for a thin lens to refract light rays, it is called the refractive power of the lens, denoted by Φ,

$$\Phi=\frac{1}{f} \tag{10-12}$$

The refractive power of a converging lens is positive, while the refractive power of a diverging lens is negative. The unit of the refractive power is D in SI units. 1 diopter is 100 degree for the definition. For example, if someone has a pair of glasses of 200 degree, the corresponding refractive power should be 2 diopter, and the focal length is $f=0.5$ m and it works as a pair of hyperopia glasses.

Example 10-3 A plano-concave lens is made of the glass with the index of refraction 1.5. It has a concave spherical front surface with a radius of curvature of 20 cm and a planar rear surface with a radius of curvature of infinity. It is placed in water. Determine the focal length in the following cases: (1) When light travels from left to right toward the lens: (2) when light travels from right to left toward the lens (Index of refraction of water is 1.33).

Solution: Assume light travels toward concave surface, with the sign convention given, we have $r_1=-20$ cm, $r_2=\infty$. Substituting it into Equation (10-9), we get

$$f=[(\frac{1.5-1.33}{1.33})(\frac{1}{-20}-\frac{1}{\infty})]^{-1}$$

The focal length is

$$f = -156.5 \text{ cm}$$

Assume light travels toward a plane, with the sign convention given, we have $r_1 = \infty$, $r_2 = 20$ cm. Substituting them into Equation (10-9), we have

$$f = [(\frac{1.5-1.33}{1.33})(\frac{1}{\infty} - \frac{1}{20})]^{-1}$$

And the focal length is

$$f = -156.5 \text{ cm}$$

The result shows that a thin lens has the same focal length, if it is placed in the same medium, no matter which surface of the thin lens faces to the light.

10.2.2 Lenses in Combination

In practical applications, most of optical instruments to form images are consisted of two or more lenses. A coaxial system, in which two or more lenses with a common axis are used in combination, is called as **lenses in combination**. To find the final image, we begin by the repeated use of the thin-lens equation. This image produced by the first lens becomes the object for the second lens. The second image by the second lens then becomes the object for the third lens, and so on. Until the final image by the last lens of the coaxial system is found.

A system, which two lenses are so close in direct physical and almost contact with each other, is called the lenses in close combination, as shown in Figure 10-6. The equation of the closely combined lenses can be expressed as a simple formula, similar to Equation (10-11).

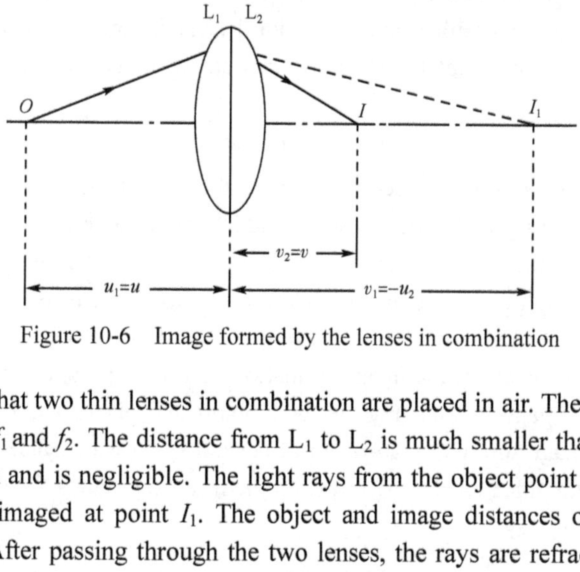

Figure 10-6 Image formed by the lenses in combination

Figure 10-6 shows that two thin lenses in combination are placed in air. The focal lengths of two thin lenses are, respectively, f_1 and f_2. The distance from L_1 to L_2 is much smaller than object distance, image distance and focal length and is negligible. The light rays from the object point O are refracted from the first thin-lens and then imaged at point I_1. The object and image distances of the first thin-lens are, respectively u_1 and v_1. After passing through the two lenses, the rays are refracted toward the axis and travel through the image point I on the right side of the combined lens. The object and image distances of the second thin-lens are, respectively, u_2 and v_2. Applying the equation for the thin-lens i.e. Equation (10-11) in L_1 and L_2, we have

$$\frac{1}{u_1} + \frac{1}{v_1} = \frac{1}{f_1}, \quad \frac{1}{u_2} + \frac{1}{v_2} = \frac{1}{f_2}$$

Assume that object and image distances of the coaxial system are, respectively, u and v, and set $u = u_1$, $v = v_2$. If d is much smaller and is negligible, $u_2 = d - v_1 \approx -v_1$, as shown in Figure 10-6. The equations above can also be rewritten as

$$\frac{1}{u}+\frac{1}{v_1}=\frac{1}{f_1}, \quad \frac{1}{-v_1}+\frac{1}{v}=\frac{1}{f_2}$$

By adding these two equations and rearranging terms, we have

$$\frac{1}{u}+\frac{1}{v}=\frac{1}{f_1}+\frac{1}{f_2} \tag{10-13}$$

Equation (10-13) can also be written as

$$\frac{1}{u}+\frac{1}{v}=\frac{1}{f} \tag{10-14}$$

where f is equivalent focal length and can be expressed by f_1 and f_2 as

$$\frac{1}{f}=\frac{1}{f_1}+\frac{1}{f_2} \tag{10-15}$$

The refractive powers of the two thin-lenses are, respectively, Φ_1 and Φ_2. The refractive power of the combined lens is denoted by Φ, and from Equation (10-15) we have

$$\Phi=\Phi_1+\Phi_2 \tag{10-16}$$

The refractive power of the system closely combined by n thin-lenses is the sum of the refractive powers of the n lenses in close contacted.

$$\Phi=\Phi_1+\Phi_2+\cdots+\Phi_n$$

Therefore, for a series of contacted thin lenses, the refractive power will be strengthened if they are the same kind; and it will be weakened if they are of different kind. After passing through two lenses in combination, if the light rays are neither converged nor diverged, the equivalent refractive power of this system of lenses is zero, which means the refractive powers of the two lenses have the same numerical value, i.e.,

$$\Phi_1+\Phi_2=0, \quad \Phi_1=-\Phi_2$$

The above equation is commonly used to measure the refractive power of a lens in diopter. For example, if a lens for the nearsighted to be measured and a known converging lens are contacted together, and the refractive power of the combination is measured as zero, i.e. the rays are neither converged nor diverged after passing through the combination, then the lens to be measured should have the refractive power of the same numerical value and of different sign as that of the converging lens.

For solving the problems about the image formations of thin-lenses, ray diagrams can be drawn to determine the location of image by knowing the focal points and planes and the center of the thin lens. Similarly, to locate the image formed by a system of coaxial spherical surfaces such as a thick lens, we make use of any two of the three special light rays to the three key points for lens and associate each of them with the corresponding ray.

10.2.3 Asymmetric Refractive System and Cylinder Lens

In geometric optics system, the plane passing through the principal axis is called **meridian plane**. The line at which the meridian plane crosses the refractive surface is called **meridian line**. For spherical lens, each meridian plane is a part of a circle with the same radius. That is, the radius of each meridian line is the same. The spherical lens is a symmetric refractive system. The refractive system of which the meridian line along each direction is different is called **asymmetric refractive system**.

Cylinder lens is one type of asymmetric refractive systems. Two surfaces of it are parts of a cylinder, as shown in Figure 10-7. There are two types of cylinder lens: Convex and concave lenses. Cylinder lens is applied in clinical and optometry to correct astigmatism. So it is necessary to know about the characters of image formed by cylinder lens.

One meridian plane looks like a cross section of a spherical lens. Light rays after passing through this meridian can be converged or diverged, as shown in Figure 10-8 (a). Another meridian perpendicular to the first one looks like a plane glass wedge, the rays travel through this meridian without any appreciable bending, as shown in Figure 10-8 (b). All rays from a point source converge at a focal line after passing through a converging cylinder lens, as shown in Figure 10-8 (c).

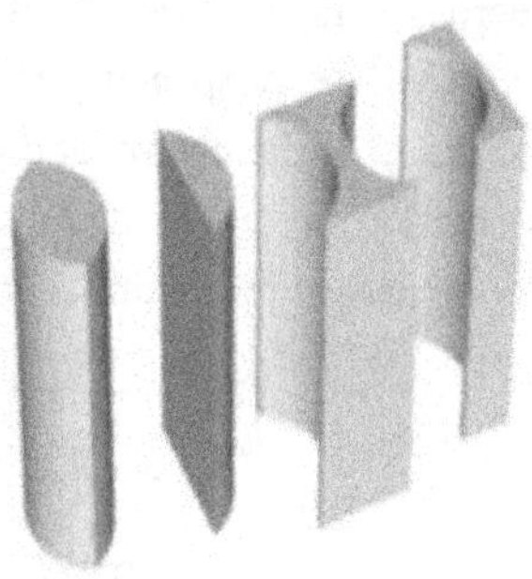

Figure 10-7 Cylinder lens

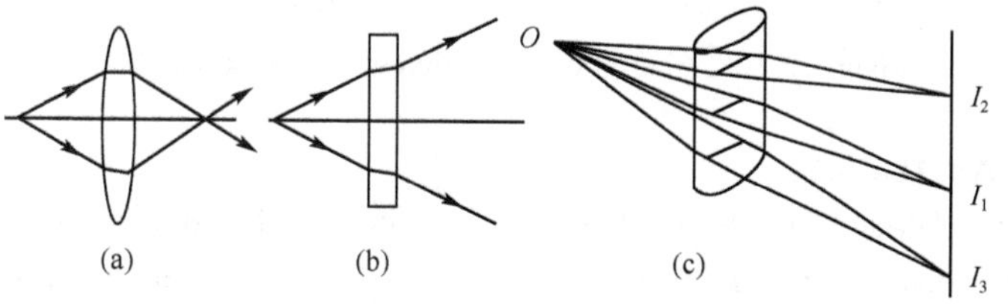

Figure 10-8 Image formed by a cylinder lens

10.2.4 Chromatic Aberration of Lens

In practice, rather than forming a sharp image theoretically, a single lens typically forms an image that is slightly out of focus. This lack of sharpness in lens is called **chromatic aberration**, which caused by numerous reasons. In this section, we will introduce the main two: Spherical aberration and chromatic aberration.

1. Spherical Aberration

When study the problem about spherical refraction, we can limit the incident rays as the paraxial rays i.e. only the rays, which are from a point lite and pass through the central part of the spherical lens, are able to converge on the axis. However, there are always abaxial rays concluded in practice. The refraction angle is bigger than the paraxial rays' when they pass through the fringe part of the lens, just as shown in Figure 10-9 (a). So the two kinds of ray can not converge on the same point after passing through the lens and refracting. What we obtain after image forming on a plane is not a luminous point, instead, it's a bright patch with blur fringe. This phenomenon is exerted by the spherical refraction, which is called the **spherical aberration**.

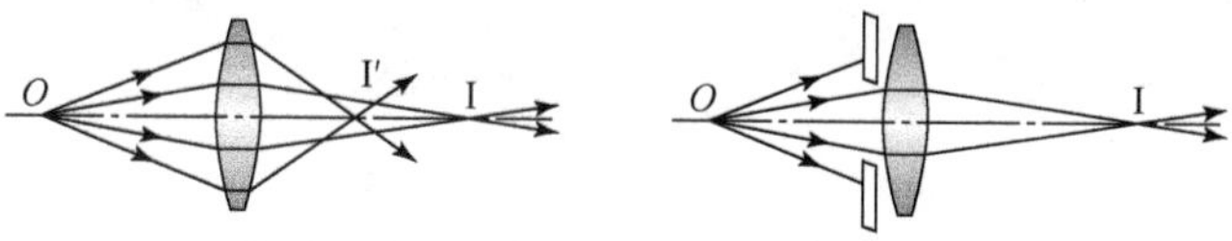

(a) Spherical lens aberration (b) Spherical lens (corrected aberration)

Figure 10-9 Spherical aberration and correction

Here are some solutions to rectify it.

(1) Place a diaphragm in front the lens, as shown in Figure 10-9 (b), which can interdict the abaxial rays and allow the paraxial ones passing through only. So we are able to gain a clear image. Owing to the rays passing through decreases, the luminance of the image fades after placing a diaphragm.

(2) Place a astigmatic lens behind the poly-lend. Because the spherical aberrations of two are opposite, such a lens group decreases the spherical aberration successfully by counteracting. However, it

decreases the dioptric strength as well.

(3) Use a special designed non-spherical lens, just as shown in Figure 10-10. The radiuses of curvature of the central and the fringe parts of it are different, which is able to maintain a good aberration correction so as to acquire the function in need. As the improvement of the fabrication process, non-spherical lens gains wild application.

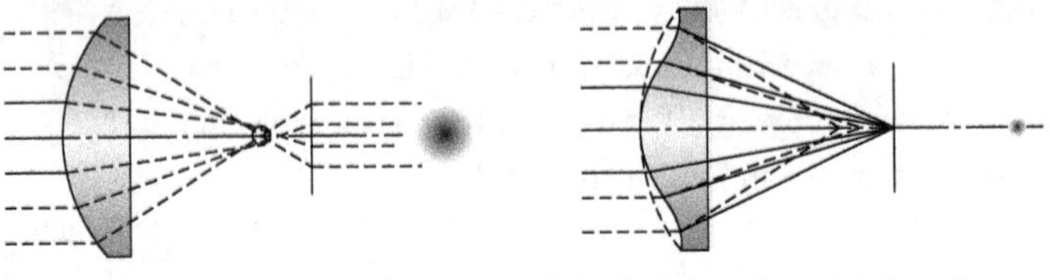

(a) Spherical lens aberration (b) Aspheric lens Corrected aberration

Figure10-10 Aberration correction by non-spherical lens

2. Chromatic Aberration

According to the Equation (10-9) we obtain that the focus distance of the thin lens is related to the refractive index of the lens material n, the radiuses of curvature r_1, r_2 of the two refractive planes and the medium of lens within. When both the radius of curvature and the medium are fixed, the optical properties of the lens are determined by the refractive index of the lens. Even the same material, the refractive index of different wavelengths of light is different. So, it's also different for the refraction of different colors of light after through the lens, as shown in Figure 10-11 (a). The white light parallel to the main optical axis is directed toward the lens, deflection of the violet light with short wavelength is more, while deflection of the red light with short wavelength is less. So rays with different wavelength cannot converge on the same point after through the lens and refraction. If the indecent rays are complex color rays, we will never obtain a luminous point in any plane, instead, it's a bright patch with blur fringe. We define the phenomenon that different wavelength cannot converge on the same point after through the lens and refraction as **Chromatic Aberration**. The thicker lens is, the more obvious the color difference is.

The chromatic aberration can be avoidable by using the point lite.

A common approach to reducing chromatic aberration is to combine the different poly and astigmatic lenses to compensate for the residual chromatic aberration of one lens by the chromatic aberration produced by the other lens, as shown in Figure 10-11 (b).

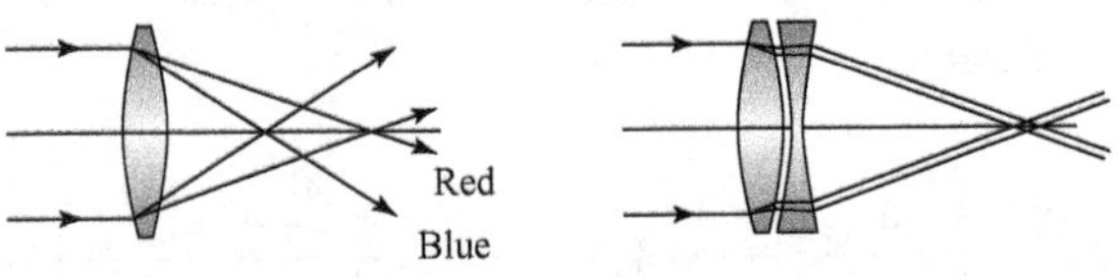

(a) (b)

Figure 10-11 Chromatic aberration lens and correction

In more sophisticated optical instruments, the lens system is more complex for it utilizes a variety of lens combinations to eliminate all kinds of aberrations to the maximum extent. When we talk about its working principles, we can simplify the lens model to replace complex systems according to the imaging law of coaxial spherical system.

10.3 Refraction of Human Eye

The human eye is an important organ to obtain information and is considered as a complex optical system, which can focus on objects located at various distances. Image principles and laws of human eye are discussed in this section from geometrical optics.

10.3.1 Anatomic Structure of the Eye

The eyeball is approximately spherical, as shown in Figure 10-12. In geometrical optics, the human eye is considered as coaxial spherical system, which can form images of the objects at different distance on the retina.

The front portion is a convex lens from the side view and is covered by a tough, transparent membrane, called the cornea and converged the light rays. The region behind the cornea is the iris, which is opaque. At the center of it is an opening called the pupil. The iris is a muscular diaphragm that not only controls the amount of light reaching the retina but also reduces chromatic aberration. Next comes the crystalline lens, a transparent and flexible tissue, double convex, which has an adjustable radius. A large part of the inner surface of the eye is covered with a delicate film of never fibers, which is called the retina. A clear liquid region among the cornea, the iris and the crystalline lens is the aqueous humor. And another jelly-like substance between lens and the retina is the vitreous humor, occupying about 80% of the total volume of the eye. The indices of refraction of both the aqueous humor and the vitreous humor are nearly equal to that of water. The main function of the aqueous humor and the vitreous humor is to fill the eye, then to keep the shape of the eye, and to reduce the vibration.

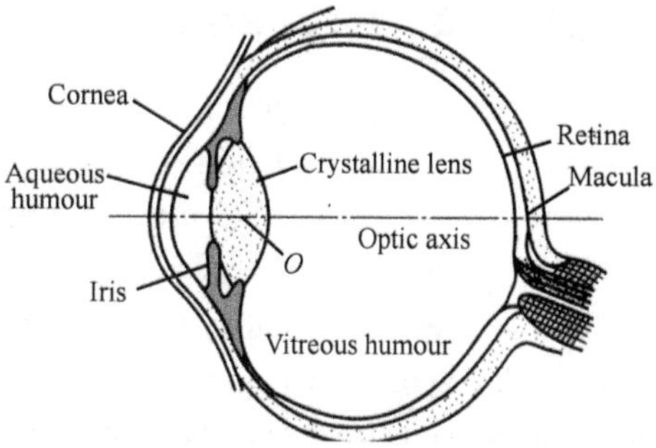

Figure 10-12 Cutaway view of human eyeball

The light rays from an object are refracted by the cornea, the iris and finally, the lens in turn to form the image on the retina. The cornea plays an important role in the lens system. It provides fine refractive power through changes in its curvature.

10.3.2 Optical Nature of the Eye

In geometrical optics, human eye can be considered as a coaxial spherical system. To simple problem human eye is simplified to a spherical surface, which is known as **reduced schematic eye**, as shown in Figure 10-13. The radius of convex interface (cornea) is r=5mm. The index of refraction in image space is 1.33. Retina is considered as the focal plane. By formula for a spherical surface, f_1=15 mm, f_2=20 mm.

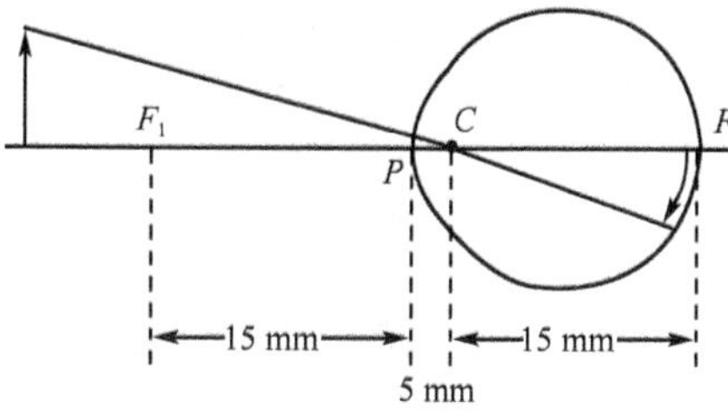

Figure 10-13 Reduced schematic eye

10.3.3 Accommodation

Compared with any other optical system, the human eye has an advantage: Images of the objects at different distance can be formed clearly on the retina. The process in which the human eye focuses on objects at different distances is called **accommodation** and occurs by changing the shape of lens.

The **far point** of the eye is the location of the farthest object on which the fully relaxed eye can focus. A person with normal eyesight can see objects very far away and thus has a far point located nearly infinity. A person who is nearsighted can focus on nearby objects but cannot clearly see objects far away. For such a person, the far point lies a few meters in front of the eye.

The point nearest the eye at which an object can be placed and generated a sharp image on the retina is called the **near point** of the eye. The ciliary muscle is fully tensed when an object at the near point. For people with normal vision, the near point is located about 10 to 12 cm. For the hyperopia, the near point is located a bit further, so they are unable to see the near objects clearly.

The shape, and therefore the focal length of the crystalline lens can be altered slightly by the ciliary muscle in order to bring into focus objects located at different distances. The process for the human eye is called accommodation. Some comfortable distance like 25 cm, a standard near point, at which a person would normally hold an object when looking at it, is known as the standard distance.

10.3.4 Resolving Power and Visual Acuity of Human Eye

The visual angle is the angle between a viewed object subtends at the fist nodal point of Gullstrand's schematic eye, as shown in Figure 10-14. The size of the image on retina depends on the visual angle. The lager the visual angle is, the larger the image is. For example, one cannot distinguish the detail of distant object, so decreasing object distance enables to distinguish the details. Experimentally when the visual angle is smaller than 1′, no matter how to move an object, one cannot distinguish two separate object points as being one object point. The corresponding shortest distance between two separate object points placed at near point is approximately 0.1mm. The minimum visual angle, which the retina can distinguish, is different for different people. The smaller the minimum visual angle is, the greater resolving power is. The **visual acuity** is expressed as the ability to distinguish an object. There are many various ways used to describe visual acuity. Before May 1990, international standard visual acuity scale, Vs, is used and defined as the reciprocal value of the minimum angle size which the retina can distinguish.

$$V_s = \frac{1}{\text{minimum visual angle of resolution}} = \frac{1}{\alpha}$$

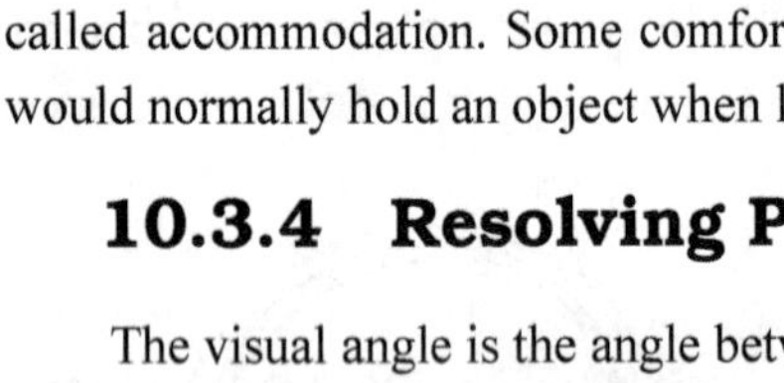

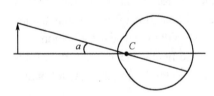

Figure 10-14 Visual angle

where the minimum angle of resolution is measured in arc minute. Recently, nation standard logarithm is another commonly used scale, V_L, expressed as the sum of 5 and the logarithm of minimum angle of resolution. The relation between V_S and V_L is

$$V_L = 5 + \lg V_S$$

The contradistinguishing of the two common types of visual acuity scales are shown as Table 10-1.

Table 10-1 Minimum angle of resolution and the two common types of visual acuity scales

Minimum angle of resolution (in arc minute)	National standard logarithm scale	International standard scale
10	4.0	0.1
5.012	4.3	0.2
1.0	5.0	1.0
0.794	5.1	1.2

10.3.5 Defects of Vision and Correction

Without accommodation, if an eye can bring rays from a distant object to form a clear image just on the retina as shown in Figure 10-15 (a), it is called **the eye with normal vision**. Otherwise it is called the eye of abnormal vision including nearsighted (myopic) eye, farsighted (hyperopic) eye and astigmatic eye.

1. Nearsightedness

Without accommodation, if the eye brings rays from a distant object to form a sharp image in front of the retina, as shown in Figure 10-15 (b), it is called the **nearsighted eye**. As the result of re-diverging, a blurred vision is formed on the retina. The far point of the nearsighted eye is the location of the farthest object on which the fully relaxed eye can focus, as shown in Figure 10-16(a). The far and near points of nearsighted eye are nearer than those of normal eye. A nearsighted person can clearly see objects that locate between the near point and the far point with accommodation.

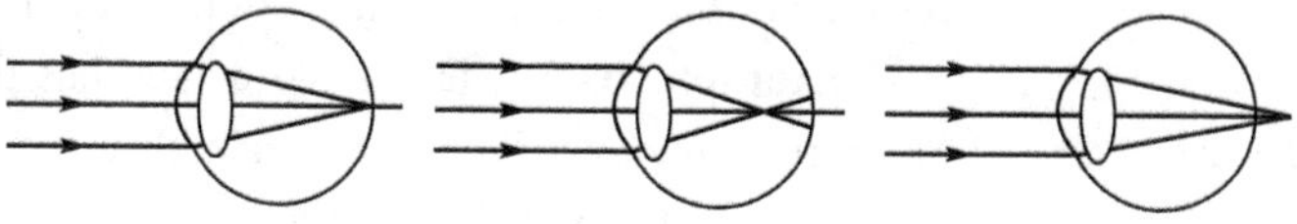

Figure 10-15 Normal eye, myopic eye and hyperopic eye

Myopia is caused by that refractive power of the eye is stronger (refractive myopia); or the lengthwise diameter of the eye is longer (axial myopia). Beside the heredity, most myopia has something with the disregard of eye healthy.

The nearsighted eye can be corrected with glasses or contacts that use diverging lenses, as shown in Figure 10-16 (b). The rays from the object diverge after leaving the eyeglass lens. Therefore, when they are subsequently refracted toward the principal axis by the eye, a sharp image is formed farther back and falls on the retina. In other words, the diverging lens is designed to transform a very distant object into the image located at the far point. Figure 10-16 (b) illustrates this transformation.

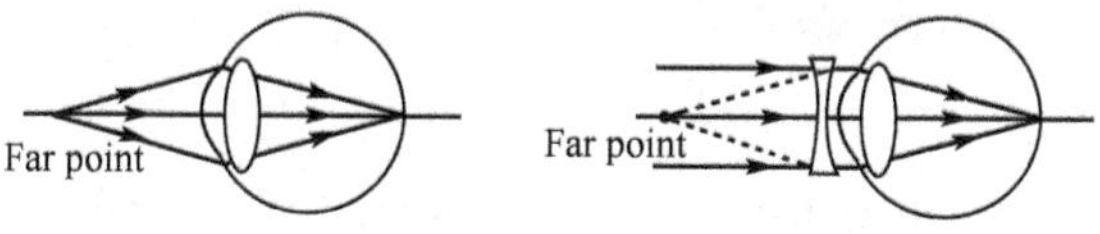

Figure 10-16 Correction of myopia

Example 10-4 A nearsighted person has a far point located 0.5 m from the eye, find the refractive power needed for the glasses to enable the person to see distant objects.

Solution: The glasses are designed to form a virtual image at the far point of the nearsighted eyes. With the glasses in front of the eyes, that person can get a clear vision. With the object and image distances of $u=\infty$ and $v=-0.5\ \mathrm{m}$, the focal length can be found as follows:

$$\frac{1}{\infty}+\frac{1}{-0.5}=\frac{1}{f}$$

We have

$$\Phi=\frac{1}{f}=\frac{1}{-0.5}=-2.0\mathrm{D}=-200\ \text{degree}$$

The value for fraction power is negative, indicating the lens is a diverging lens.

2. Farsightedness

Without accommodation, the eye brings rays from a distant object to form a sharp image behind the retina causing blurred vision, as Figure 10-15 (c) shows, and is called **farsighted eye**. When a farsighted eye tries to focus on distant objects, the eye accommodates and shortens its focal length as much as it can. Whereas the near point of a "normal eye" is located about 25 cm from the eye, the near point of a farsighted eye may be considerably farther away than that.

The reason for generating hyperopia is that refractive power of the eye is weaker (refractive hyperopia); or the lengthwise diameter of the eye is shorter (axial hyperopia). Hyperopia has something with heredity, and except that, the eyes of most babies are immature and behave as hyperopia.

Farsightedness can be corrected by placing a converging lens in front of the eye. The lens refracts the light rays more toward the principal axis before they enter the eye. Consequently, when the rays are refracted even more by the eye, they converge to form an image on the retina, as Figure 10-17 illustrates. The near point of hyperopia is more distant than that of a normal eye. The converging lens is designed to form a virtual image at the near point of the farsighted eye.

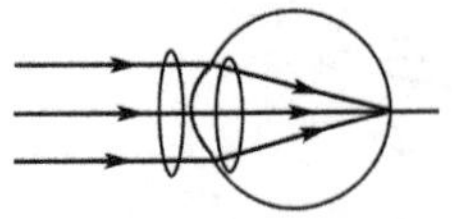

Figure 10-17 Correction of hyperopia

Example 10-5 A farsighted person has the near point located 1.0 m from the eyes. For obtaining a clear view of an object located 0.25 m from the eyes, what kind of glasses should be used and what should be the degree of that pair of glasses?

Solution: The function of the lens is to form an image of the object at the near point of the eye. With the object and image distances $u = 0.25$ m and $v = -1.0$ m, the focal length can be determined as follow:

$$\frac{1}{0.25} + \frac{1}{-1.0} = \frac{1}{f}$$

We have

$$\Phi = \frac{1}{f} = 3\text{D} = 300 \text{ degree}$$

The value of the refractive power is positive, indicating the lens is a converging lens to correct the farsightedness.

3. Astigmatism

The cornea of the normal eye and the refractive surface of crystalline lens should be a part of a sphere and a symmetric system. So the light rays originating from a single point source are focused to a single point even for a farsighted eye and a nearsighted eye, although an image can not be formed on the retina. **Astigmatism** is caused by uneven curvature of the cornea. The radius of each meridian line is not the same. The eye is asymmetrical. Rather than a single point, an astigmatism lens typically form an image that is a short line. As a result, the image becomes a little blur.

The correction for astigmatism is to wear the cylinder lens to correct the refractive power of the abnormal meridian plane. However it is hard to correct vision well by wearing a pair of glasses because of difficulties in measurement and correction. Another correction is to wear rigid gas permeable contact lens. The principle of correction is that tear lens is formed between glasses and cornea to compensate the irregular shape of cornea. As a result, the vision is corrected.

Presbyopia is a common phenomenon as getting old. The reason for presbyopia is that the crystalline lens would decrease deformability after it hardens. As a result, the ability for adjusting an eye decrease, the range of adjusting is being reduced, and the far point moves far away gradually. Then presbyopia happens. Usually it can be corrected by using convex lens properly.

10.4 Medical Applications of Geometrical Optics

10.4.1 Magnifying Glass

In order to observe small or distant objects, we usually bring the objects closer to eyes for increasing the visual angle and letting the enlarged images form on the retina. Since the ability of the adjustment of human eye is limited and the object distances are usually not less than the near point of the eye, it is necessary to use the aid of optical instruments for observing small or distant objects. As shown in Figure 10-18, a converging lens, known as the magnifying glass, is placed in front of the eye to obtain larger visual angle.

When utilizing the magnifying glass to observe objects, we often place the object on somewhere within the focal point and near the focus. Then an enlarged, upright image is generated on the same side of the object. Rays from the object can form a sharp image on retina after traveling through the magnifying glass. That is the principle for a magnifying glass.

An important physical quantity describing the lens magnification is the line magnification. As shown in Figure 10-19, suppose the length of the observed object is AB and it transforms into $A'B'$ amplified by the magnifying glass. The ratio of the image length and the object length is called the line magnification, donated by m.

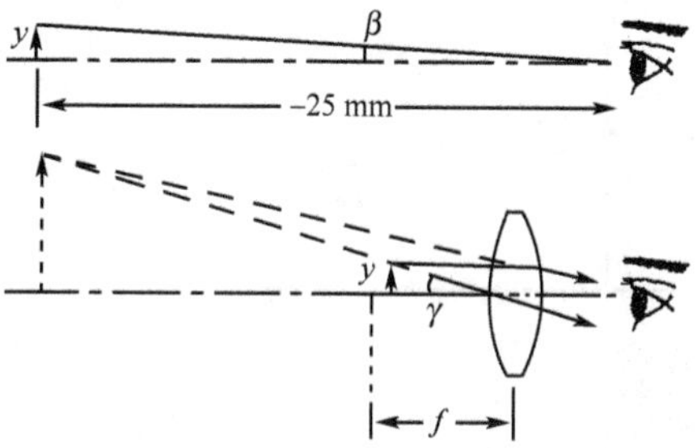

Figure 10-18 A magnifying glass

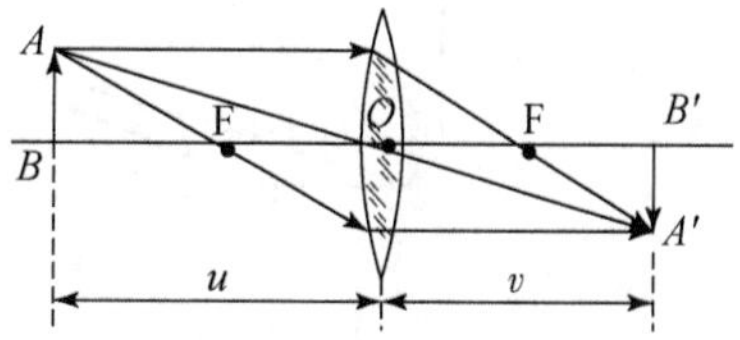

Figure 10-19 Line magnification

Drawing two light through the focus and light through the optical heart, it’s obtained:

$$m = \frac{A'B'}{AB} \tag{10-17}$$

The **angular magnification** is an important parameter of an optical instrument to describe the ability of magnification. As shown in Figure 10-18, without the magnifying glass, the angular size of an object is β when the object is placed at the near point located 25 cm from the eye. While when the same object is placed inside the focal point of the lens, the magnifying glass produces an enlarged, virtual image of the object and the angular size of the image is γ. Angular magnification α of a magnifying glass is the ratio of the angular size of the final image produced by the magnifying glass to the reference angular size of the object observed without the magnifying glass.

$$\alpha = \frac{\gamma}{\beta} \tag{10-18}$$

For a small object, its size y is so short and the angles of γ and β are so small as well, the approximate expressions for small angles will be

$$\gamma \approx \tan\gamma = \frac{y}{f}, \quad \beta \approx \tan\beta = \frac{y}{25}$$

Substituting them to Equation (10-18), we have

$$\alpha = \frac{y/f}{y/25} = \frac{25\ \text{cm}}{f} \tag{10-19}$$

where the unit of the focal length of a magnifying glass f is cm. Equation (10-19) shows that the angular magnification α is inversely proportional to the focal length of a magnifying glass. The smaller the focal length of a magnifying glass is, the larger the angular magnification is. In fact the focal length of a magnifying glass can not be too short since it is too hard to make a lens with much shorter focal length. For that kind of lens, the chromatic aberration is obvious. The angular magnification of a single magnifying glass is usually less than 3 times while that of a sheet magnifying glass, consisting of many concentric lenses, can reach dozens of times.

10.4.2 Microscope

1. Imaging Principle

The microscope is an important optical instrument in biology and medicine, which is often used to increase the visual angle and to enable us to observe much smaller objects. A general microscope usually consists of two converging lenses, as shown in Figure 10-20. The left lens L_1 of a microscope with shorter focal length is called the objective, and the right one L_2 with longer length is called the eyepiece.

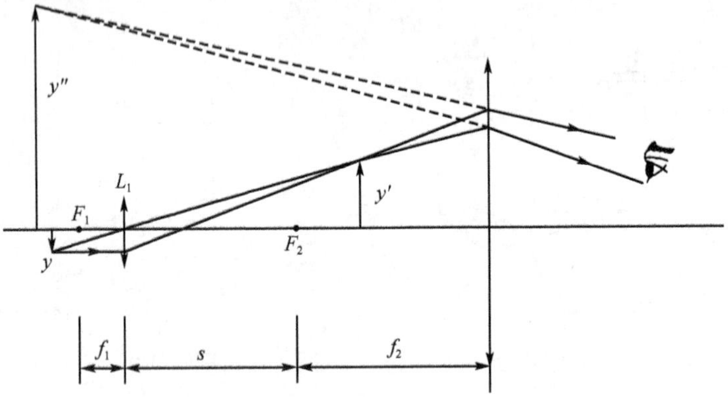

Figure 10-20 Optical path of the microscope

An objective produces an enlarged, real, inverted image y' of an object y placed outside the focal point of the objective. By adjusting the eyepiece makes the first image produced by the objective fall inside the focal point of the eyepiece. So the eyepiece produces an enlarged, virtual, final image y'', as shown in Figure 10-20. To see an object by the microscope, the angular magnification of a microscope is much larger than that of a magnifying glass. Practically, the eyepiece and objective consist of many lenses.

2. Angular Magnification of a Microscope

The angular magnification of such a microscope is the ratio of the angle γ produced by a microscope to the angle β produced by the object held at a distance of 25 cm.

$$M = \frac{\gamma}{\beta} \approx \frac{\tan\gamma}{\tan\beta}$$

Exactly. γ is the angular size of the final image and β is the reference angular size of object seen without a compound microscope.

By substituting $\tan\gamma \approx \frac{y'}{f_2}$, $\tan\beta = \frac{y}{25\ \text{cm}}$ into the equation above, we get

$$M = \frac{y'}{f_2} \cdot \frac{25}{y} = \frac{y'}{y} \cdot \frac{25\ \text{cm}}{f_2}$$

where f_2 is the focal length of the objective, and y'/y is linear magnification, denoted by m. $25/f_2$ is the angular magnification of the eyepiece, denoted by α . So the **angular magnification** of a microscope can also be written as

$$M = m \cdot \alpha \tag{10-20}$$

Equation (10-20) shows that the magnification of a compound microscope is the product of the linear magnification of the objective and the angular magnification of the eyepiece. There are usually some kind of objectives and eyepieces for choice and different magnification is gotten by using different devices.

3. Resolving Power of a Microscope

In geometrical optics, if the aberration of a microscope has been corrected, every point of the object being viewed has its corresponding image. But practically, to increase the magnification of a microscope, the objective is considered as a small circular opening for shorter focal length and smaller lens' size. According to the theory of diffraction, at very high magnifications with transmitted light, point objects are seen as fuzzy discs surrounded by diffraction rings. These are called Airy disks together with a series of concentric bright rings around. The object being observed can be seen as consisting of many material points which have different brightness and different locations. Each material point produces its own diffraction spot on the image plane of the lens. Zf the distances between material points are very close, the diffraction spots of material points are also very close and overlap each other, the details of the object will blurred. Therefore, too much diffraction limits the ability to resolve fine details. Resolution, denoted by Z, is expressed as the shortest distance between two separate points in a microscope's field of view that can still distinguished as distinct entities. Its reciprocal is called the **resolving power** of a microscope, determining the degree of detail that is visible, and depends on the objective used. Microscope resolution is generally calculated using the following equation formulated by Abbe.

$$Z = \frac{0.61\lambda}{n\sin\beta} \tag{10-21}$$

where n is the refractive index of the intervening medium between object and objective, λ is the wavelength of light used, β is the included angle of the objective, and $n\sin\beta$ is the numerical aperture of the objective, denoted by N. A.

Based on the Abbe Equation (10-21), one of the methods to improve resolution is that the light with shorter wavelength should be used to illuminate the specimen. So fluorescence microscopes, ultraviolet microscopes and electron microscopes have the higher resolutions based on that. The other way to increase the numerical apertures N.A is to increase n or β. This is the reason for using the oil immersion objectives.

10.4.3 Medical Endoscopes

The total internal reflection can occur only when light travels from a medium with the larger index of refraction toward a medium smaller index of refraction, i.e., $n_1 > n_2$ and the angle of incidence is bigger than the critical angle i.e., $i_1 > i_c$.

The angle of incidence is the critical angle i_c when the angle of refraction is $i_2 = 90°$. The critical angle is given by

$$i_c = \arcsin\left(\frac{n_2}{n_1}\right) \tag{10-22}$$

Optical fiber is made of glass or plastic smaller than 10 μm in radius and has a core of higher index and a cladding of lower index.

A step-index fiber has a core index of n_1 and a cladding index of n_2 ($n_2 < n_1$), as shown in Figure 10-21. Any light ray is incident on the fiber face at the angle of incidence φ such that the refracted ray in the core of the fiber is incident on the cladding at angle of incidence i. When $i = i_c$, total internal reflection happens.

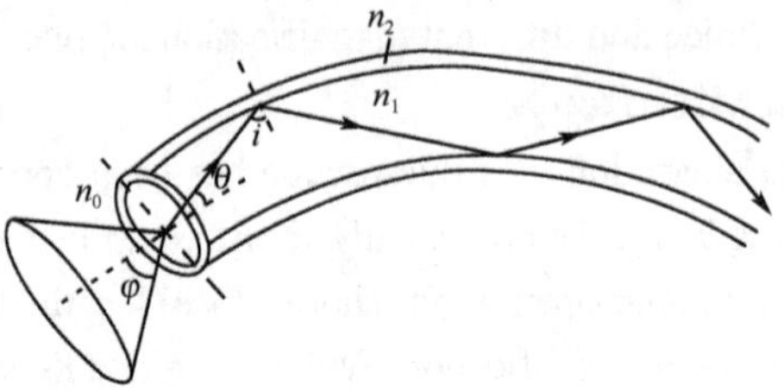

Figure 10-21 Optical conduction in a fiber

When the light fibers are bundled up together in an ordered array, pictures can be transmitted from one of its end to the other. An image element input at one end of a fiber produces the same image output at the far end of the fiber. The bundled fibers have been used widely in the variety of medical applications, the corresponding equipment include gastroscopes, oesophagoscopes, duodenoscopes, uteroscopes, cystoscopses, choledochoscopes, arthroscopes, angioscopes, and so on.

A Brief Summarization of This Chapter

(1) Refraction on a spherical surface

1) Formula of refraction on a spherical surface (only for the light rays near and parallel to the principal axis)

$$\frac{n_1}{u}+\frac{n_2}{v}=\frac{n_2-n_1}{r}$$

The sign conventions: The object distance and the image distance are both positive when the object and the image are both real, and they are both negative when the object and the image are both virtual. The radius of curvature is positive when incident light ray strikes toward the convex surface and negative when incident light ray strikes toward the concave surface.

2) Refractive power

$$\Phi=\frac{n_2-n_1}{r}$$

The first focal length:

$$f_1=\frac{n_1}{n_2-n_1}r$$

The second focal length:

$$f_2=\frac{n_2}{n_2-n_1}r$$

3) Spherical surfaces in combination: For the light rays near and parallel to the principal axis, the image for spherical surfaces in combination can be formed by the repeated use of the simple equation for a spherical surface.

(2) Lens

1) Thin lens equation

$$\frac{1}{u}+\frac{1}{v}=\frac{n-n_0}{n_0}\left(\frac{1}{r_1}-\frac{1}{r_2}\right)$$

If the thin lens is placed in air, the thin lens equation

$$\frac{1}{u}+\frac{1}{v}=(n-1)(\frac{1}{r_1}-\frac{1}{r_2})$$

Gauss formula for a thin lens

$$\frac{1}{u}+\frac{1}{v}=\frac{1}{f}$$

2) Refractive power of a lens: It is measured in diopters and is given by

$$\Phi=\frac{1}{f}$$

3) Equivalent focal length and refractive power for lens in combination

$$\frac{1}{f}=\frac{1}{f_1}+\frac{1}{f_2},\quad \Phi=\Phi_1+\Phi_2$$

(3) Dioptrics of human eye

1) Reduced schematic eye is considered as a spherical surface. The radius of convex surface is $r=$ 5 mm. The index of refraction of material in image space is 1.33. Retina is considered as the focal plane of the system. The first and the second lengths are $f_1=15$ mm, $f_2=20$ mm, respectively.

2) Nearsightedness can be corrected by wearing eyeglasses or contacts made of diverging lenses.

3) Farsightedness can be corrected by using converging lenses.

4) Correction for astigmatism: To wear cylinder lens to correct the refractive power of the abnormal meridian plane.

(4) Magnifying glass and microscope

1) Angular magnification of magnifying glass

$$\alpha=\frac{y/f}{y/25}=\frac{25\text{ cm}}{f}$$

2) Angular magnification of a microscope

$$M=m\cdot\alpha$$

3) Resolving power of a microscope

$$Z=\frac{0.61\lambda}{n\sin\beta}$$

Exercises 10

10-1. In the image formation of the refraction on a single spherical refractive interface, what are the sign conventions for the object distance, the object distance and the radius of curvature?

10-2. A transparent material sphere with radius R is placed in air. What is the index of refraction of the material so that parallel rays which enter the front surface of the sphere focus on the back surface?

10-3. The interface between some liquid (n_1=1.3)and glass (n_2=1.5)is a part of a sphere. An object in the liquid is located 40 cm left of the interface. Then its virtual image is located 32 cm front of the interface. Determine the radius of the interface and which material lies at the convex surface.

10-4. Cornea is considered as a spherical surface with radius 7.8 mm, behind which the index of refraction of the medium is 4/3. If the image locates 3.6 mm behind cornea, where is the location of pupil?

10-5. The material inside of the plano-convex lens has an index of refraction of 1.5. Its focal length in air is 50 cm. Determine the radius of convex surface of the lens.

10-6. One end of a glass rod (n=1.5) is convex surface with radius 2 cm. A point object is placed 8 cm on the principal axial in front of the end of the rod, find the location of image. If it is placed in a liquid (n=1.6), find the location of image, and determine whether the image is real or virtual.

10-7. A converging lens (f=15cm) is located 5cm to the left of a diverging lens (f=−10cm). The light rays travel through the converging lens, then the diverging lens. The final image is located 15cm to the front of the converging lens. Where is the object located?

10-8. A plano-concave lens is made up of glass (n=1.5). The front face of the lens is a plane, the rear face of the lens is a concave surface with radius r=0.2 m. The lens of which a concave surface is filled with water (plane-convex lens is made of water), is placed in air. Determine the refraction power and focal distance (the index of refraction of water is 4/3).

10-9. The eyeglasses of person A is +2.0 D, while that of person B is −4.0 D. Who is myopic and who is hyperopic? Where is the far point of the nearsighted person and where is the far point of the nearsighted person?

10-10. A nearsighted person has a far point located only 0.5 m from his eyes. Determine the refractive power of contact lenses that will enable him to see distant objects clearly.

10-11. A farsighted person has a near point located 0.5 m from the eyes. Obtain the refractive power of the glasses that can be used to see an object at a distance of 0.25 m from the eyes.

Chapter 11 Fundamental of Quantum Mechanics

Wave theories of light explain the phenomena such as interference, diffraction, polarization, etc. perfectly. And it succeeds in explicating the nature of light, that is, the nature of electromagnetic wave. But in the experimental investigations of thermal radiation, photo electric effect and other regularities, it encounters difficulties. In 1900, a German physicist Max Planck proposed the hypothesis of energy quantum, which successfully explained the experimental laws of thermal radiation. In the enlightenment of this hypothesis, Albert Einstein put forward the photon hypothesis, with which the experimental laws of photoelectric effect is explained successfully. In the year of 1923, the explanation of the experimental law of Arthur Compton Effect in terms of photons confirmed the correctness of the photon theory. Moreover, in 1924, French physicist Louis de Broglie came up with the idea that any entity particle has the wave-particle duality in nature. Based on this, Erwin Schrödinger and Werner Heisenberg et al. founded the system of quantum mechanics, which extends the physics investigations from macroscopic field into microcosmic field. As the development of physics, the researches of atomic and molecular spectrums have been deepening continuously, which have provided clearer evidences in identifying the microstructure of matters as mighty tools. It has been found that the factors such as the wavelength of light either absorbed or emitted under any conditions are essentially connected with the structural characteristics of the matters. The connection can be revealed by spectroscopy, and spectroscopy has been widely used in chemical and medicinal analyses.

In this chapter, the corpuscular property of light will be explicated with the explanation of experimental laws of thermal radiation and photoelectric effect, and then the wave particle duality of light will also be proved. It will be elaborated that particle entities have wave-particle duality by the electronic diffraction experiment which confirmed the hypothesis brought up by Louis de Broglie. We will mainly focus on the introduction of the uncertainty principle that reflects the motional laws in microscopic space. Then we will also emphasize on the presentation of the regularity of hydrogen atomic spectrum, Niels Bohr's theory of hydrogen atom and the physical interpretations of the four quantum numbers. Finally, we will give a brief introduction to the atomic spectrum and the molecular spectrum; at the same time we will summarize the principle of laser in the aspects of its production, feature, applications, and so on.

11.1 Thermal Radiation

11.1.1 Radiant Exitance and Absorptance of a Radiating Object

The phenomenon that any object at the temperature above absolute zero radiates energy in the form of electromagnetic wave is called the **thermal radiation**, which is caused by the thermal motion of charged particles within the object. Total energy radiated from the unit surface per unit time is called as the **radiant exitance**, denoted by M and its unit is W/m^2. The value of M is the function of the temperature T namely $M = M(T)$.

Experiments show that thermal radiation spectrum consists of a continuous distribution of total light spectrum. The energy of electromagnetic wave within a unit range of wavelength near the wavelength λ radiated from unit surface per unit time is called the **monochromatic radiant exitance**. Apparently, monochromatic radiant exitance is the function of thermodynamic temperature T and the wavelength λ, denoted by $M(\lambda, T)$ whose unit is W/m^3. Thus the value of $M(T)$ can be described by the integral in all wavelengths range:

$$M(T) = \int_0^{\infty} M(\lambda, T)d\lambda \tag{11-1}$$

Any object can never exist in isolation. As it's radiating, the object absorbs energy emitted by the surroundings constantly. When the energy radiated is equal to the energy absorbed, the radiation approximate to the dynamic equilibrium which means the temperature remains unchanged. We define the ratio of the energy absorbed and the energy radiated corresponding to a particular wavelength as the **monochromatic absorptance**. It is the function of the temperature of the object T and the incident wavelength λ, denoted by $\alpha(\lambda,T)$. The monochromatic absorptance of an object should be less than 1, because it only absorbs part of the radiate energy incident on its surface and the rest of the energy is reflected or transmitted. The object that can absorb all the radiation incident completely, or, the object which has a monochromatic absorptance of $\alpha(\lambda,T)=1$ for any wavelength is called the **absolute black body**, or **black body**. It is an ideal model.

11.1.2 Kirchhoff Radiation Law

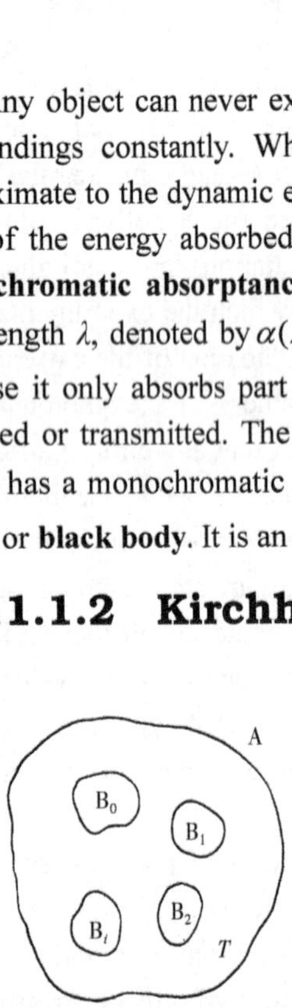

Figure 11-1 Objects in a container with a constant temperature

Suppose there are several different objects B_0, B_1, ⋯, B_i, as shown in Figure 11-1, in the thermostat A at the temperature T. In the state of equilibrium, all of them are at the same temperature. So during a time interval, for each object the energy emitted and the energy absorbed must be equal. This state is called the **equilibrium thermal radiation** state. It is deduced theoretically by Gustar Robert Kirchhoff which indicates that in this state, the ratio of the monochromatic radiant exitance and the monochro matic absorptance of any object for the same wavelength has the same value. Furthermore the value of this ratio is equal to the radiant exitance of the black body for the wavelength at the same temperature, i.e.,

$$\frac{M_1(\lambda,T)}{\alpha_1(\lambda,T)} = \frac{M_2(\lambda,T)}{\alpha_2(\lambda,T)} = \cdots = \frac{M_i(\lambda,T)}{\alpha_i(\lambda,T)} = \frac{M_0(\lambda,T)}{\alpha_0(\lambda,T)} \tag{11-2}$$

where $M_1(\lambda,T)$, $M_2(\lambda,T)$, ⋯, $M_i(\lambda,T)$, and $\alpha_1(\lambda,T)$, $\alpha_2(\lambda,T)$, ⋯, $\alpha_i(\lambda,T)$ in the equation above represent the specific values of the monochromatic radiant exitances and absorptances of B_1, B_2, ⋯, B_i respectively. Assume that B_0 is a black body, and $\alpha_0(\lambda,T)=1$, $M_0(\lambda,T)$ is the maximum one, so the black body is called the full radiator. When the equilibrium state is maintained, although the temperature remains unchanged, there are still heat exchanges among the objects. It is merely the case that for any object the energy absorbed and the energy emitted in per unit time and on per unit area have the same value, and the greater the radiant exitance, the larger the absorptance. To sum up, in the state of equilibrium thermal radiation, the ratios of monochromatic radiant exitances and monochromatic absorptances of any objects are the same and equal to the monochromatic radiant exitance of the black body at the same temperature $M_0(\lambda,T)$, and the ratios have nothing to do with the properties of the objects. This conclusion is called **Kirchhoff radiation law**.

11.1.3 Radiation Laws for the Black Body

In the nature, the absorptance of any object is less than 1, so there isn't any black body at all. But the following model can be regarded as a black body approximately. Let's open a tiny hole on a hollow cavity of any shape made from non-transparent materials, as shown in Figure 11-2. If electromagnetic radiations enter into the cavity from the hole, after being reflected for many times by the inner wall, nearly all of the incident energy is absorbed. So we can take this cavity with a hole as an ideal black body. If this black body is heated and maintained with a certain temperature *T*, the radiation out of the tiny hole is the radiation emitted by the black body at the temperature *T*. For the electromagnetic radiations of various wavelengths emitted from the hole, they can be separated by the spectrometer and the radiation energies of different wavelengths during a unit time can also be measured separately. If we change the temperature and repeat the above experiment, we can get the distribution curves of the monochromatic radiant exitance of the black body versus the wavelength at different temperatures, as shown in Figure 11-3. With these experimental curves, the following two experimental laws for the radiation of the black body can be concluded.

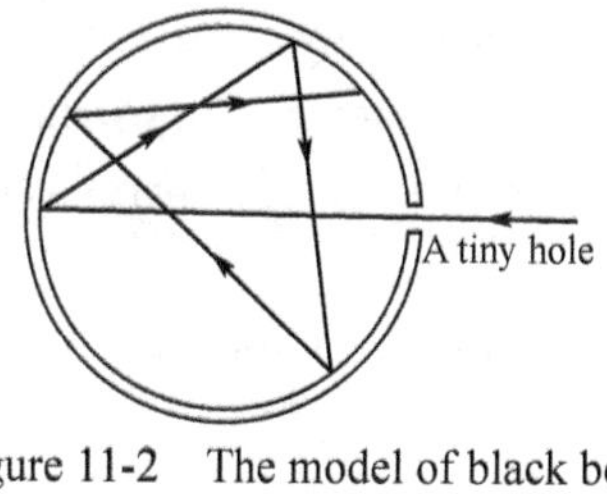

Figure 11-2 The model of black body

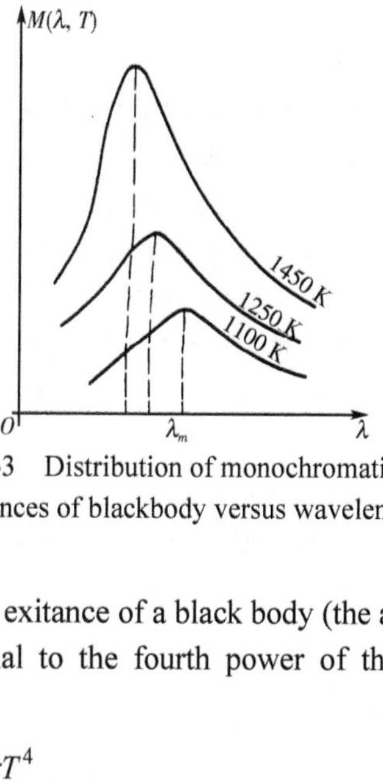

Figure 11-3 Distribution of monochromatic radiant exitances of blackbody versus wavelength

1. Stefan-Boltzmann Law

From experiments Josef Stefan drew a conclusion that the radiant exitance of a black body (the area under the distribution curve, as shown in Figure 11-3) is proportional to the fourth power of the thermal dynamic temperature *T*, i.e.

$$M_0(T)=\int_0^{\infty} M_0(\lambda,T)\mathrm{d}\lambda=\sigma T^4 \tag{11-3}$$

where $\sigma=5.67\times10^{-8}\,\mathrm{W/(m^2\cdot K^4)}$ is the **Stefan constant**. Ludwig Boltzmann derived the same conclusion on the basis of theory of thermal dynamic, so this result is called **Stefan-Boltzmann law** which is only fit to the radiation of black bodies.

2. Wien's Displacement Law

It can be concluded form this set of the experimental curves shown in Figure 11-3 that for any distribution curve, there is a maximum of the monochromatic radiant exitance and there is a corresponding wavelength, i.e., the peak wavelength λ_m; as the temperature increases this wavelength λ_m will shift towards the direction of shorter wavelength. Wien pointed out that the peak wavelength of λ_m is inversely proportional to the temperature *T*, i.e.

$$\lambda_m T=b \tag{11-4}$$

where the constant b=2.897×10^{-3}m · K is called **Wien constant**; and this relation is called **Wien's**

displacement law.

The regularities of the radiation of the black body have been widely used in modern technology and daily life, such as in modern cosmology, infrared remote sensing, infrared tracking, optical measurement of high temperature, and so on.

11.1.4 Planck Quantum Hypothesis

In order to explain the radiation laws of the black body, many scientists attempted to deduce the function relationship of the experimental distribution curves of the monochromatic radiant exitance of the black body versus the wavelength as shown Figure 11-3, by classical physical theories, however, they all did in vain. Until 1900, Planck provided the revolutionary hypotheses, i.e., the hypothesis of quantization of energy which could interpret the radiation laws of the black body successfully. Its contents are as follows.

①An irradiator is supposed to be composed of many charged linear harmonic oscillators which radiate electromagnetic wave and exchange energy with the electromagnetic field around as they are oscillating. Each harmonic oscillator has a different frequency and emits or absorbs the radiation of a mono-wavelength, thus all of the harmonic oscillators emit or absorb the radiation of the continuous wavelengths.

②Each linear harmonic oscillator can only remain in a series of particular discrete energy states, in which the corresponding energy can only be the integral multiple of a minimum energy. If the minimum energy is ε, then the energy of the harmonic oscillator can only be one of the discrete values ε, 2ε, 3ε, 4ε, $\cdots$, $n\varepsilon$. Where n is positive integer called **quantum number**, ε is the **energy quantum**, or simply the **quantum**. So the energy of the oscillator is in a discontinuous quantized state. For an oscillator, when it emits electromagnetic waves to the outside or absorbs energy from surroundings, its energy can only leap from one of the quantum states to another.

③The energy quantum ε is proportional to the frequency of linear harmonic oscillator ν, that is

$$\varepsilon = h\nu \tag{11-5}$$

where h is called Planck constant $h=6.63\times10^{-34}\text{J}\cdot\text{s}$.

Based on the hypotheses mentioned above, Planck derived the empirical equation for the radiation of the black body:

$$M_0(\lambda,T)=\frac{2\pi hc^2\lambda^{-5}}{e^{\frac{hc}{k\lambda T}}-1} \tag{11-6}$$

where c represents the velocity of light, $c=3\times10^8\,\text{m/s}$, and k is Boltzmann constant, $k=1.3810\times10^{-23}\text{J/K}$. This equation is in complete agreement with the experimental results of the radiation of the black body, meanwhile, on the basis of which we can also derive the result of Stefan-Boltzmann law and Wien's displacement law. These facts verified the correctness of the Planck's hypothesis, since then, a new epoch of modern physics—quantum theory began.

11.2 Photoelectric Effect and Compton Effect

11.2.1 Photoelectric Effect

When a beam of light with a certain frequency irradiates on the surface of metal, there will be electrons escaped from the surface of the metal. This phenomenon is called the **photoelectric effect**; and these electrons are called **photoelectrons**. The phenomenon that there are photoelectrons escaped out from the metal surface is called the external photoelectric effect. Besides, light can also penetrate into some objects (such as semi-conductors, crystals), and cause the inner atoms releasing electrons, while, those electrons will still remain inside the object so as to increase its electro-conductivity. This phenomenon is called internal photoelectric effect.

1. Experimental Regularities of Photoelectric Effect

The schematic diagram for the study of external photoelectric effect is shown in Figure 11-4. There is an anode A and a cathode K in the vacuum glass vessel, where the cathode is metal plate. Now let's put the power through two poles. Meanwhile, a beam of light with a certain frequency irradiates on the cathode, if there are electrons escaped from the cathode, then photoelectrons will move towards the anode under the action of the electric field. At the same time there is electric current flowing through the circuit. The current is called the **photocurrent**. We can measure the magnitude of the photocurrent by the galvanometer. After analyzing the experiment results, the following regularities can be summarized.

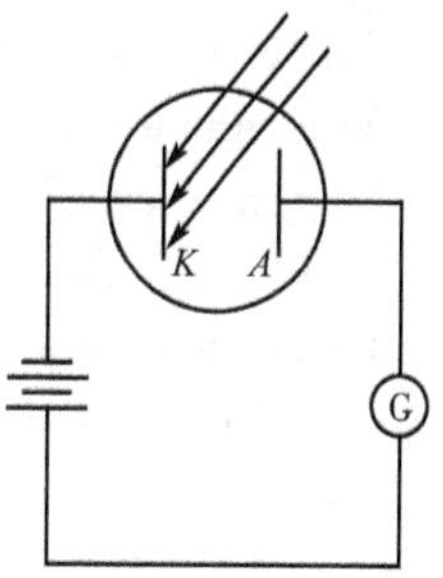

Figure11-4 Schematic diagram of photoelectric effect experiment

(1) The magnitude of photocurrent is proportional to the intensity of incident light.

(2) Initial kinetic energy of any photoelectron escaped from the cathode K moving towards the anode A is related only to the frequency of incident light and has nothing to do with its intensity.

(3) For a particular metal, there is not photocurrent, only when the frequency of incident light is bigger than a special magnitude, and this frequency is called threshold frequency, also known as red limit. If the frequency of the incident light is below the threshold frequency, there will never be photoelectrons escaped from the metal, no matter how intense the light is and how long the irradiated time is.

(4) As long as the frequency of incident light is above the threshold frequency, the photoelectrons can be observed almost instantaneously while the surface is irradiated by the light (generally speaking the delay time is less than 10^{-9} s) , regardless the intensity of the light.

2. Einstein's Equation of Photoelectric Effect

(1) Einstein's theory of photon: In order to explain the experimental regularity of photoelectric effect, Albert Einstein proposed a hypothesis related to the nature of light based on the Planck quantum hypothesis of energy. Einstein believed that light is the particle flow with the speed of light, and these light particles are called light quantum, or simply photons. If the frequency of the light is ν, the energy of each photon should be $\varepsilon = h\nu$, photons with different frequencies has different energies, while the light intensity is determined by the photon numbers through per unit area in per unit time. According to the mass-energy relation in relativity, Einstein also pointed out that the relation between the momentum of a photon and the corresponding wavelength of light can be described as follows:

$$p = \frac{h\nu}{c} = \frac{h}{\lambda} \tag{11-7}$$

This is what we called **Einstein's theory of photon**. Apparently, Einstein's theory of photon revealed the corpuscular property of light.

(2) Einstein's equation of photoelectric effect: According to Einstein's theory of photon, when light with the frequency of ν (greater than the threshold frequency) irradiating on the surface of a metal, each photon can only interact with one electron in the metal, and each electron can only absorb the whole

energy of a single photon $h\nu$ at a time. During the process one part of the energy act as the work function of the electron's escaping out from the metal surface A, and the rest of energy transform into the kinetic energy of the moving photoelectron $\frac{1}{2}mv^2$, which can be expressed as

$$h\nu = \frac{1}{2}mv^2 + A \tag{11-8}$$

Equation (11-8) is Einstein's equation of photoelectric effect. We can get from Equation (11-8) that the initial kinetic energy is dependent only on the frequency of light and is independent of the intensity of the light. When the intensity of light increases, the number of photons increases as well, thus the number of photoelectrons escaped from the metal surface per unit time will also increase. Then there are more photons rushing towards the anode plate per unit time. So we can know that, the greater the intensity of light, the larger the photocurrent will be. If the frequency of the incident light is not big enough, namely, the energy of a photon is less than the work function for the metal; there won't be any electron escaping out from the metal surface. There won't be photoelectric effect, until $h\nu \geqslant A$, so the threshold frequency is $\nu_0=A/h$. When light irradiates on the metal surface, an electron can absorb all of the energy of a photon at a time and this process is in the instant without time accumulation. Thus, Einstein's theory of photon can fully explained the experimental regularities of photoelectric effect.

11.2.2 Compton Effect

1. Compton Effect

In 1923, when Arthur Holly Compton was studying the scattering phenomenon of X-ray penetrating through materials such as paraffin, graphite, metals and so on, he found that among the scattered rays, besides the rays with the same wavelength of the incident ray λ_0, there are scattered rays with the wavelengths of $\lambda > \lambda_0$. This phenomenon is called **Compton effect**. In 1926, after lucubrating the experimental results about the Compton effect, our Chinese physicist Youxun Wu pointed out that the change of wavelength of a scattered ray $\Delta\lambda$ is only associated with the magnitude of scattering angle (the angle between the direction of incident ray and the direction of the scattering ray) , and has nothing to do with the wavelength of incident ray or the scattered material.

The schematic diagram of Compton experiment is shown in Figure 11-5. After passing through the diaphragm D, a beam of X-ray with the wavelength of λ_0 irradiates on and is scattered by a scattering object S. The wavelength of different scattered ray can be measured by the X-ray spectrograph C.

By analyzing the results of a huge amount of experiments, Compton equation was found:

$$\Delta\lambda = \lambda - \lambda_0 = 2K\sin^2\frac{\theta}{2} \tag{11-9}$$

where $K=2.43\times10^{-12}$m is **Compton wavelength** which is the change of wavelength when the scattering angle is a right angle.

By means of Einstein's theory of photon, Compton explained the Compton effect perfectly. He considered that the energy of roentgen photon is great enough, but the nuclear bound forces for outer electrons in atoms especially in light atoms are quite week, so the electrons can be looked as free electrons approximately. The scattering of X-ray can be seen as the result of the elastic collisions between photons and free electrons. During the collision, a photon deliver part of its kinetic energy to an electron, so the energy of the scattered photon is reduced, then its frequency decreases and the wavelength increases accordingly.

2. Derivation of Compton Equation

According to Einstein's theory of photon, the photon has the energy of $E = h\nu$. By Einstein's mass-energy relation $E=mc^2$, we can get the mass of a photon moving at the speed of c:

$$m = \frac{h\nu}{c^2}$$

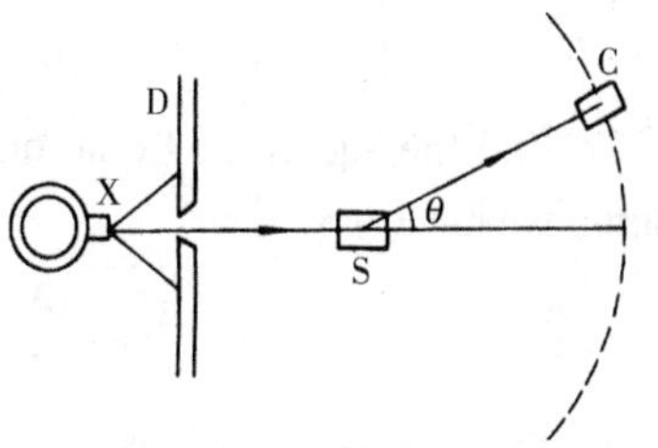

Figure 11-5 Schematic diagram of Compton effect experiment

The theory of relativity indicates that the relationship between the rest mass of an object m_0 and the mass m as it is moving at the velocity of v is

$$m = \frac{m_0}{\sqrt{1-\frac{\upsilon^2}{c^2}}} \tag{11-10}$$

Owing to that a photon is always moving at the speed of light c, we can conclude from Equation (11-10) that, the rest mass of a photon must be zero.

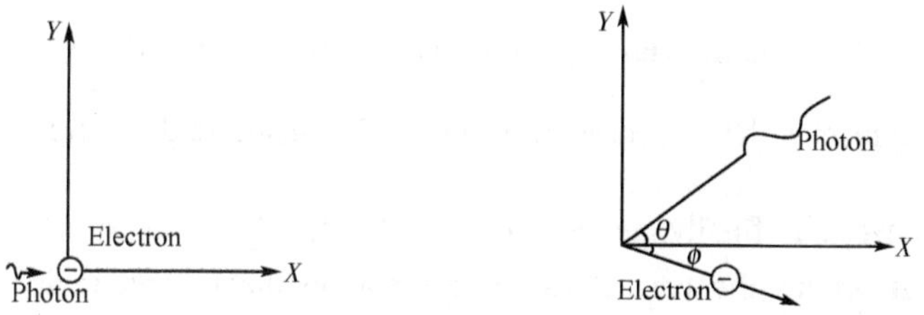

Figure 11-6 The collision of a photon and an electron

Since a photon has the mass of m when it is moving at the speed of light c, the momentum of the photon should be

$$p = mc = \frac{h\nu}{c} = \frac{h}{\lambda}$$

It just accords with Equation (11-7).

Now let's discuss the case in which there is an elastic collision between a photon with the energy of $h\nu$ and a free electron at stationary, as shown in Figure 11-6. Based on the laws of conservation and conversion of energy, we can get

$$m_0c^2 + h\nu_0 = mc^2 + h\nu$$

that is

$$mc^2 = h(\nu_0 - \nu) + m_0c^2 \tag{11-11}$$

where m_0 and m represent the stationary mass and the motion mass of the electron respectively; ν_0 and ν represent the frequencies of the photon before and after the elastic collision with the electron.

According to the law of conservation of momentum we can also get

$$\frac{h\nu_0}{c} = m\upsilon\cos\phi + \frac{h\nu}{c}\cos\theta \tag{11-12}$$

and

$$0 = -m\upsilon\sin\phi + \frac{h\nu}{c}\sin\theta \tag{11-13}$$

To solve the simultaneous Equation (11-12) and Equation (11-13) and eliminate ϕ, we have

$$m^2v^2c^2 = h^2\nu_0{}^2 + h^2\nu^2 - 2h^2\nu_0\nu\cos\theta \tag{11-14}$$

To find the square of Equation (11-11) , and then subtract Equation (11-14) from the result, after settling, we have

$$m^2c^4(1-\frac{v^2}{c^2}) = m_0{}^2c^4 - 2h^2\nu_0\nu(1-\cos\theta) + 2m_0c^2h(\nu_0-\nu) \tag{11-15}$$

To find the square on both sides of Equation (11-9) , and multiply the result by c^4, we have

$$m^2c^4(1-\frac{v^2}{c^2}) = m_0{}^2c^4$$

To substitute it into Equation (11-15) , we have

$$\frac{c}{\nu} - \frac{c}{\nu_0} = \frac{h}{m_0c}(1-\cos\theta)$$

that is

$$\Delta\lambda = \lambda - \lambda_0 = \frac{2h}{m_0c}\sin^2\frac{\theta}{2} \tag{11-16}$$

Comparing it with the experimental Equation (11-9) , we can get the theoretical value of K, i.e. $K = \dfrac{h}{m_0c}$, where m_0 represents the rest mass of electron. To substitute the corresponding quantities with the known constants, we can finally get $K = 2.43 \times 10^{-12}$ m, which conforms to the value from the experimental results. It proves the correctness of the photon theory and indicates further **the wave-particle duality** of light.

11.3 Wave-Particle Duality

11.3.1 De Broglie Wave

Light has both wave and corpuscular properties. The corpuscular property presents only as the integrity when the photon exchanges the momentum and the energy. A photon can't be interpreted as a particle which has the same motion characteristics as what in the classical mechanics. For example, a particle has a certain position and momentum at any moment, and has a definite track, etc. during the whole motion process. In macroscopic, the wave property and corpuscular property of light is inconsistent, but they are in concomitant in microscopic field. Just on different conditions, light behaves as the wave or particle behavior. In other words, light has the wave-particle duality.

In 1924, inspired by the process of cognition of the wave-particle duality of the light, de Broglie put forward that the wave-particle duality is not only the feature of light but also the essence of any object particles. In optics, the expressions of $\varepsilon = h\nu$ and $p = h/\lambda$ connect the quantities of ν and λ which represent the wave property of light with the quantities of ε and p which represent the corpuscular property of light quantification. Thereupon, de Broglie supposed that the above relational expressions should be suitable for any object particles. When an object particle with the mass of m is moving at the velocity of v, we have the following relational expressions:

$$\lambda = \frac{h}{p} = \frac{h}{mv} \tag{11-17}$$

$$\nu = \frac{\varepsilon}{h} \tag{11-18}$$

Such wave connected with the matter is called **de Broglie wave** or matter wave. Equations (11-7) and Equation (11-18) are called de Broglie relational expressions.

11.3.2 Experiment of Electron Diffraction

The validity of hypothesis of matter wave and de Broglie relational expressions could be demonstrated by the experiment of electron diffraction carried by Davisson and Germer. The diagram of experimental apparatus is shown as Figure 11-7 (a). Under the action of the electric field with the voltage of U, the electrons sent from the filamentary cathode K pass through a slit to form a beam of electrons and project onto the nickel single crystal. The glancing angle of the beam of electrons to the surface of the crystal is ϕ. The electrons reflected from the crystal surface are collected by the current collector B to form a current, and the value of current I is detected by the galvanometer G. In the experiment the glancing angle keeps constant. By changing the voltage U and measuring the corresponding I, we can draw the relation curve of I-$\sqrt{U}$ as shown in Figure 11-7 (b).

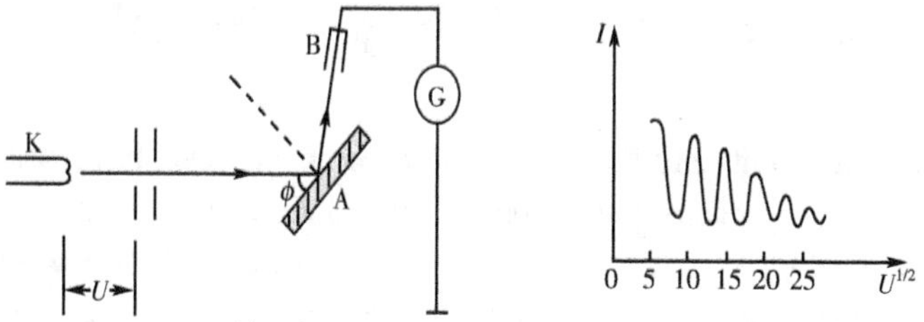

(a) (b)

Figure 11-7 Schematic diagram of the experiment of electron diffraction

Experiments indicate that the value of current I doesn't increase continuously with the increase of the acceleration voltage U. Only when the voltage equals some fixed values, the current I appears the corresponding maximum values. We can't explain this experimental phenomenon in terms of the corpuscular property of electrons, because the reflection of electrons on the surface of the crystal should obey the law of reflection and the whole beam of electrons should be collected into B. The change of accelerating voltage could only cause the change of the velocity of electrons and shouldn't cause any undulatory change of the current I. But in terms of the wave property of object particles we can explain the phenomenon as: The reflection of the electrons on the crystal surface A is similar to the scattering of the roentgen ray; only when the relation among the wavelength λ, the glancing angle ϕ and the lattice constant of the nickel single crystal d complies to Bragg equation (similar to the film interference equation in optics)

$$2d\sin\phi = k\lambda \qquad k = 1, 2, 3, \cdots \tag{11-19}$$

The beam of electrons will comply to the law of reflection, otherwise, the electrons will be scattered in all directions. If the voltage is changed, the velocity of the electrons varies as well. According to the equation below, we can find the corresponding wavelength of the electron wave

$$\lambda = \frac{h}{mv} \tag{11-20}$$

The work done by electric field on some electron U_e transformed into its kinetic energy, i.e.

$$\frac{1}{2}mv^2 = U_e \tag{11-21}$$

Substitute it into Equation (11-20) , we have

$$\lambda=\frac{h}{mv}=\frac{h}{\sqrt{2mU_{\mathrm{e}}}}=\frac{1.225}{\sqrt{U}}\times10^{-9}\ \mathrm{m} \qquad (11\text{-}22)$$

Substitute Equation (11-22) into Equation (11-19) then we have

$$2d\sin\phi=k\frac{1.225}{\sqrt{U}}\times10^{-9}$$

The equation above indicates that in the case when ϕ, d are constant, the change of the voltage will cause the change of the wavelength of de Broglie wave of these electrons. For some fixed voltages, if Bragg equation could just be satisfied, the maximum values of current will be produced. Experiments have proved that the calculated values of voltage derived by the equation above conform to the experimental results, which means the de Broglie hypothesis is correct.

Many experiments also demonstrate that apart from electrons, other microscopic particles such as neutrons, atoms and molecules have also the wave property. This shows that de Broglie equation is an essential equation for uncovering the wave-particle duality of microscopic particles.

11.4 Uncertainty Principle

Large number of experiments prove that all microscopic particles have wave-particle duality. In classical mechanics, particles of macroscopic motion move along certain tracks, and the moving state of any particle can be described by its position and momentum on the track at any moment. While, for the microscopic particles with the wave-particle duality, whether can we describe its motion with a definite coordinate and definite momentum at the same time?

Next, let's give an illustration with the experiment of single slit diffraction of electrons, as shown in Figure 11-8.

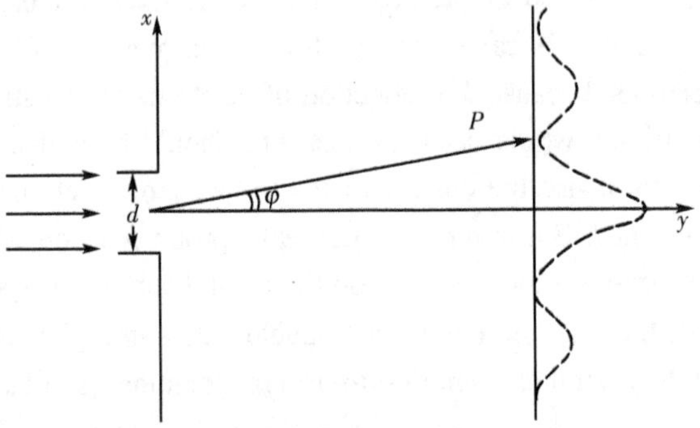

Figure 11-8 Single slit diffraction of electrons

A beam of electrons is assumed to project onto the slit with the width of d along y axis. After passing through the single slit this beam of electrons is diffracted, and the diffraction pattern of electrons on the observing screen can be shot. The diffracting minimum condition for the wavelength of the matter wave of the electrons λ, the width of the slit d and the diffraction angle φ should follow the equation:

$$d\sin\varphi=k\lambda \qquad (k=1,2,3,\cdots)$$

For the first order of minimum (dark fringe) , $k=1$ and

$$d\sin\varphi=\lambda$$

According to the wave property, the uncertainty of position coordinate in x direction for some electron is equal to $\Delta x = d$ at the position of the slit; according to the corpuscular property, the x component of the momentum of this electron would be confined to a range of variation Δp_x .

For the first dark fringe

$$\Delta p_x = p\sin\varphi \tag{11-23}$$

To substitute $\sin\varphi = \frac{\lambda}{d}$, $\Delta x = d$ and de Broglie relation $p = \frac{h}{\lambda}$ into Equation (11-23) we have

$$\Delta p_x \cdot \Delta x = h$$

Because the electron can present in other higher orders of diffraction fringes, the uncertainty may ever be greater, so we have

$$\Delta p_x \cdot \Delta x \geqslant h \tag{11-24}$$

If Equation (11-24) is generalized in other coordinate directions, then it should be the form of

$$\Delta x \cdot \Delta p_x \geqslant h, \quad \Delta y \cdot \Delta p_y \geqslant h, \quad \Delta z \cdot \Delta p_z \geqslant h \tag{11-25}$$

These relational expressions are called **Heisenberg uncertainty relation** which is stated as: **For a particle, the product of the uncertainty of its position in a particular direction and the uncertainty of the component of its momentum in this direction can never be smaller than Planck constant.**

The uncertainty relation indicates that the uncertainty of the coordinate and the uncertainty of the momentum of microscopic particle are in inverse proportion to each other. The narrower the slit is, i.e., the smaller the uncertainty of the coordinate Δx of a particle, the bigger the uncertainty of the momentum p_x will be. It is impossible for the particle's position and momentum to have the certain values simultaneously. If the position of a particle is measured accurately enough, its moving direction couldn't be determined perfectly; and if its momentum is measured precisely, its position can't be determined at the moment. This is the inevitable conclusion of the wave-particle duality of the microscopic particles. Therefore, for the microscopic particles, the concept of the rack is meaningless.

In quantum mechanics, the uncertainty relation expressed with Equation (11-25) can be deduced as the uncertainty relation of the momentum and the time. The uncertainty of energy is denoted by ΔE and the uncertainty of time is denoted by Δt, we can get

$$\Delta E \cdot \Delta t \geqslant h$$

The uncertainty relation is a fundamental objective regularity which is based on the wave-particle duality. It is the reflection of the natural characteristics of the microscopic particles, and is not caused by the defects of the apparatus' accuracy and the measuring methods. The uncertainty relation revealed the principles of motion in the microscopic world more truly.

11.5 Hydrogen Spectral Series and Bohr's Theory

11.5.1 Regularity of Hydrogen Spectral Series

As the development of physics, it is realized that the atomic spectrum is bright line spectrum. After a long-term accumulation of experimental results, it is found that many spectra emitted by scorching elements are bright line spectra, and for a certain spectral line, the wavelength of it is fixed. For the spectral lines, they are not in succession, or to say, they are separated and arranged in several spectral series.

To observe the spectral lines emitted by the hydrogen discharging in a low pressure discharge tube with a spectroscope, it can be found that hydrogen spectrum is a bright line spectrum composed of many separated spectral lines, and moreover the wavelengths of this spectral lines follow a certain principle. In 1885, Johann Jakob Balmer summarized a simple formula to generalize the wavelength of each spectral line in the spectrum first, which is named **Balmer Formula** later.

$$\frac{1}{\lambda}=R\left(\frac{1}{2^2}-\frac{1}{n^2}\right) \tag{11-26}$$

where $n=3, 4,\cdots$; and $\frac{1}{\lambda}$ is called the **wave number** in the spectroscopy, which represents the number of complete waves in a unit length; R is Rydberg constant, its experimental value is R=1.097×10^{7}m^{-1}. Balmer spectral series of hydrogen is shown in Figure 11-9. And the spectral lines marked in the diagram H_α, H_β, H_γ are measured with the spectroscopy, among them H_α is a bright red line and H_β, H_γ, H_δ represent cyanine, blue and violet lines respectively, and the rest of the lines are in ultraviolet region.

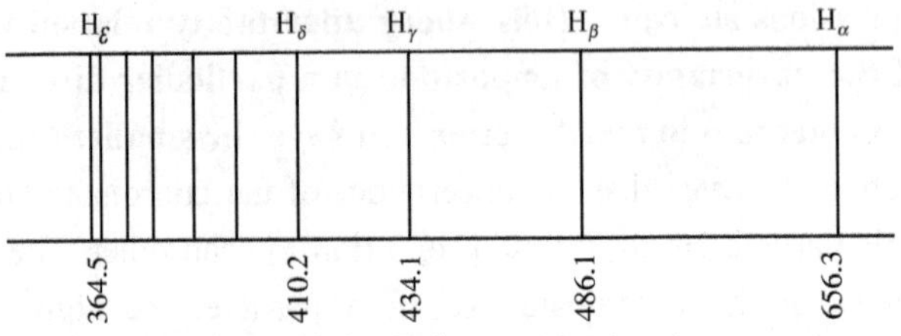

Figure 11-9 Balmer spectral series

Since then, during the years of 1915-1924, Theodore Lyman, Friedrich Paschen, August Herman Pfund, and Frederick. Brackett, etc. found some new spectral series of hydrogen successively in the ultraviolet region and infrared region and their names were used to name these spectral series. The wavelengths of the spectral lines in these spectral series can be calculated with the following similar equations.

$$\frac{1}{\lambda}=R(\frac{1}{1^2}-\frac{1}{n^2}) \qquad n=2, 3,\cdots\text{(Lyman series)}$$

$$\frac{1}{\lambda}=R(\frac{1}{3^2}-\frac{1}{n^2}) \qquad n=4, 5,\cdots\text{(Paschen series)}$$

$$\frac{1}{\lambda}=R(\frac{1}{4^2}-\frac{1}{n^2}) \qquad n=5, 6,\cdots\text{(Brackett series)}$$

$$\frac{1}{\lambda}=R(\frac{1}{5^2}-\frac{1}{n^2}) \qquad n=6, 7,\cdots\text{(A. H. Pfund series)}$$

The equations above can be integrated into one generalized equation, which is known as Rydberg formula

$$\frac{1}{\lambda}=R(\frac{1}{k^2}-\frac{1}{n^2}) \qquad n=k+1,\ k+2,\cdots \tag{11-27}$$

where k is positive integer, as it is 1, 2, 3, 4, 5 the equation corresponds to the equations for Lyman, Paschen, Brackett and A. H. Pfund series. So Equation (11-27) is also called the **generalized Bamler formula**.

In a conclusion, the wavelength of each spectral line in each spectral series of hydrogen atom can be generalized by such a simple equation, and its calculated value is just consistent with the experimental result, which must reflect some kind of regularity inside the hydrogen atom. The equation reveals that:

The wave number corresponding to each spectral line can be expressed with the difference of two items, and the value of each item is only determined by a certain integer, i.e.

$$\frac{1}{\lambda}=T(k)-T(n)$$

For each spectral series, $T(k)$ is fixed and $T(n)$ is variable. $T(k)$ and $T(n)$ are called spectral terms.

At that time, this regularity was not acceptable and comprehensible to the public, so it was called the puzzle of Balmer Formula. As the development of science and technology, it has been explained in theory gradually.

11.5.2 Bohr's Theory of Hydrogen Atom

In 1911, Ernest Rutherford proposed the nucleus structural model of atom according to the experiment of the scattering of α-particles, which states that an atom is composed of a nucleus and several electrons rotating around the nucleus. Although this model could give the perfect explanations to some of the experimental results, still, it encountered difficulties when comes to the explanation of atomic spectrums. According to the classical electromagnetic theory, an electron orbiting around the nucleus should have a centripetal acceleration and should radiate electromagnetic wave continuously. Therefore, the energy of the electron should decrease gradually, which should result in the approach of the electron to the nucleus. Finally, the electron would fall into the nucleus and be annihilated. Thus, atoms should be an unstable system, and the spectrums radiated should be continuous. But as the demonstrations of experiments, any atom is a steady system; moreover, the atomic spectrums are line spectrums.

For giving a reasonable explanation, in 1913, Niels Bohr abandoned some classical conceptions and brought the idea of quantum into the theory of the atomic structure. He proposed his hypothesis that successfully explained the regularity in hydrogen spectral series. This is called Bohr's theory of the hydrogen atom. Bohr's postulates are as follows.

①For an atom there exist a series of stable states. In these states the atom has the decided energies and doesn't radiate any electromagnetic wave. These states are simply called **stationary states**. In these states, the orbital angular momentum of the rotation of an extra-nucleus electron about the nucleus L must be the integer times of $h/2\pi$ which is expressed as

$$L=mvr_{\mathrm{n}}=n\frac{h}{2\pi} \qquad (n=1,2,3,\cdots) \tag{11-28}$$

where m, v, r_{n} represent the mass, velocity, orbital radius of the electron respectively; h is Planck constant and n is called the quantum number.

②Atoms emit or absorb electromagnetic wave with the fixed frequency as long as the electron makes a transition from one stationary state with energy level of E_n to another of E_k in an atom. The frequency of the photon, which is radiated or absorbed, is determined by the following equation

$$\nu=\frac{E_n-E_k}{h} \tag{11-29}$$

This equation is called frequency condition. Bohr worked out the orbital radius and energy levels of hydrogen atom and was rather successful in explaining the regularities of spectral series of hydrogen atom based on the postulates above.

For the purpose that taking the hydrogen atom and hydrogen-like atoms into account at the same time, supposing the nucleus charge number is Z, electron with the mass of m and the electric quantity of e is moving on an orbit with the radius of r_n at the velocity of v. The centripetal force is provided by electrostatic Coulomb force between nucleus and electron. It is expressed as

$$\frac{1}{4\pi\varepsilon_0}\cdot\frac{Ze^2}{r_n^2}=m\frac{v^2}{r_n} \tag{11-30}$$

To solve the simultaneous Equation (11-28) and Equation (11-29) and eliminate v, we can get

$$r_n=\frac{\varepsilon_0 n^2 h^2}{m\pi Ze^2} \quad (n=1, 2, 3\cdots) \tag{11-31}$$

When $Z=1, n=1$, we can get the minimum orbital radius, which is **Bohr radius**, generally denoted by a_0, so we have

$$a_0=\frac{\varepsilon_0 h^2}{\pi e^2 m}=5.29\times10^{-11}\text{m}$$

In this way, Equation (11-31) can also be rewritten as

$$r_n=\frac{n^2}{Z}a_0 \quad (n=1, 2, 3\cdots) \tag{11-32}$$

The order of magnitude of a_0 conforms to the experimental result.

The total energy of the atom E_n should be the algebraic sum of the kinetic energy of the electron and the potential energy between the electron and the nucleus when its electron is on the orbit with quantum number n. If the electric potential energy while the electron is at infinity (i.e. $r_n=\infty$) is zero, then

$$E_n=\frac{1}{2}mv^2-\frac{Ze^2}{4\pi\varepsilon_0 r_n}$$

From Equation (11-30) we can see that

$$\frac{1}{2}mv^2=\frac{Ze^2}{8\pi\varepsilon_0 r_n}$$

So when quantum number is n, the total energy is

$$E_n=-\frac{Ze^2}{8\pi\varepsilon_0 r_n}=-\frac{mZ^2e^4}{8\varepsilon_0^2 n^2 h^2} \quad (n=1, 2, 3\cdots) \tag{11-33}$$

Because it is defined that the potential energy between the electron and the nucleus is zero when the distance between the electron and the nucleus is infinity, the electron is in the bounded state, therefore the total energy of the whole atom must be negative. When $n=1$, the energy is the minimum and the corresponding state of the atom is called the **Ground State**. In this way, we can work out the energy of ground state of hydrogen atom E_1, that is

$$E_1=-2.18\times10^{-18}\text{ J}=-13.6\text{ eV}$$

The value is just equal to the ionization energy of hydrogen atom as the experimental result. Equation (11-33) can also be written as

$$E_n=-13.6\frac{Z^2}{n^2}\text{ (eV)} \tag{11-34}$$

An atom gets the minimum energy when it is in the ground state. When the electron is on one of the outer orbits ($n>1$), the energy of the atom will be in one of the corresponding states which has the energy higher than the energy of the ground state, and these states are all called the **excited states**. As an electron jump from the orbit with the quantum number of n to another orbit with quantum number of k, according to the second postulate of Bohr's theory, we can determine the frequency of the corresponding photon of the transition radiation.

$$\nu = \frac{E_n - E_k}{h} = \frac{me^4 Z^2}{8\varepsilon_0^2 h^3}(\frac{1}{k^2} - \frac{1}{n^2}) \qquad (n > k)$$

and we have

$$\frac{1}{\lambda} = \frac{\nu}{c} = \frac{me^4 Z^2}{8\varepsilon_0^2 h^3 c}(\frac{1}{k^2} - \frac{1}{n^2}) = RZ^2(\frac{1}{k^2} - \frac{1}{n^2}) \qquad (11\text{-}35)$$

where

$$R = \frac{me^4}{8\varepsilon_0^2 h^3 c} = 1.097 \times 10^7 \text{ m}^{-1}$$

This value conforms to the result of R detected by experiments, so the theoretical foundation for Rydberg constant and the theoretical explanation of the generalized Balmer formula were found.

For the hydrogen atom, whose $Z = 1$, from Equation (11-35) we can get

$$\frac{1}{\lambda} = R(\frac{1}{k^2} - \frac{1}{n^2})$$

Thus, the regularity of hydrogen spectral series was perfectly explained. Lyman series ($k = 1$) is produced when electrons of atoms jump from the outer orbits to the most inner first orbits of atoms; likewise, Balmer series is produced, when electrons of atoms jump to the second orbits of atoms; similarly, when electrons of atoms jump to the third orbits of atoms, Paschen series is produced; and so forth.

These spectral line series produced as electrons' transitions among their orbits can also be described by the energy levels in Figure 11-10. Each directed line corresponds to a spectral line, and we can calculate the respective frequency of the spectral line according to the energy levels corresponding starting and ending of the directed line. At some moment, one hydrogen atom can only emit one spectral line. While many electrons can emit many different spectral lines simultaneously. For the situation that numerous of atoms are excited at the same time, we can observe the whole spectrum. From the experimental results we can find that the intensities of different spectral lines are different, which indicates that at some moment, the number of atoms for radiating some special spectral line is different from others.

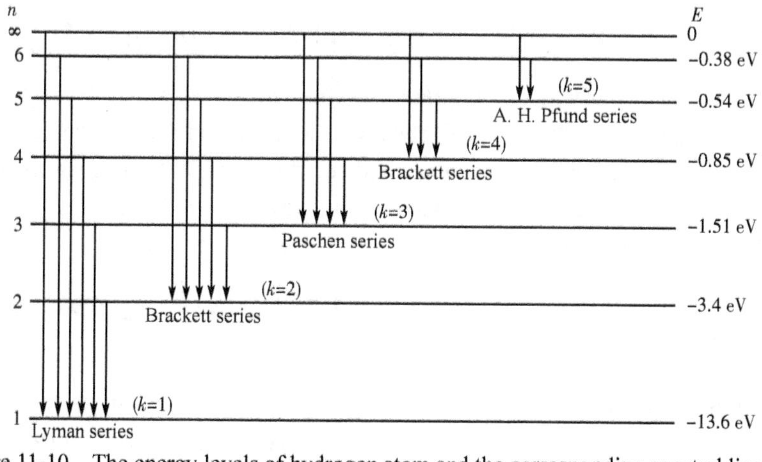

Figure 11-10 The energy levels of hydrogen atom and the corresponding spectral line series

11.6 Four Quantum Numbers

Bohr introduced the quantum hypothesis into classical physics. Though this theory can explain the regularity of the hydrogen spectral series rather perfectly, but its result can merely be extended to hydrogen-like ions, which around a nucleus there is only one electron orbiting. For other more complex atoms or molecules, Bohr's theory can't be applied successfully, and its limitation is embodied. Until 1926, Schrödinger proposed the mechanics system for studying the motion of microscopic particles-wave mechanics, which laid a groundwork for quantum mechanics. In quantum mechanics the motional states of the electrons in an atom are mainly determined by four quantum numbers, as stated as follow.

11.6.1 Principal Quantum Number

It can be derived from the theory of quantum mechanics that the energy states of hydrogen atoms are several discrete values determined by the equation below:

$$E_n = -\frac{me^4}{8\varepsilon_0^2 h^2}\cdot\frac{1}{n^2} \qquad (n = 1, 2, 3, \cdots) \qquad (11\text{-}36)$$

where n is called the **principal quantum number**. This expression is in complete agreement with the equation deduced by Bohr's Theory.

We usually divide the distribution of electrons in an atom into several shells. Electrons with the same principal quantum n are in the same shell. When the principal quantum number n is assigned respectively as one of these integers 1, 2, 3, 4, 5, 6, the corresponding shells are identified respectively by these letters K, L, M, N, O, P.

11.6.2 Angular Momentum Quantization and Angular Quantum Number

If L represents the angular momentum of an electron orbiting around a nucleus, as the researches of quantum mechanics, the value of L can only be some of the definite discrete values, rather than an arbitrary one, which indicates that the angular momentums of electrons is also quantized. And these discrete values are

$$L = \sqrt{l(l+1)}\frac{h}{2\pi} \qquad [l = 0, 1, 2, 3, \cdots, (n-1)] \qquad (11\text{-}37)$$

The quantum number l is called the **angular quantum number**, which decides the value of the quantized angular momentum. The different electrons with different angular momentums should be in the different moving states. The electrons on the same shell could have different angular momentums, which correspond to different moving states. One of the moving states of l = 0, 1, 2, 3, 4, 5, or 6 is usually denoted by one of the corresponding states of *s*, *p*, *d*, *f*, *g*, *h*, or *i*.

11.6.3 Space Quantization and Magnetic Quantum Number

In classical mechanics, the angular momentum is a vector quantity, and its spatial orientation is arbitrary. But in terms of quantum mechanics the angular momentum can only take a series of specific directions as an electron orbiting around a nucleus, so its spatial orientation is quantized as well. That is called **space quantization**. Thus, the component of the angular momentum in a particular direction (such as along the z axis or the direction of the external magnetic field) can only take a series of discrete values which are

$$L_z = m\frac{h}{2\pi} \qquad (m = 0, \pm 1, \pm 2, \cdots, \pm l) \tag{11-38}$$

where the quantum number m is called the **magnetic quantum number**. The component of the angular momentum L_Z takes different values, which indicates that the angular momentum of the electron has the different spatial orientations and the electron is in different moving states as well. The electron with a fixed angular momentum may have $2l+1$ different spatial orientations corresponding to $2l+1$ different moving states.

11.6.4 Electron Spin Quantization and Spin Magnetic Quan tum Number

It is proved with theories and experiments that, for the electrons in the atoms apart from orbiting around the nuclei, they also spin around their own axes. Similar to the angular momentum of an electron orbiting around the nucleus, the spin angular momentum of the electron is also quantized and it can be expressed as the following expression

$$L_s = \sqrt{s(s+1)}\frac{h}{2\pi}, \quad s = \frac{1}{2} \tag{11-39}$$

Here, the quantum number s is called the **spin quantum number**. Spin angular momentum component along the external magnetic field (z axis) is

$$L_{sz} = m_s\frac{h}{2\pi}, \quad m_s = \pm\frac{1}{2}$$

where m_s is called the **spin magnetic quantum number**.

To sum up, for any electron in an atom, its moving state is determined by the four quantum numbers mentioned above. In quantum mechanics, these four quantum numbers are decided by solving the Schrödinger equation, rather than the figments. Meanwhile with the theory discussed above, it also points out that the electrons in an atom are distributed to different shells according to the different quantum states, and which in turn proves the periodic law of elements, i.e., electrons is arranged on the shells periodically. In this way, the periodic law of elements is improved to the level of the quantum theory, and the foundation for the research of atomic spectrum is established.

11.7 Atomic Spectrum and Molecular Spectrum

11.7.1 Atomic Spectrum

Atoms in excited states will emit photons and form spectra. The photons corresponding to a certain spectral line in a spectrum are emitted as the atoms jumping from higher energy levels to relatively lower levels. Several bright lines are formed by the photons emitted by a large amount of atoms; and these bright lines form the **atomic emission spectrum** and it is also called the **bright line spectrum**. Atomic emission spectrum is formed when the valence electrons are excited to get a transition to an outer orbit corresponding to some empty energy level and then have some transitions among the outer orbits corresponding to some empty energy levels or jump back to its original state. The energy differences between different levels corresponding to the states when electrons are on different outer shells are smaller, so the frequencies of the spectral lines produced by the transitions of the electrons should be lower. Generally, the wavelengths of the spectral lines are in the region of visible light or in the near-infrared or near-ultraviolet bands.

Atomic absorption spectrum is formed as a valence electron absorbs a photon and is excited to some higher energy level. When an incandescent light with a continuous spectrum passing through some special steams or gases, for certain wavelengths in the spectrum, the corresponding photons are absorbed numerously, that will lead to a series of dark lines in the continuous spectrum which is called **atomic absorption spectrum**, or **dark line spectrum**. For example, the dark-line spectrum of the sun is formed as the self-emitted continuous spectrum is absorbed by its incandescence outer gas layer. The wavelengths of the bright line spectrum of the some element must be equal to the wavelengths of its dark-line spectrum. The reason is that these two kinds of spectrums are both formed by the transitions between pairs of corresponding energy levels in the same kind of atoms. But the lines in the dark line spectrum are far less than the lines in the bright line spectrum. The reason is that atoms are normally in the ground state, and the dark lines in the dark line spectrum are only formed by the transitions from the ground state to the excited states, rather than the transitions among various excited states.

Since each element has its own particular bright line spectrum and dark line spectrum, we can detect the existence of an element or the elementary composition in some absorber from the distribution of its spectral lines. That is exactly the essential principle of spectrographic analysis. It is not necessary to measure all of its spectral lines in the identification of certain element. We only need to find some of its most obvious and typical lines for determining the existence of such element. Also, we can identify the metal elements in liquid samples by means of atomic absorption spectrum. For example, in the examination to some body to detect if there is the lead poisoning or not, we can take his urine or blood as absorber then according to its absorption spectrum to determine whether there is lead. In medical applications the widely used atomic spectrum analysis is carried out by drying, ashing and vaporizing biological samples into gases. The spectrum analysis is far more accurate and sensitive than the chemical analyses, and it can identify the mass of trace elements up to 10^{-9} gram.

11.7.2 Molecular Spectrum

Compared with the atomic spectrum, the molecular spectrum is much more complex. As for the range of wavelengths, molecular spectra can be divided into far infrared spectrum, mid-infrared spectrum, near infrared spectrum, visible spectrum and ultraviolet spectrum. The schematic diagram of molecular spectrum is as shown in Figure 11-11. A spectral band (I) consists of several separated spectral lines; a spectral band group (II) consists of several spectral bands; a molecular spectrum (III) consists of several spectral groups. As the arrangement of these spectral lines is too dense to distinguish the lines clearly with common instruments, so a cluster of spectral lines is considered as a continuous spectrum band. Hence the molecular spectrum is also called the **band spectrum**. This is the difference between the atomic spectrum and the molecular spectrum in shape.

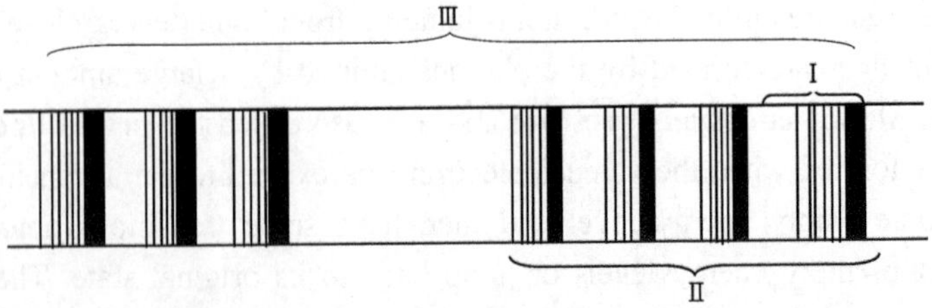

Figure 11-11 Schematic diagram of molecule spectrum

The complexity of the molecular spectrum depends on the complicated moving states inside molecules. For the sake of simplicity, let's take diatomic molecules as an example to discuss. The motions inside a molecule can be described as three forms: ①The rotation of the molecule around an axis; ②the vibration among the atoms to compose the molecule; ③the motions of the electrons among the energy levels of stationary states. The energies of these three kinds of motions make up the total energy of the molecular E:

$$E = E_{\mathrm{r}} + E_{\upsilon} + E_{\mathrm{e}}$$

where E_{r}, E_v, E_{e} are molecular rotational energy, atomic vibration energy and the electronic energy of stationary states. However, these energies are all quantized.

Molecules emit photons as they transit from a higher energy of E_2 to a lower energy state of E_1, likewise, they absorb photons as they transit form the lower energy state E_1 to the higher energy state E_2. The energy of an emitted or absorbed photon is

$$h\nu = E_2 - E_1 = \Delta E_{\mathrm{r}} + \Delta E_v + \Delta E_{\mathrm{e}}$$

where ΔE_{r}, ΔE_v, ΔE_{e} represent respectively the changes of the rotational energy, the vibration energy and the energy of electrons during the molecular transition. Usually, ΔE_{e} is in 1-20 eV; ΔE_v is in 0.05-1 eV and ΔE_{r} is in 0.0001-0.05 eV. The energy levels of a molecule also overlap with each other. As the transitions of electrons among the stationary states in the molecule, the vibration state and rotational state will vary too. These are the reasons that lead to the complexity of the molecular spectrum.

Among the changes of the energies, the change of stationary energy of the electrons ΔE_{e} is the biggest, so it determines the region of the spectral band group; while the change of vibration energy ΔE_v is much smaller than ΔE_{e}, its change can only cause the change of position of each spectral band in the band group; and the change of the rotational energy ΔE_{r} is the smallest one, it decides the fine structure of the spectral band (the position of each spectral line in the spectral band). Because ΔE_{r} is so small, the spectral lines are so dense to form a spectral band. Summing up, on the energy levels of the electrons in the molecules there are superimposed vibration energy levels and rotational energy levels, which is the primary cause why the molecular spectrum is more complicated than the atomic spectrum.

Usually, the absorption spectrum is adopted in molecular spectrum analysis. That is because during the heating or discharging processes, a lot of molecules, especially the molecules with the complex structures would decompose if the emission spectrum were adopted, so we can't get the corresponding real spectrum. However, the entire process of absorption spectrum analysis is performed at room temperature. It does not change the molecular structures of the measured sample. Analogue to the atomic absorption spectrum, molecular absorption spectrum bands are less than molecular emission spectrum, this is because most molecules are in the ground state at room temperature. Molecular absorption spectrum analysis, especially ultraviolet and infrared absorption spectrum analyses and researches have been widely used in the scientific researches such as the analyses of Chinese herb medicines' components and so on.

11.8 Laser and Its Applications

Laser is the abbreviation of light amplification by stimulated emission of radiation, also known as laser light. Laser is a wonderful coherent light obtained by stimulated radiation that lead to a constant enlargement to light, which is produced on the basis of the theory of stimulated radiation put forward by Einstein in 1916. The device for producing laser is called laser device (or optical master) . In this section, we will give a brief introduction to the principle to generate laser, the particular property of laser and its applications in medicament.

11.8.1 Principle to Generate Laser

As a beam of light passing through an object, parts of the photons would be absorbed, which results in the transition of atoms from some lower energy level of E_k to an excited state with a higher energy level of E_n. An atom in the excited state will spontaneously jump back to the lower energy level from higher energy level, and the energy difference between the two levels would radiate in the form of a photon. This process is called the **spontaneous radiation**. The spontaneous radiation will produce photons with corresponding frequency of $\nu = \dfrac{E_n - E_k}{h}$, whose vibration directions, propagation directions, and initial phases are all independent of each other. Because there are a large amount of atoms and molecules in a light source, they emit photons irrelatively and independently in every direction, and this kind of light is the normal natural light.

For atoms in higher energy levels, under the inducing action from the external photons with certain frequency coincident in the conditions above, there will be the transition of atoms from higher energy levels to lower energy levels and the radiation of photons with identical features with the external photons. This kind of radiation is called the **stimulated radiation**, whose characteristics are: The vibration direction, vibrating frequency, propagation direction and phrase of the emitted photons are the same as the external photons'. By the stimulated radiation the number of the photons in the emitted light is much larger than the photons in the incident light; therefore we can say that the light is "amplified". This shows that **the stimulated radiation is the important basis to form laser**.

According to the law of Boltzmann distribution, at thermal equilibrium most of atoms in objects are in ground state. To realize stimulated radiation and make it in the dominative situation, the first thing is that there must be far more atoms in higher energy levels than in lower energy levels. This kind of state is just contrary to the normal distribution at thermal equilibrium, so it is called the population inversion, and the population inversion is the prerequisite condition to realize the light amplification by stimulated emission of radiation.

To realize the population inversion, firstly we need to supply energy to the working substance from the outside constantly, so that after absorbing the energy as many atoms in the working substance as possible will be excited and jump from the lower levels to the higher levels continuously. This process is called as the **excitation**, and also called as **pumping**. The working substance in current laser is commonly stimulated by optical excitation or gas discharge excitation. Secondly, the energy level structure of the working substance must be appropriate so as to meet the need that the average lifetime of the atoms in higher level must be long enough. These energy levels are called the **metastable state energy levels**. The average lifetime for atoms to stay in higher energy levels are 10^{-9} s, but the average lifetime for the atoms to stay in the metastable state is much longer, it can even be over 1000 000 times, i.e., the lifetime can be up to a few tenths of a second. In this case, because of the excitation from the outside and the existence of the working substance with the metastable state, more atoms of the working substance are in the metastable state energy level. In this way, the population inversion as the condition to produce laser is realized. A kind of three-level structure which can represent the population inversion is shown in Figure 11-12. Where A represents ground state, B and C are excited states therein B is the metastable state. By absorbing photons, discharging or collisions, the atoms are stimulated from state A to state C.

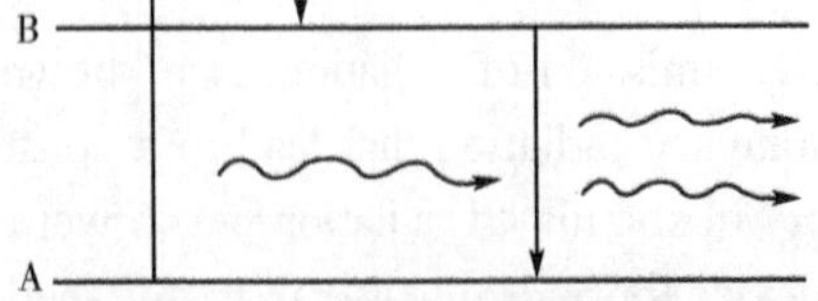

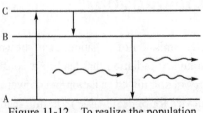

Figure 11-12 To realize the population inversion by a metastable state

In a short time, the atoms will jump to state B from state C spontaneously. But state B is a metastable state, atoms can stay in state B for a long time and not jump back to state A quickly. In this way, there will be a great increase in the number of atoms in state B, then the population inversion between state B and state A is realized. As the spontaneous radiation goes on, the atoms from state B jump back to state A and emit photons. When these photons meet the atoms in state B, the stimulated radiation will be induced.

The conditions above are not enough for generating laser. The original photons which cause the stimulated radiations come from the spontaneous radiations, but the directions and phases of the photons produced by spontaneous radiations are irregular. These irregular photons induce the stimulated radiations and generate the light waves amplified in intensities, and these light waves will propagate in all directions and have the different phases of themselves. In order to produce a laser with good directionality and intense coherence, it is necessary to choose the light signal with a certain propagation direction and a certain frequency as the first priority of amplification and inhibit the rest signals. Therefore, a completely reflecting mirror (such as the mirror with the reflectivity more than 99.9%) and a partially reflecting mirror (such as the mirror with the reflectivity of 90%) should be placed parallel at the both ends of the working substance respectively, and the mirrors should be perpendicular to the axis of the working substance. In this way, the working substance and the two mirrors construct an optical resonant cavity together. Usually the photons diverged from the axis of the optical resonant cavity will soon escape from the cavity, and can't come into contact with the working substance again. Meanwhile, photons moving along the direction of the axis will stay in the cavity and move back and forth along the axis continuously by means of the reflections of the two mirrors. Photons moving in cavity will continually encounter excited particles and induce stimulated radiations. Finally, the number of photons moving along the direction of the axis will increase constantly in the resonant cavity and form an intense beam of light with the completely same propagating direction and the common phase. After outputting through the partially reflecting mirror it was the laser. Therefore, the optical resonant cavity is one of the necessary conditions in the formation of laser. It is used for maintaining the optical oscillation and optical amplification and obtaining an excellent monochromatic light beam. According to the view of wave, only when the length of the resonant cavity is equal to integer times of half wavelength of the light, this corresponding light with the specific wavelength can form a strengthened superposition as a stable standing wave after moving back and forth for a circle. Meanwhile, the material and the thicknesses of the reflecting films coated on the mirrors should also meet the condition that they should be reflection increasing films for the light wave with the specific wavelength, i.e., they should ensure the light to have the greatest reflection.

11.8.2 Laser Devices

According to the difference of working substances laser devices can be roughly divided into four types: Solid laser devices, liquid laser devices, gas laser devices, and semiconductor laser devices. First, let's take the ruby laser as an example to introduce the structure of a laser device briefly.

The working substance in the ruby laser is a ruby rod made of aluminum oxide crystal doped with small amount of chromium ions; and the chromium ions replace some of the aluminum ions in the crystal. The two end faces of the crystal rod are polished exquisitely and kept parallel extremely. The silver is coated on one end face with a thicker thickness to form a completely reflecting mirror, while the other end face is coated with a thinner thickness to form a partially reflecting mirror whose light transmittance is about 1%-10%, and it was from the end that the laser is let out. This whole structure constructs a resonant cavity. Outside the cavity there is a pulse xenon lamp as the optical excitation, also known as the "pumping", which emits intense blue-violet light and yellow-green light, which can stimulate chromium ions to the excited states during every spark of several milliseconds and leading to the formation of population inversion. The structure diagram of the ruby laser is as shown in Figure 11-13.

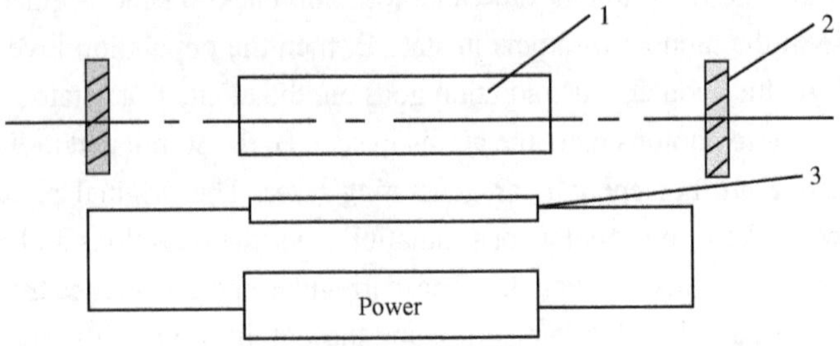

Figure 11-13 Schematic diagram of the structure of a ruby laser

1. A ruby rod; 2. A partially reflecting mirror; 3. A xenon lamp

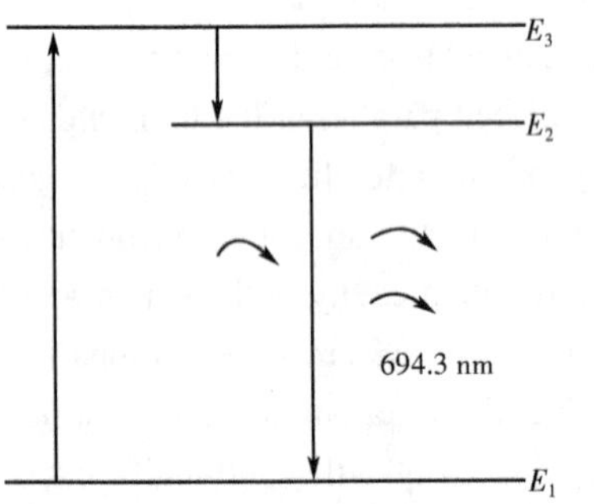

Figure 11-14 Schematic diagram of energy levels of the ruby laser

Figure 11-14 is a schematic diagram of the energy levels of a ruby laser, where E_1 is the ground state and E_2 is a metastable state. A large amount of chromium ions in the state of E_1 are stimulated onto the level E_3 as the ruby rod is irradiated by the xenon lamp. The average lifetime of chromium ions on the energy level E_3 is very short (about 10^{-9} s) , hence it emitted spontaneously onto the energy level E_2 from E_3 rapidly. And the average lifetime on the energy level E_2 is about 3 ms. Consequently, there is population inversion between energy levels E_2 and E_1. Thereafter, by a stimulated emission, a red laser with the wavelength of 694.3 nm is produced.

There are many different types of laser devices with different outputting energy or power, which are continuous output mode and pulsed output mode. Helium-neon laser is a gas laser whose working substance is neon atoms. Helium atoms only constitute the auxiliary material which helps the neon atoms realize the population inversion by transmitting energy. The shell of the laser tube is made of glass in the middle of it there is a capillary for discharging. Two reflecting mirrors at the both ends of the tube construct a resonant optical cavity, as shown in Figure 11-15.

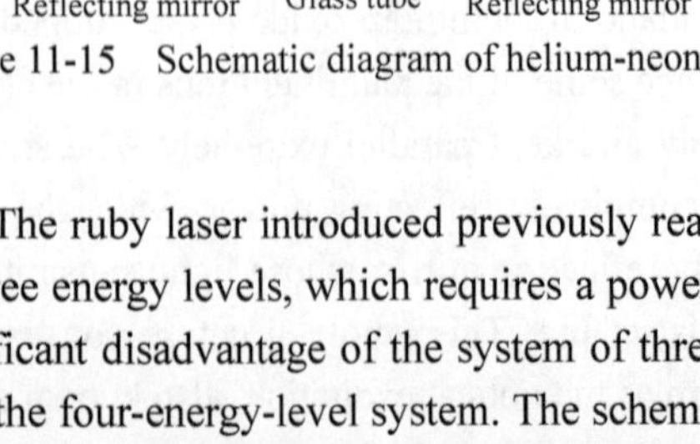

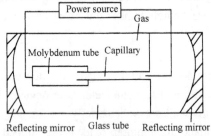

Figure 11-15 Schematic diagram of helium-neon laser

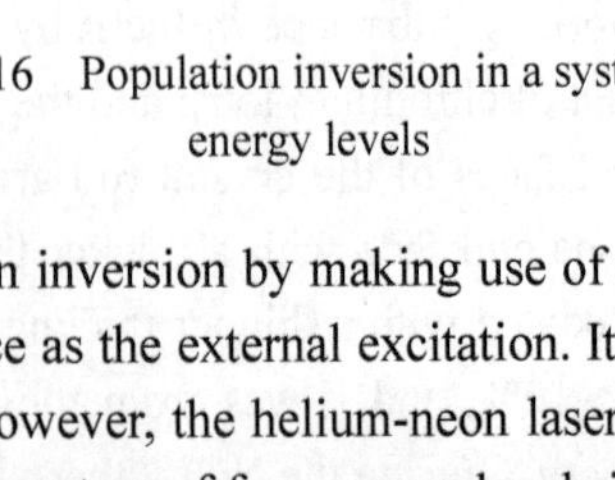

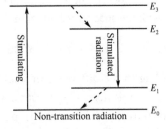

Figure 11-16 Population inversion in a system of four energy levels

The ruby laser introduced previously realizes the population inversion by making use of the system of three energy levels, which requires a powerful pumping source as the external excitation. It is also the significant disadvantage of the system of three energy levels. However, the helium-neon laser is the one with the four-energy-level system. The schematic diagram of the system of four energy levels is shown in Figure 11-16. In the system, the population inversion is realized between E_2 and E_1. At room temperature, the number of atoms on E_1 is very little, so the realization of population inversion in the system of four energy levels is easier than that in system of three energy levels. There are other lasers such as neodymium glass laser, neodymium-doped yttrium aluminum garnet (Nd: YAG) glass laser and carbon dioxide laser. All of them are the lasers with the system of four energy levels.

Table 11-1 lists the simple statuses and applications of several commonly used lasers in medicine.

Table 11-1 Lasers commonly used medicine

Working substance	Working style	Wavelength (μm)	Output energy or power	Main applications
Ruby	Pulse	0.6943	0.05-500 J	Ophthalmology, clinical research
CO_2	Continuous	10.6	15-300 W	Dermatology, surgery, medical oncology, radiation or burning
He-Ne	Continuous	0.6328	1-70 mW	Acupuncture, surgery, dermatology, gynecology, obstetrics and irradiation
He-Cd	Continuous	0.4416	9-120 mW	Body surface tumor, fluorescence diagnosis
N_2	Pulse	0.337	0.4-1 mJ	ENT, dermatology, basic research

11.8.3 Characteristics of Laser

Compared with ordinary light sources, laser has the following characteristics.

1. Good Directionality

Taking advantage of the effect of optical **resonant** cavity, the laser output is in parallel transmission. The order magnitude of the divergence angles of the laser beams output from ordinary lasers are at 10^{-3} rad. Therefore, the directionality of the laser is very good. Owing to this, laser can be used in the aspects such as radar, positioning, guiding and communication, etc.

2. High Intensity

Due to the good directionality of laser, its energy can be focused in a narrow beam, so its intensity is extremely high. It can be used in crystal cutting, welding and drilling, and it can also be used in surgical operations, etc.

3. Good Monochromaticity

There must be a wavelength coverage for any light emitted from any monochromatic light source, which is represented by the width of the spectral line. The narrower the spectral line width is, the better the monochromaticity of this light will be. Before the invention of laser, the monochromaticity of krypton lamp was the best one and the width of spectral line is about 10^{-4} nm, while, the width of the spectral line of the helium-neon laser is only about 10^{-8} nm. Therefore, the monochromaticity of laser is very good so as to be used as a standard for length measurement.

4. Good Coherence

As the laser is composed of photons with the same frequency, the same phase and vibration direction, the laser is coherent light. For a light with the best monochromaticity emitted from an ordinary light source, after being split into two beams, the two wavelets could produce the interference only within the optical path difference (OPD) of several 10 cm. But the optical path difference for the interference produced by laser can be up to several 10 km. Therefore, the laser is an ideal coherent light source that can be used for precision measurement and holography.

11.8.4 Applications of Laser in Medicine and Pharmacology

Laser has many advantages: It can be controlled as a narrow beam of light, it has the short pulse period, it can be orientated easily, and so on. These advantages just fit for the requirements of medical science. First laser can be applied in ophthalmology. The laser with highly focused intensity can penetrate through the eyeball to reach fundus oculi without any damage to the forepart tissues. Hence, laser can be used in the treatments like the welding of retinal detachment, the closure of retinal tears, the operation of iris resection, and so on. The ruby laser is commonly applied in ophthalmology; meanwhile, Ar^+ laser and the He-Cd laser with blue-green light can be easily absorbed by hemoglobin and is better for the treatment of fundus oculi diseases.

In the surgery treatments, lasers with high-power such as the neodymium doped yttrium aluminum garnet (Nd: YAG) laser, the carbon dioxide laser and so on are used as the laser scalpels in operations, for they can produce the power at the magnitude order of 100 W. This application has shown the great advantages in tumor resection, for it can help close the blood vessels, reduce bleeding in the process of organ resection. Lasers with middle or low power have a better effect in anti-inflammatory and the promotion to epithelial growth. And they have the great advantages in the remove of skin color spots, moles, warts and other blemishes, so as to become the wonderful cosmetic appliances. Highly focused laser can also be made into acupoint-irradiated laser needle, with the apparent curative effects and the features of being harmless and painless for patients, it is one of the examples of Chinese medicine acupuncture instruments' reformations.

Because the laser generated by the YAG (yttrium aluminum garnet) laser and the laser of 1.06 μm generated by the neodymium glass laser can be transmitted in optical fibers, combined with the endoscopy, they can be used for the treatment of bleeding in gastric ulcer and stomach aneurysm resection. Some successful experiences have been achieved in the treatments of various skin diseases by the irradiation of Nitrogen molecular ultraviolet laser and the diagnoses of tumors by the utilization of fluorescent beam.

With the aid of an inverted microscope we can destroy specific parts inside a cell by laser, and that has provided a powerful tool in the research of the mechanisms of cell metabolism and division.

Lasers have also been used in the identifications and analyses of herbal medicines, such as Raman spectroscopy analysis of the effective ingredients of herbal medicines and the identifications of authenticity and quality of Chinese herbal medicines with laser beams.

As the development of science and technology, the applications of laser in medicine and pharmacology are still extending. Staffs and patients should pay attention to the protection of eyes in the use of laser. For the laser with higher intensity and its energy are concentrated, even the reflected light could cause effects to human body, so we should pay special attention to the precaution of laser.

A Brief Summarization of This Chapter

(1) Definitions of the radiant exitance $M = M(T)$, monochromic radiation exitance $M = M(\lambda, T)$ and integral relation between them

$$M(T) = \int_0^{\infty} M(\lambda, T)\mathrm{d}\lambda$$

(2) Two experimental laws of the radiation of the black body:

Stefan-Boltzmann Law

$$M_0(T)=\int_0^{\infty} M_0(\lambda,T)\mathrm{d}\lambda = \sigma T^4$$

Wien's Displacement Law

$$\lambda_m T = b$$

(3) Planck's hypothesis of quantization of energy first proposed the concept of energy quantum $\varepsilon=hv$, laid the

foundation of quantum physics.

(4) The content of Einstein's theory of photon and the equation of photoelectric effect

$$h\nu = \frac{1}{2}mv^2 + A$$

(5) the wave-particle duality of microscopic particles, and de Broglie equation satisfied for material particles

$$\lambda = \frac{h}{p} = \frac{h}{mv}, \quad \nu = \frac{\varepsilon}{h}$$

(6) Uncertainty principle

$$\Delta x \cdot \Delta p_x \geqslant h, \quad \Delta y \cdot \Delta p_y \geqslant h, \quad \Delta z \cdot \Delta p_z \geqslant h, \quad \Delta E \cdot \Delta t \geqslant h$$

(7) Regularity of hydrogen atomic spectrum

Hydrogen atomic spectrum is the line spectrum composed of several separated spectral line groups, which follow the Rydberg formula:

$$\frac{1}{\lambda} = R(\frac{1}{k^2} - \frac{1}{n^2}) \qquad (k = 1, 2, 3, \cdots; \ n = k+1, \ k+2, \cdots)$$

where k determines the spectral line group, and n determines each spectral line.

(8) The hypotheses in Bohr's theory for hydrogen atom: The hypothesis of stationary state, the hypothesis of quantum theory of orbital angular momentum and the hypothesis of transition; the Bohr radius can be derived from them

$$a_0 = \frac{\varepsilon_0 h^2}{\pi e^2 m} = 5.29 \times 10^{-11} \text{m}$$

(9) Four quantum numbers: According to the theories of quantum mechanics they determine the moving states of electrons, they are principle quantum number n, angular quantum number l, magnetic quantum number m and electron spin magnetic quantum number m_s.

(10) Atomic spectrums and molecular spectrums contain emission spectrums and absorption spectrums, where an atomic spectrum is the line spectrum and a molecular is the complex band spectrum.

(11) The production of laser: The stimulated emission is the important basis to form laser, and the population inversion is the prerequisite to realize the light amplification by stimulated emission of radiation, while the optical resonant cavity is the necessary condition to produce laser.

(12) The characteristics of laser are: High intensity, good directionality, good monochromaticity and good coherence.

Excises 11

11-1. Determine the ionization energy of the hydrogen atom.

11-2. Try to calculate the energy of the hydrogen atom in ground state.

11-3. Determine the de Broglie wavelength of an electron with the kinetic energy of 500 eV.

11-4. Try to determine the longest and the shortest wavelengths in Balmer series in hydrogen spectrum.

11-5. Try to determine the corresponding frequencies of the highest and the lowest frequency spectral lines in Brackett series.

11-6. If the hydrogen atoms in the ground state are bombarded by the electrons with the energy of 12.5 eV, which spectral lines could be produced?

11-7. If the power of radiation from per unit surface of a black body is 5.67 W/cm^2, what is the surface temperature of the black body?

11-8. What is the wavelength of the photon radiated, if the electron in a hydrogen atom jumps from the state of $n = 5$ to the state of $n = 2$?

11-9. When the peak wavelength corresponding to the maximum monochromatic radiant emittance in the spectrum of a black body is 400 nm, what is the temperature of the blackbody approximately?

11-10. In hydrogen atoms, as the electrons jump from the state of $n=4$ to the ground state, what is the number of spectral lines in all the possible spectral series?

11-11. When $l=3$, what are the possible values of the magnetic quantum number m for a hydrogen atom? And what are the corresponding components of the angular momentums in the direction of the external magnetic field?

11-12. As the electron in a hydrogen atom is in the state of $n=3$, what are the possible values of angular quantum number corresponding to the state? And what are the corresponding angular momentums?

11-13. Suppose the speed of an electron is measured to be 200 m/s with the precision of 0.1%. What is the uncertainty in determining the position of the electron?

11-14. If the spin quantum number of the electron is $s=1/2$, what is the spin angular momentum of the electron? And what are the possible values of the components of the spin angular momentum along with the direction of the external magnetic field?

11-15. A bullet with the mass of 10 g is flying at the speed of 1000 m/s. Determine:

(1) Its de Broglie wavelength;

(2) What is the uncertainty of the speed , if the uncertainty of the position of the bullet is measured to be 0.10 cm.

11-16. According to the Bohr theory, For a hydrogen atom in the state of $n = 2$, what are the orbiting radius, linear velocity and the angular momentum of its electron? And what is its total energy?

11-17. If the stars like the sun can be looked as black bodies, and the peak wavelengths of some stars are measured as: for the sun $\lambda_m = 0.55\ \mu m$, for the Polaris $\lambda_m = 0.35\ \mu m$ and for the Sirius $\lambda_m = 0.29\ \mu m$. Try to determine their surface temperatures.

11-18. For a human erythrocyte with the diameter of 8 μm, the thickness of 2-3 μm, and the mass of 10^{-13} kg, it is supposed that the uncertainty of its location is 0.1 μm. Try to calculate the uncertainty of its speed.

11-19. In the cases when the wavelengths of the incident lights are respectively $\lambda_0 = 400\ nm$ and $\lambda_0 = 0.05\ nm$, if the scattering angle is $\theta = \pi$, calculate the wavelength change of Compton effect $\Delta\lambda$ and the ratio $\Delta\lambda/\lambda$.

11-20. The accelerating voltage in the television picture tube is 9 kV, and the diameter of muzzle of the electric gun is 0.1 mm, determine the uncertainty of the transverse component of the velocity as electrons are shot out from the electric gun. Could these electrons be looked as classical particles?

11-21. In a uniform magnetic field with the magnetic induction of $B = 0.025\ T$, an α-particle is moving along the circular orbit with the radius of $R = 0.83\ cm$. Determine:

(1) The de Broglie wavelength of this α-particle;

(2) The de Broglie wavelength of a small ball with the mass of $m = 0.1\ kg$ and with the same speed as the α-particle's.

11-22. According to Bohr theory, the diameter of the orbit of the electron inside a hydrogen atom in ground state is about 10^{-10} m, and the speed of the electron is about 2.18×10^6 m/s . Suppose the coordinate uncertainty of an electron inside a hydrogen atom is 10^{-10} m, try to determine the speed uncertainty of the electron.

11-23. Photons with the wavelength of $\lambda = 0.2\ nm$ are scattered by the electrons in a piece of graphite, if we take the observation in the direction with an angle of 90° to the incident direction. Determine:

(1) The change of the wavelength of the scattered light $\Delta\lambda$;

(2) The kinetic energy of a recoil electron. It is supposed that the electron can be looked as static before the scattering.

11-24. Compared with the atomic spectrum, what are the features of the molecular spectrum? And what are the reasons to form these features?

11-25. Population inversion is the prerequisite to cause the realization of the stimulated radiation in the operation of the laser. Then, how to realize the population inversion in a ruby laser?

Chapter 12 X-Rays

In 1895, Wilhelm Conrad Röntgen, a German physicist, discovered the invisible but highly penetrating rays when he was performing the discharge experiments of rarefied gases. For not knowing what those emanations were, Röntgen named the rays he found after the term X-ray. Only three months after the publication of Röntgen's findings, X-rays were applied to clinical application. Now there have been new developments of medical applications of X-rays in diagnosis and treatment. And application method of X-rays has become one of the most important parts in medical field.

In this chapter we will introduce the properties of X-rays and its generation principles, X-ray spectrum, the attenuation law and medical applications of X-rays.

12.1 Properties of X-rays

In 1912, Max von Laue discovered the diffraction of X-rays by crystals. It revealed that X-ray is a form of electromagnetic wave. Laue also measured the wavelengths of X-rays. X-rays are electromagnetic radiations with very short wavelengths, and just like γ rays emitted from the nucleus, X-rays are also high-energy photons. Apart from a varieties of common characteristics of electromagnetic waves, X-rays have many other properties.

12.1.1 Ionizing Function

X-rays enable the atoms and molecules to be ionized. This may result in the conduction of gases to electricity and induce various biological effects. The function of ionization can be used in measuring the intensity of X-rays and treating certain diseases.

12.1.2 Fluorescence Function

When the atoms and molecules, which are excited by X-rays jump back to the ground states and release their excess energies, the fluorescence will be emitted. Some excited states of the atoms or molecules are metastable, so after being irradiated, the fluorescence may be emitted continuously for a while of time. Fluorescence function has been used in medical fluoroscopy for forming the image of X-rays penetrated through the human body.

12.1.3 Penetrating Effect

X-rays have different penetrating abilities to different materials. Researches suggest that the degree of absorption depends on the wavelength of X-ray beam, the atomic number and the density of the substance. The shorter the wavelength of the X-ray is, the lower the absorption of the substance to it and the greater its penetrating ability will be. In medicine, X-rays can be used in the fluoroscopy and the radiography by taking advantage of the penetrating effect and the different extents of absorption in different materials.

12.1.4 Actinic Function

X-rays can cause many actinic reactions in many substances. For example, X-rays can affect sensitively negative film in the same way as light rays do. In medicine, negative films are commonly used to record the images of photosensitive effects.

12.1.5 Biological Effect

The principle of the biological effect is that the cells of creature tissues may be damaged, halted, or even be killed by undergoing the ionization and the excitation. For different sensitivities to X-rays of different cells of creature tissues, the damage degrees are different. On one hand, X-rays can be used to kill the cancer cells dividing rapidly. On the other hand, X-rays may damage the normal tissues. So those who deal with X-ray should take necessary protections.

12.2 X-ray Generator

Figure 12-1 is a diagram of an X-ray generator. The major components are the X-ray tube and the high voltage generator. Two conditions for generating X-rays: High-speed electrons and a metal target used as the appropriate obstacle. The electrons are slowed down and deflected by the atoms of the target. The kinetic energy of the electrons is converted directly into the energy of the X-ray radiation.

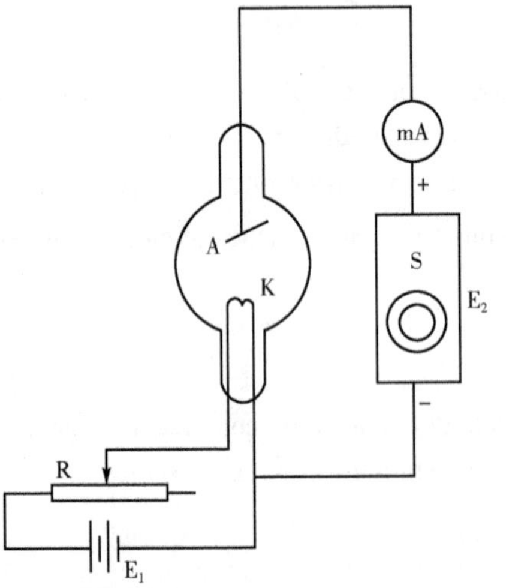

Figure 12-1 Sketch map of an X-ray generator

The X-ray tube is a vacuum glass tube. It contains two electrodes: An **anode** A, which collects the high velocity electrons as a target and is made of tungsten (or molybdenum), and a **cathode** (filament) , which is usually made of tungsten. As shown in Figure 12-1, the filament is operated at 10 V supplied by the power E_1. Electric current flows through the filament, so that it is heated and emits electrons. The current of a few amps, which is called the filament current, can be adjusted by the resistor R. A high DC voltage of 10^3-10^6 V is generated between the cathode and the anode by the high-voltage power E_2, which is called the **tube voltage**, can be adjusted by the rotary knob S. The hot electrons emitted from the cathode are strongly attracted to the anode by the action of the electric field built between the cathode and the anode. The stream of electrons is the **tube current**. When the electrons with high speed collide onto the tungsten target (anode) , X-radiation is produced.

12.3 Hardness and Intensity of X-rays

The **hardness** refers to the penetrating ability of a beam of X-ray, which depends on its wavelength. The shorter the wavelength is, the larger the energy of the X-ray photons, the greater the penetrating ability, and the higher the hardness of the X-ray will be. It is usually used to treat deep tissues. On the contrary, the longer the wavelength is, the smaller the energy of the X-ray photons, the poorer the penetrating ability, and the softer the X-ray will be. It is suitable for the fluoroscopy and epidermis treatments.

The hardness of the radiation is dependent on the voltage across the X-ray tube. The higher the voltage of the tube is, the greater the kinetic energy of the electrons that strike the target, the greater the energy of the X-ray photons, and the harder the X-ray will be. Therefore, in medical field the tube voltage is usually used to measure the hardness of X-rays produced by the X-ray tube. Table 12-1 gives the classification of hardness of X-rays, the corresponding tube voltage, the minimum wavelength and the main applications.

Table 12-1 Classification of hardness of X-rays

Hardness	Tube voltage (kV)	Minimum wavelength (nm)	Applications
Very soft	5-20	0.25-0.062	Photography for soft tissue and therapy for epidermis
Soft	20-100	0.062-0.012	Fluoroscopy and photography
Hard	100-250	0.012-0.005	Therapy for deep tissue
Very hard	over 250	0.005 or shorter	Therapy for very deep tissue

The **intensity** of a beam of X-ray is defined as the radiation energy of the X-ray penetrating perpendicularly through a unit area per unit time.

$$I=\sum_{i=1}^{n} N_i h\nu_i = N_1 h\nu_1 + N_2 h\nu_2 + \cdots + N_n h\nu_n$$

where $N_1, N_2, \cdots, N_n$ are respectively the numbers of photons which have different energies of $h\nu_1, h\nu_2, \cdots, h\nu_n$. As the tube current is increased, the number of electrons produced is increased. With the increasing number of electrons, the number of X-ray photons produced by colliding target of anode will be increased, so the intensity of X-ray is also heightened. When the tube voltage is increased, the energy of each X-ray photon will be increased. In fact, for getting the X-ray with proper hardness, the tube voltage should be first determined according to the application. The intensity of the X-ray is only determined by the tube current when the tube voltage is a constant. In consequence, the intensity of the X-ray in medical applications is commonly expressed by the tube current in milliamperes.

12.4 Diffraction of X-rays

12.4.1 Wave Properties of X-rays

X-ray is a form of electromagnetic wave with the wavelength range of 0.01-10 nm, much shorter than the visible light. Since X-ray is an electromagnetic wave, its interference and diffraction should be observed. However, diffraction effects can not be observed when X-rays penetrates through an optical grating with the grating constant in the range of 10^{-6}-10^{-5} m, which is much longer than X-rays. The diffraction effects may be observed only when the grating constant is matched to the wavelength of X-rays.

In 1912, Max von Laue suggested that the regular array of atoms in a crystal could act as a three-dimensional diffraction grating for X-rays. The corresponding experimental device is as shown in Figure 12-2. A collimated beam of X-ray is incident on a crystal. The X-ray beam passing through the crystal is irradiated on a photographic negative film. At the center of the film a dark spot is formed by the X-ray beam which directly hit the film along the straight line. There are also a number of spots symmetrically distributed around the center, and this distribution is called the Laue pattern. This phenomenon is the diffraction of the X-ray by the crystal. It confirms that X-rays are electromagnetic waves.

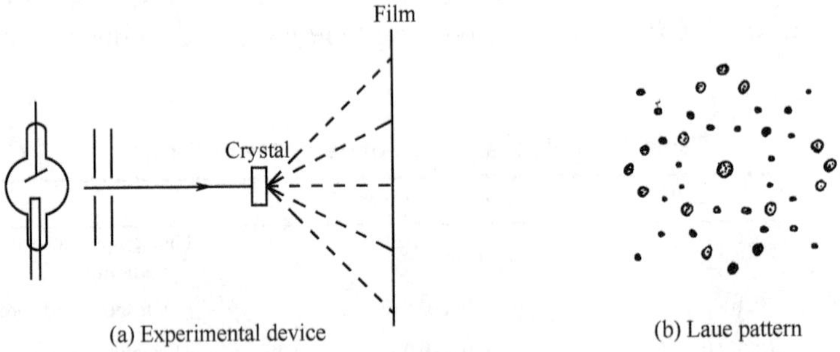

Figure 12-2 The diffraction of X-ray

12.4.2 Bragg Equation

A piece of crystal is composed of a set of particles (atoms, molecules, or ions) arranged in an ordered pattern, so it is a natural diffraction grating. When a beam of X-ray is incident on an array of particles of a crystal, every particle could be looked as a center for radiating a wavelet. For the array of particles, the wavelets should be emitted in all directions. This phenomenon is called the **scattering**. The diffracted beams will be intensified in certain directions corresponding to constructive interference for the wavelets reflected from layers of atoms in the crystal. Figure 12-3 shows the diffraction of X-ray by a piece of crystal. The dark pots refer to the particles in a crystal. The distance between two adjacent planes is d. An incident X-ray beam makes an angle θ with one of the planes. The beam of X-ray will be scattered by the particles on any planes. The interference peak can only be measured in the direction following the reflection law. As is shown in Figure 12-3, beam 1 is reflected from the upper plane and beam 2 is reflected from the lower plane. The path difference between the two beams is

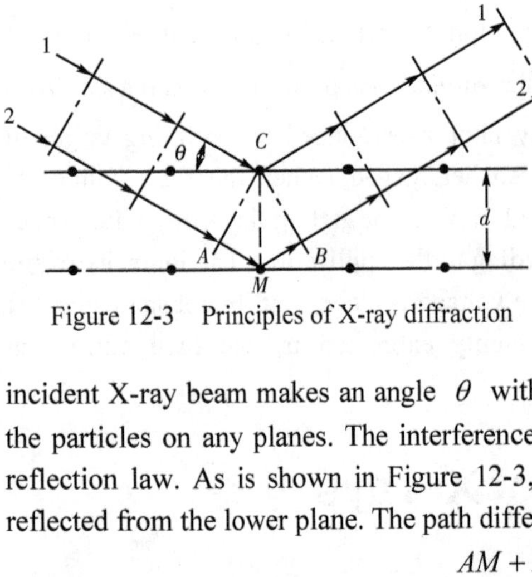

Figure 12-3 Principles of X-ray diffraction

$$AM + BM = 2AM = 2d\sin\theta$$

Hence, the condition for constructive interference is

$$2d\sin\theta = k\lambda \ \ (k = 1, 2, 3, \ \cdots) \tag{12-1}$$

Equation (12-1) is called **Bragg equation**. The angle θ can be measured experimentally. We call it the **grazing angle**. Where, d is the spacing between the particles, and also called **lattice constant**. If one of the quantities: The lattice constant d or the wavelength of X-ray is measured, the other one can be determined. In this way, both the X-ray spectrum analysis and crystal structure analysis could be achieved. In biomedicine researches, this method can also be used to investigate the fine structures of organisms, such as cells and proteins, etc. Nowadays, it has been developed into an independent scientific discipline, which is called X-ray structure analysis.

12.4.3 X-ray Spectrograph

Figure 12-4 is the diagram of principles of X-ray spectrograph. A beam of X-ray is incident on the crystal grating through the lead shielding slit B. By the rotating of the crystal C, the angle θ is changed, and X-rays with different wavelengths will be strengthened in different certain directions. When the angle θ satisfies Bragg equation (12-1) , the strength of X-rays scattering from the crystal is the maximum. Correspondingly, the photographic sensitivity of the film DE will be the strongest. Because X-rays have different wavelengths, there will be different corresponding angles θ s. Thus a series of sensitive stripes arranged by the wavelengths is formed, namely X-ray spectrum.

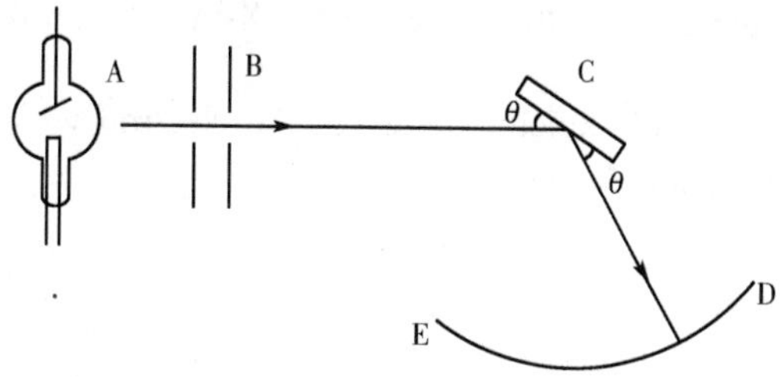

Figure 12-4 Principles of X-ray spectrograph

12.5 X-ray Spectra

The X-ray produced from an X-ray tube is not monochromatic. It consists of a broad continuous spectrum of different wavelengths, within which there are a number of sharp lines of specific wave lengths, as is shown in Figure 12-5. The former is called the **continuous X-ray spectrum**, while the latter is called the **characteristic X-ray spectral lines**.

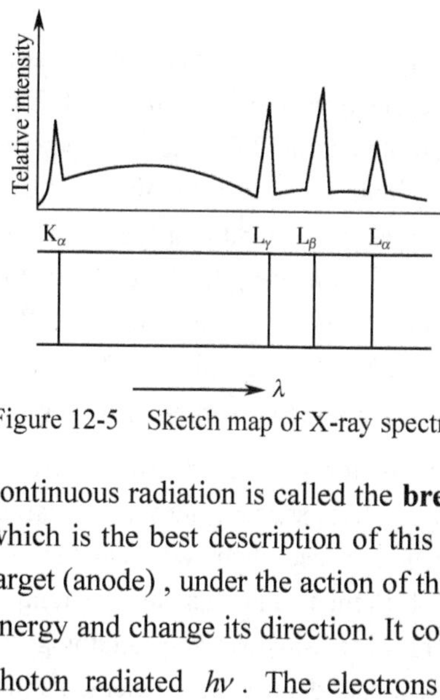

Figure 12-5 Sketch map of X-ray spectra

12.5.1 Continuous X-ray Spectrum

When the high-speed electrons are slowed down by the atoms of the target (anode) , they convert a part of their kinetic energy into the energy of the X-ray photons radiated. This continuous radiation is called the **bremsstrahlung**. It's from the German word for "**braking radiation**", which is the best description of this process. When an electron with high speed collides onto the metal target (anode) , under the action of the strong electric field of the nucleus, the electron will lose its kinetic energy and change its direction. It converts some of its kinetic energy ΔE_k into the energy of the X-ray photon radiated $h\nu$. The electrons moving along different tracks have varying distances form the corresponding nuclei, so there will be different changes of the velocities and different values of the kinetic energy lost ΔE_k. In this way, the X-ray photons with different energies are produced. So the bremsstrahlung interactions generate X-ray photons with a continuous spectrum of energy. Let's suggest U as the tube voltage and e as the electric quantity of the electron. The kinetic energy of the electron arriving at the anode is equal to the work done by the electric force in the tube, so $eU = \frac{1}{2}mv^2$. It may undergo several interactions with the atoms of the target before the electron loses all of its kinetic energy. The value of kinetic energy lost for any given interaction can vary from zero up to the entire kinetic energy of the electron, i.e., 0- eU . X-ray photons with different energies, or X-rays with different wavelengths are emitted to form a continuous spectrum as the consequence of the collisions of numerous electrons. There is a short wavelength limit recorded on the side of short wavelength in the continuous spectrum, it is called the **minimum wavelength** (or short wavelength limit) , denoted with symbol λ_0 .

Accordingly, the energy of the X-ray photon is the maximum ($\frac{hc}{\lambda_0}$). Obviously, the maximum energy is the whole kinetic energy of the electron which is transformed into a single X-ray photon in a single collision. So that

$$\frac{1}{2}mv^2 = eU = \frac{hc}{\lambda_0}$$

$$\lambda_0 = \frac{hc}{e} \cdot \frac{1}{U} \tag{12-2}$$

where h is Planck's constant and c is the speed of light in the vacuum. Equation (12-2) shows that the minimum wavelength λ_0 is inversely proportional to the tube voltage U. The larger the tube voltage U, the shorter the minimum wavelength λ_0, the greater the energy of the X-ray photon, and the stronger the penetrating power.

12.5.2 Characteristic X-ray Spectrum

When a high-speed electron bombards the target, it may knock an inner-shell electron of the atom out, as a result the atom is excited. The vacancy is then filled with an electron from an outer shell. This transition results in the emission of an X-ray photon with the energy of the energy difference between the two shells. Electrons in outer shells have much higher average energy than those in inner shells. Hence the photons emitted in such transitions correspond to a type of X-ray radiation with higher energy and shorter wavelength. If the electron is knocked out from the K (or L) shell, the X-rays emitted are called the characteristic radiations of K (or L) series. Figure 12-6 shows the K_α, K_β and K_γ lines result from the transitions in which the vacancies of K-shells of the excited atoms are filled respectively by electrons from different outer shells. These spectral lines are so called characteristic X-ray spectral lines because their wavelengths are related to the nature of the target element and indicate the unique characteristics of the target element. In recent years, the technology of microanalysis has been developed. It can identify all the elements in a compound sample by taking advantage of the characteristic X-rays excited by a very fine beam of electrons incident on the sample. This technique has been used in medical research. For instance, the wavelengths of the K_α and K_β lines of tungsten are 0.021 nm and 0.018 nm, while those of molybdenum are 0.071 nm and 0.069 nm. The energy differences between the inner orbits and the outer orbits in the atoms are proportional to the atomic numbers. Thus, the higher the atomic number, the shorter the wavelengths of the characteristic X-ray lines.

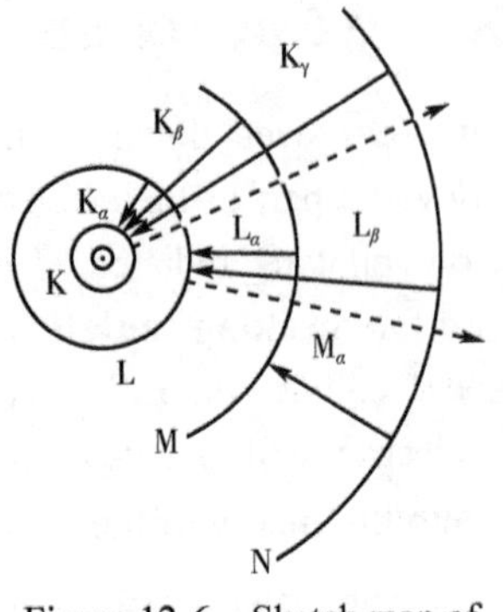

Figure 12-6 Sketch map of atomic shells and characteristic radiations

It should be mentioned that, X-rays emitted by a medical X-ray tube are mainly composed of continuous X-rays and the characteristic X-rays distributed among them are so few. However, we can determine the atomic structure of inner shells by studying the characteristic X-ray spectra of various elements, just as that we can determine the atomic structure of outer shells by studying the optical spectra. The study of the characteristic X-ray spectra is very helpful to know the shell structures of atoms and is also very useful when analyzing the chemical elements.

12.6 Attenuation of X-rays

The intensity of a beam of X-ray traveling along the incident direction decreases because of the interaction with some atoms when it passes through some materials. This is called the attenuation of X-ray. The attenuations of X-rays have two different manners: One is that the energy of the X-ray photons is absorbed and converted to other forms of energy; the other is that the X-ray photons are scattered by the atoms of the material and deviated from the original direction. In the latter case, although X-ray photons are not absorbed, the number of X-ray photons in the original direction is reduced. The absorption and the scattering of X-rays are two different ways in which X-rays are attenuated by a material.

Suppose that I_0 is the intensity of an X-ray perpendicularly incident on a material and I is the intensity of the X-ray after penetrating through the material with the thickness of d. From experimental and theoretical conclusions it has been found that the intensity I decreases exponentially with the distance penetrated d:

$$I = I_0 e^{-\mu d} \tag{12-3}$$

where μ is the linear attenuation coefficient which depends on the material and the energy of the X-ray photon. If the unit of the thickness d is m, then the unit of μ is m^{-1}. Table 12-2 shows some linear attenuation coefficients of bone and muscle.

Table 12-2 Linear attenuation coefficients of bone and muscle

X-ray photon energy (keV)	μ (bone) (m^{-1})	μ (muscle) (m^{-1})	X-ray photon energy (keV)	μ (bone) (m^{-1})	μ (muscle) (m^{-1})
20	496	73.0	60	47.7	19.6
30	168	34.2	100	32.3	16.7
40	88.4	24.9	150	27.0	14.7
50	60.3	21.4	200	24.4	13.5

The main component elements of the muscle tissue of a human body are H, O and C. Bone is composed mainly of calcium phosphate [$Ca_3(PO_4)_2$]. And the atomic numbers of the element Ca and the element P are greater than those of any other elements in muscle tissue. Thus, the value of the linear attenuation coefficient of bone is bigger than that of the muscle tissue. So the shadows corresponding to the bones can be formed on a photographic plate or a fluorescent screen more clearly. The thickness of a material which reduces the exposure rate by one-half is called the **half-value thickness**, or half-value layer (HVL), denoted with $d_{1/2}$. We can therefore determine the relationship between $d_{1/2}$ and μ by Equation (12-3). Suppose that $d_{1/2}$ is the thickness and $I = \frac{I_0}{2}$ is the transmitted intensity. Equation (12-3) then gives the half-value thickness as

$$d_{1/2} = \frac{\ln 2}{\mu} = \frac{0.693}{\mu} \tag{12-4}$$

which is inversely proportional to the linear attenuation coefficient. The value of half-value thickness depends on the material and the energy of the X-ray photon. For instance, the HVL of aluminum is 7 mm and that of lead is 0.1 mm corresponding to the X-ray photon of 50 keV. And the HVL of aluminum is 18.6 mm and that of lead is 0.3 mm corresponding to the X-ray photon of 150 keV. Lead is the most commonly used shielding material because of its high-attenuation properties.

12.7 Medical Applications of X-rays

X-rays have been applied widely in medicine. In summary, the applications can be divided into three aspects: In treatment, in drug analysis and in diagnosis.

12.7.1 Applications in Treatments

X-rays are mainly used to treat cancers. The mechanism is that ionization effect on human tissue can induce biological effects, stop the cell metabolism and damage the biological tissue especially to the cells that are rapidly dividing. Nowadays, X-rays have certain curative effects for some skin diseases and certain types of cancers. The X-ray stereotactic radiotherapy system (SRS) was developed in the 1980s. If a high dose of X-rays is fully focused on the infected part and the edge of this part would be cut down as a knife. So it is vividly called X-knife. SRS is operated by the rotation of the X-ray beam in a circle around the patient's tumor combining with the rotation or translation of the bed. Generally speaking, X-rays have intense energy to damage cancer cells. But different cancer cells have different X-ray sensitivities. X-rays are not commonly used to treat the insensitive cancers. In the process of treatment, hardness and intensity of the X-ray depend on the extent of the disease and other factors. An appropriate exposure dose, which would kill all of the cancer cells without causing permanent damage and serious complications to normal tissues, is especially important. X-rays may also cause damage to normal tissues and even induce cancers. So it is necessary to take protective measures to avoid any unnecessary exposure.

12.7.2 Applications in Medicine Analyses

In the research of Chinese medicine, X-ray diffraction is used to analyze the structures of the active components and to seek their substitutes. It plays a major role in protecting the natural environment. There are two important methods.

(1) X-ray diffraction (XRD) : It is the main method used to study the phases and crystal structures of substances. When a certain substance undergoes diffraction analysis, the substance produces different degrees of diffraction phenomena, under the effect of X-ray. The composition, crystal structure, type of molecular bonding and molecular geometry of this substance determine its distinctive diffraction pattern. If the material is a mixture, the diffraction pattern can be obtained from the superimposed diffraction effect of all components. X-ray diffraction provides a great deal of pattern information, and it is stable, reliable and recordable. Based on it we can make a qualitative analysis of the substance. By the analyses of *rhizoma gastrodiae* and its fake, fleece-flower root and its similar product, medicinal indianmulberry root and its similar product, and other proprietary Chinese medicines, a better identification has been achieved.

(2) X-ray fluorescence (XRF) : XRF is a non-destructive analysis of sample by scanning qualitatively with a spectrometer. The method is: To put the sample into an XRF spectrometer, make a qualitative scanning as routine test, observe the species of elements from the scanogram, and then make the qualitative and quantitative analysis according to the contents of elements and the intensities of spectral lines shown in the figure. XRF is used to make elemental analyses of keel, gypsum, oyster, Glauber's salt, talc and other minerals.

12.7.3 Applications in Diagnoses

1. Fluoroscopy and Radiography

X-ray can be used to check the interior of the human body because of the different attenuations by different organizations. For example, the intensities of X-ray penetrated through different parts of the human body have significant differences because bone has a greater linear attenuation coefficient than muscle. Shadows with different darkness produced on a fluorescent screen or a photographic plate can be observed. The former is called the fluoroscopy, while the latter is called the radiography. There are two specific types of radiographies.

(1) Soft X-ray radiography: Soft X-rays usually refer to the low energy X-rays with the tube voltage less than 40 kV. The absorption by photoelectric effect is the predominant interaction mechanism in the soft X-ray absorption. Because of the significant differences of soft X-ray absorptions in different organizations, images of fat, muscle, gland and other soft tissues with similar densities it can form sharp contrast on photographic plates. This method is usually used to check female breast diseases. Clear images of breast gland tissue, connective tissue, fat, blood vessel and other fine structures, other mammary gland diseases and even the tumor edge, could be achieved.

(2) High-kV X-ray radiography: High-kV X-rays refer to the X-rays with high energy of the tube voltage more than 120 kV. In this case, Compton scattering is the predominant interaction between X-rays and soft tissue. So it becomes easy to observe soft tissues overlapping upon the bone, fine structures of bone itself and gas filling lumen. Chest X-ray examination is very common. X-rays with the tube voltage of 140-150 kV will be used to take a chest radiograph. The texture or inflammation of the lung can be identified from the shadow on ribs. And the shadows of mediastinum, trachea and bronchia can also be observed easily in spite of the overlap with sternum and spine.

The degree of fracture, tuberculosis lesions, the location and size of tumor, organ shapes, and the location of foreign bodies, etc. can be clearly seen on fluoroscopy or radiography. Fluoroscopy can provide an observation lasting for a while, so that the movement of organs can be observed. It is better to have both position resolution and contrast resolution of radiography. And radiographs can be permanently preserved. If the difference of linear attenuation coefficient between the organ and its surrounding tissues is small, some contrast agent may be used to improve the contrast and make the image clearer. For example, in the examination for intestines and stomach disorders the patient need to swallow barium sulfate ($BaSO_4$) which would adhere to the stomach lining. So the images of intestines and stomach can be shown with X-ray irradiation. X-rays can damage biological tissues. Too much exposure of X-rays can cause leukemia, keratosis, and hair loss, etc. Thus, X-ray operators should take necessary protections and have regular health checks. Lead screens, leaded glass, leaded rubber dresses and gloves are all commonly used protective articles.

2. Digital Radiography and Digital Subtraction Angiography

(1) Digital Radiography: It is a technically forming digital image which would then be converted into analog images. The advantages include enhanced images, less radiation exposure to the patient and the ability to store and transfer, etc.

(2) Digital Subtraction Angiography: DSA, developed on the basis of analog subtraction angiography, is a diagnostic method utilizing the combination of digital signal processing and traditional angiography. The principles are as follows.

1) Time Subtraction Angiography: The image of blood vessels filling with some contrast agent can be formed by subtracting the same other parts of two different digital images of the same area. First, an image of bone including the blood vessels is acquired, and the other image can be obtained with injecting

contrast agent into the blood vessels. Then the image of blood vessels is ultimately formed by subtracting the first image from the later image by means of image processing. As the two images are respectively produced at different time, this principle is named as time subtraction angiography.

2) Energy Subtraction Angiography: First two images of the same area are obtained by X-ray irradiations with two different energies. And then the image of blood vessels with the excluded bones and soft tissues can be formed by digital processing and "subtraction".

3. Computed Tomography

Computed tomography (CT) is a new technology which has been developed rapidly in recent years. The principle is based on the attenuation properties of X-rays by materials. For example, a layer of tissue is divided up into four small cubes, called **voxels**. Suppose that d is the side length of each voxel and μ_1, μ_2, μ_3 and μ_4 are their linear attenuation coefficients. The X-rays with certain wavelength are incident on the four cubes along different directions. Suppose that I_0 is the incident intensity and I_1, I_2, I_3 and I_4 are the transmitted intensities, as shown in Figure 12-7. The transmitted intensity of X-rays after penetrating through the voxel with the linear attenuation coefficient of μ_1 is given by Equation (12-3).

$$I_0 e^{-\mu_1 d}$$

And the transmitted intensity of X-rays after penetrating through the voxel with the linear attenuation coefficient of μ_3 can be then derived by the expression of

$$I_1 = I_0 e^{-\mu_1 d} e^{-\mu_3 d} = I_0 e^{-(\mu_1+\mu_3)d}$$

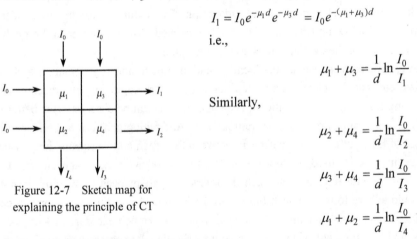

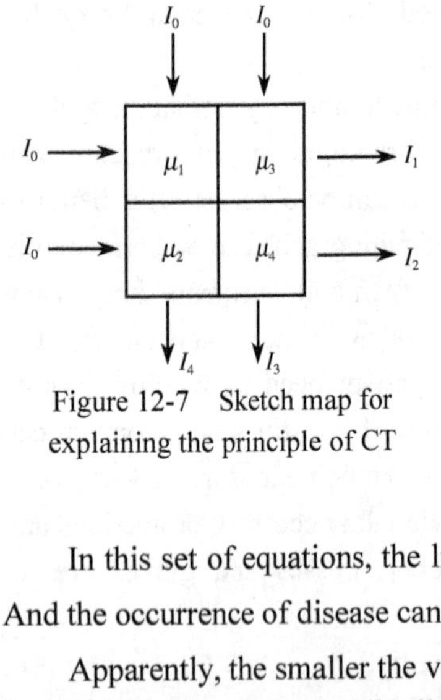

Figure 12-7 Sketch map for explaining the principle of CT

i.e.,

$$\mu_1 + \mu_3 = \frac{1}{d}\ln\frac{I_0}{I_1}$$

Similarly,

$$\mu_2 + \mu_4 = \frac{1}{d}\ln\frac{I_0}{I_2}$$

$$\mu_3 + \mu_4 = \frac{1}{d}\ln\frac{I_0}{I_3}$$

$$\mu_1 + \mu_2 = \frac{1}{d}\ln\frac{I_0}{I_4}$$

In this set of equations, the linear attenuation coefficients of μ_1, μ_2, μ_3 and μ_4 can be solved. And the occurrence of disease can be determined with the change and the contrast of μ.

Apparently, the smaller the volume of each voxel is, the higher the accuracy of the measurement will be. A layer of tissue is usually divided into $160 \times 160 = 25600$ voxels. The side length and thickness of a voxel are 1.5 mm and 8 mm respectively. When a narrow beam of X-rays produced by X-ray tube passes through the filter plate, the long-wave part is filtered out and the transmitted X-rays with a narrower wavelength range are achieved. The intensity of the beam of X-rays penetrated through the absorber is recorded by the detector D. As shown in Figure 12-8, with the translation of the X-ray source, the scan along the straight line is going on. Meanwhile, the detector D will keep on translating synchronously with the X-ray source. Hundreds of data (e.g. 240 data), which represent the intensities of X-rays penetrated through the absorbers, can be recorded continuously by the detector during each scan.

Then the X-ray source and the detector are rotated by an angle of 1° for a second scan and another 240 data are recorded, until the rotation goes through 180°. So a total of $180 \times 240 = 43200$ intensity values are obtained. In other words, we have 43200 linear equations. The computer collects all the information from the detector then solves the attenuation coefficients of the voxels quickly. This set of data is fed into a computer and the image of the cross section can be formed on the fluorescent screen for the observation and the photography. The tiny difference between the attenuation coefficients of small volume units can be detected because of the high measurement accuracy.

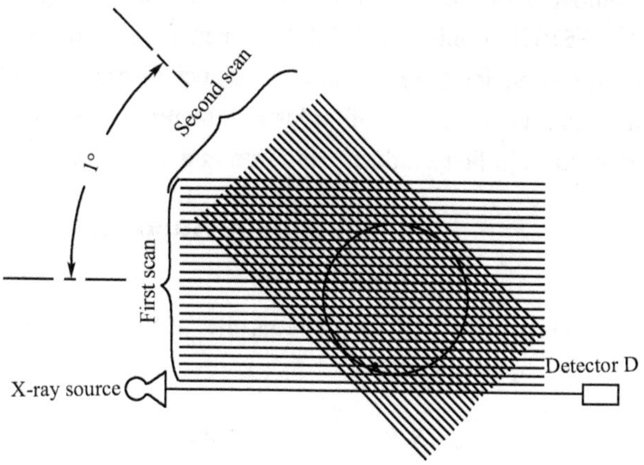

Figure 12-8 Sketch map of CT scanning

The technology of CT has been developed rapidly since 1972. By now it has experienced five generations. X-ray sources have undergone many developments from single-beam and multi-beam of the first-generation to sectored beam and till electron-beam of the fifth-generation. Scanning modes have undergone many developments from translations and rotations of the source and the detector to only the rotation of the source. Now it has no motion of the both. X-ray detectors have been developed from the single-detector to the multi-detector of the fifth-generation which can collect the scanning data in an array. The time for each scan has been shorten to 50 ms from 4 or 5 min. CT could only be used to examine the head in static state at the beginning, but now it has been developed gradually to perform dynamic checks and nondestructive examinations of the whole body. Taking advantage of new type CT, we can obtain the 3D images of varieties, such as multidimensional reconstruction and CT angiography etc.

In recent years, the important developments of CT are the popularity of the spiral CT and the application of the multi-slice spiral CT. The CT scanners, including low-grade scanner, adopt the slip ring and the spiral scanning. And the detectors are made from solid materials with low afterglow and high detection efficiency. This indicates that the conventional CT scanners have been updated from plane scan to spiral scan.

Here are some new CT technologies.

(1) Compton Scattering CT: CST has been successfully used to detect the defects on metal surfaces, aluminum castings and nonmetallic structures. It is mainly used to test some enormous and heavy objects or extend systems, such as airport runways, building components and other concrete buildings.

(2) Nuclear Magnetic Resonance CT: Because of the harmlessness to human body of radio waves, NMR CT is used to detect the functions and situations of the internal organs, which leads to the revolutionary changes of medical diagnosis and life science researches.

(3) Positron Emission Tomography CT: The conception of PET CT is dependent on the principle that some radionuclides (e.g. ^{11}C, ^{13}N, ^{15}O, ^{18}F, etc.) emit positrons rather than gamma rays directly. The distribution patterns of radionuclides and changes showed on PET-CT images can be used to detect the distributions of saccharides, acids and proteins in organisms, simulate the metabolic process and diagnose the special pathologies.

(4) Microwave CT: It has a strong ability to recognize soft tissues such as muscle and fat according to their remarkable differences of conductivities. Some electric constants of the human tissues are related to the temperature, so microwave CT can be used to convert temperature changes in vivo to images.

Compared with X-ray CT, microwave CT can distinguish cancers easily and is much safer in application.

(5) Ultrasonic CT: UCT has been used in ultrasonic imaging of breast and other soft tissues and becomes an important method to detect diseases such as breast cancer. In addition, it is also used in nondestructive testing of industrial materials and in high-tech fields or in the departments such as aerospace, military industry and iron and steel enterprises etc.

A Brief Summarization of this Chapter

(1) Intensity of X-rays: The energies of X-rays penetrating perpendicularly through a unit area per unit time, denoted by symbol I,

$$I = \sum_{i=1}^{n} N_i h\nu_i = N_1 h\nu_1 + N_2 h\nu_2 + \cdots + N_n h\nu_n$$

Where $N_1, N_2, \cdots, N_n$ are respectively the numbers of photons which have energies of $h\nu_1, h\nu_2, \cdots, h\nu_n$.

(2) Bragg equation: $2d\sin\theta = k\lambda,\quad k = 1, 2, 3\cdots$, where θ is the grazing angle.

(3) The attenuation of X-rays: Suppose that I_0 is the intensity of X-rays perpendicularly incident on a material along the vertical direction and I is the intensity of X-rays after penetrating through the matter with the thickness of d. From experimental and theoretical results it has been found that the intensity I decreases exponentially with the distance traveled d: $I = I_0 e^{-\mu d}$, where μ is the linear attenuation coefficient which depends on the material and the energy of the X-ray photon. If the unit of thickness d is m, the unit of μ is m^{-1}.

(4) Half-value thickness (layer) : $d_{1/2} = \dfrac{\ln 2}{\mu} = \dfrac{0.693}{\mu}$

Exercises 12

12-1. What is the maximum energy and the shortest wavelength of an X-ray photon emitted from an X-ray tube with the tube voltage of 100 kV?

12-2. The ratio of the HVLs of two materials is $1:\sqrt{2}$. What is the ratio of their linear attenuation coefficients?

12-3. There is a loss of 10% in intensity when a certain X-ray beam penetrates through the fat with the thickness of 1 mm. What is the percentage of the intensity after penetrating through the thickness of 3 mm?

12-4. If the HVL of aluminum for the X-ray with certain wavelength is 3.00 mm, what is the linear attenuation coefficient of aluminum?

12-5. For the X-ray with certain wavelength, the linear attenuation coefficient of lead is $1.32\times10^4\ m^{-1}$ and that of aluminum is $2.6\times10^{-5}\ m^{-1}$. Determine the thickness of the aluminum protecting plate, which has the same shielding effect of the lead protecting sheet with the thickness of 1 mm?

12-6. If a layer of copper with the thickness of 4.0 mm can reduce the intensity of a certain monochromatic X-ray beam to 1/10 of its original value, try to determine the linear attenuation coefficient and the HVL of copper.

12-7. How many HVLs are needed to reduce the intensity of an X-ray beam to 1% of its original value?

12-8. The linear attenuation coefficient of lead for the X-ray of 15.4 Å is 2610 cm^{-1}. If the intensity of the penetrated X-ray is 10 % of its original value, what is the thickness of the lead plate needed?

Chapter 13 Fundamental of Nuclear Physics

Nuclear physics is a branch of physics that studies the structures, properties and the inter-conversions of atomic nuclei. The research achievements of nuclear physics have provided many applications in medicine. The combination of nuclear technology and medicine has constituted the nuclear medicine. In this chapter, we will mainly introduce some basic properties of nuclei, nuclear decay regularity, and the principle of nuclear magnetic resonance.

13.1 Composition of the Nucleus

The atomic nucleus consists of two kinds of nucleons: **Protons** and **neutrons**. The mass of the nucleus is measured in **unified atomic mass units** u. 1 u is defined as one twelfth of the mass of an unbound neutral atom of ^{12}C. The value is

$$1u = \frac{0.012}{N_A} \times \frac{1}{12} = 1.660565 \times 10^{-27}\ \text{kg}$$

where the constant N_A is called the **Avogadro constant** and equals to 6.022×10^{23} entities per mole. Masses of micro particles are often expressed in terms of the atomic mass unit u. For example, the masses of proton and neutron can be given respectively by m_p= 1.007276 u, m_n= 1.008665 u. The total number of nucleons (protons and neutrons) in the nucleus is called its **mass number** A. The atomic nuclei of different kinds which have specific numbers of protons and neutrons are commonly called the **nuclides**. Conventionally, a nucleus of certain kind or so-called a nuclide is denoted by the symbol X, with a superscript for the mass number A on the left and a subscript for the proton number Z on the left, written as ${}_Z^AX$, e.g., ${}_1^1H$, ${}_8^{16}O$, etc.

A proton is positively charged with the electric quantity corresponding to the electric quantity of an electron, but the neutrons carry no charge. The force that binds protons and neutrons together in the nucleus, despite the electrical repulsions among the protons, is a strong interaction called the nuclear force. This force does not depend on the charges and it has short acting range of the order of the nuclear dimension within 10^{-15}m. Different nuclides have different number of protons and neutrons. A neutron hasn't any net electric charge, so the number of charges in a nucleus is identical with the number of protons Z (atomic number) .

13.2 Radioactivity and the Decay Law

We've acknowledged more than 2600 different nuclides now and about 90% are unstable. These unstable nuclides are called **radioactive nuclides**. Radioactivity is the phenomenon that an unstable nucleus emits spontaneously some rays and transfers to a new nuclide. This transforming phenomenon is called the nuclear decay or the **radioactive decay**.

13.2.1 Decay Law

All decays obey the same statistical law: The number of the nuclei decayed $-dN$ in the time interval

t to $t+dt$ is proportional not only to the time interval dt, but also to the number of the nuclei N i.e.,

$$-dN = \lambda N dt \tag{13-1}$$

where the constant λ is called the **decay constant**. It is the decay probability per unit time for a single radioactive nucleus, which relates to the properties of the nuclide. For the same nuclides, λ remains constant, for a different kind of nuclides, it has a different value. The value of λ for any isotope determines that the rate for which that isotope will decay. If N_0 represents the number of radioactive nuclei that haven't decayed at $t = 0$, by integrating to Equation (13-1) we have

$$N = N_0 e^{-\lambda t} \tag{13-2}$$

This is called the **decay law**. The radioactive decay is conversely exponential. The quantity of some nuclides may decay via two or more different processes simultaneously. In general, these processes have different probabilities of occurring, and thus occur at different rates with different decay constants $\lambda_1, \lambda_2, \cdots, \lambda_n$. And the total decay constant is given by the sum of the decay constants, i.e., $\lambda = \lambda_1 + \lambda_2 + \lambda_3 + \cdots + \lambda_n$.

13.2.2 Mean Life

Although the exact while for an individual atomic decay of a single nuclide cannot be predicted, it's measurable that the time period during which a given number of some kind of nuclides are decayed out. This quantity is called the **mean life**, denoted by τ. Suppose at the moment of $t = 0$ the number of the nuclei in the sample is N_0, and at the moment of t the number of the nuclei in the sample is N; the number the radioactive nuclei delayed during t to $t + dt$ is $-dN = \lambda N dt$, so the lifetime of these delayed nuclei should be t. In this way, the mean lifetime of the N_0 nuclei is

$$\tau = \frac{1}{N_0}\int_{N_0}^{0} dN \cdot t = \frac{1}{N_0}\int_0^{\infty} -\lambda N dt \cdot t = \frac{-\lambda}{N_0}\int_0^{\infty} N_0 e^{-\lambda t} \cdot t dt = \frac{1}{\lambda} \tag{13-3}$$

That is, the mean life is the reciprocal of the decay constant. The larger decay constant is, the faster the number of nuclei is and the shorter the mean life is.

13.2.3 Half-life

Another quantity to describe the decay rate is the **half-life** which is defined as the time required for one half of the radioactive nuclei in a given sample to decay and is expressed by $T_{1/2}$. Setting $t = T_{1/2}$ and $N = N_0 / 2$ in Equation (13-2) gives

$$\frac{N_0}{2} = N_0 e^{-\lambda T_{1/2}}$$

$$T_{1/2} = \frac{\ln 2}{\lambda} = \frac{0.693}{\lambda} \tag{13-4}$$

Combining it with Equation (13-2), we get

$$N = N_0 \left(\frac{1}{2}\right)^{t/T_{1/2}}$$

This is another form of decay law. Some examples of half-life and types of decays are shown in Table 13-1. Where the units of half-life are respectively: Year (a), day (d), hour (h), minute (min), second (s), and so on.

Table 13-1 The half-lives and types of decays of some nuclides

Nuclide	Half-life	Type of decay	Nuclide	Half-life	Type of decay
$^{3}_{1}H$	12.33 a	β^-	$^{125}_{53}I$	60 d	EC, γ
$^{11}_{6}C$	20.4 min	β^+ (99.75%) EC (0.24%)	$^{131}_{53}I$	8.04 d	β^-, γ
$^{14}_{6}C$	5730 a	β^-	$^{222}_{86}Rn$	3.8 d	α, γ
$^{32}_{16}P$	14.3 d	β^-	$^{226}_{88}Ra$	1600 a	α, γ
$^{60}_{27}Co$	5.27 a	β^-, γ	$^{238}_{92}U$	4.5×10^{-9} a	α, γ

13.2.4 Radioactivity

Radioactivity is measured with the quantity of activity, or the number of nuclides decayed in a unit time. Highly radioactive means the number of decays happened is very high in per unit time.

The **radioactivity** or **activity** of a radioactive sample is defined as the number of nuclides decayed per second. It is denoted by A, then

$$A = -\frac{dN}{dt} = \lambda N$$

From Equation (13-2) , we get

$$A = \lambda N_0 e^{-\lambda t} = A_0 e^{-\lambda t} = A_0 \left(\frac{1}{2}\right)^{t/T_{1/2}} \tag{13-5}$$

where $A_0 = \lambda N_0$ is the initial activity when $t = 0$. Therefore, the activity of a radioactive sample decreases with the same rate exponentially as the number of radioactive nuclei.

The SI unit of activity is **Becquerel**, denoted by Bq, and defined as $1\text{Bq} = 1$ decay/s. The traditional unit of activity is the **curie**, denoted by Ci, and defined as $1\,\text{Ci}=3.7\times10^{10}\text{Bq}$. For it is a large number of decays per second, the activity is usually expressed in the smaller multiples of: 1×10^{-3} Ci = 1 millicurie, or 1×10^{-6} Ci = 1 microcurie.

Example 13-1 A person is injected intravenously with salt water containing radioactive ^{131}I for thyroid scanning. 0.5 ml of injection should be taken when it was just produced. If it has been stored for 16 days since being produced, find the suitable volume of this injection for doing the same scanning. The half-life of ^{131}I is 8 d.

Solution: From

$$A = A_0 \left(\frac{1}{2}\right)^{t/T_{1/2}}$$

we get the relationship between the concentrations of C and C_0

$$C = C_0 \left(\frac{1}{2}\right)^{t/T_{1/2}}$$

then at $t = 16\text{d}$

$$A = A_0 \left(\frac{1}{2}\right)^{t/T_{1/2}} = A_0 \left(\frac{1}{2}\right)^2 = \frac{A_0}{4}$$

Because the concentration has been decreased, to keep the same activity so as to reach the medical needs, the volume of injection should be increased due to concentration is inversely proportion to the volume of the solution, i.e.,

$$\frac{V}{V_0} = \frac{C_0}{C} = (2)^{t/T_{1/2}} = 4$$

It indicates that 2 ml of the solution is to inject now.

13.3 Radiation Dose and Radiation Protection

13.3.1 Radiation Dose

1. Exposure

The exposure is the quantity of electric charge ionized in one unit mass of air by X-rays or gamma rays as they penetrate a collecting volume. It is defined as

$$X = \frac{\mathrm{d}Q}{\mathrm{d}m} \tag{13-6}$$

where $\mathrm{d}m$ is the mass of dry air and $\mathrm{d}Q$ is an absolute value of the total ions charges that is of any kind (either positively charged or negatively charged). The SI unit for exposure is C/kg, and its traditional unit is **roentgen**, denoted by R, $1\,\mathrm{R}=2.58\times10^{-4}\,\mathrm{C/kg}$.

2. Absorbed Dose

The effects of ionizing radiation are very complicated. But all effects of the radiation are assumed to be directly proportional to the amount of the energy absorbed. The **absorbed dose** is defined as the energy absorbed by one unit mass of material, and denoted by *D*, so the **absorbed dose** is expressed as

$$D = \frac{\mathrm{d}E}{\mathrm{d}m} \tag{13-7}$$

Its unit is Gy, $1\,\mathrm{Gy}=1\,\mathrm{J/kg}$.

3. Dose Equivalent

Though there may be the same amount of energy absorbed by one unit mass of biological tissue from types of radiations, the abilities for those radiations to produce biological effect differ from each other considerably. The **dose equivalent** reflects the recognition of differences in the effectiveness of different radiations to inflict over all biological damages. The dose equivalent is denoted by *H* and is defined as

$$H = Q \cdot D \tag{13-8}$$

where *Q* is the relative biological effectiveness or the **quality factor**, as shown in Table 13-2. The greater the *Q*, the more effective the radiation. The SI unit for dose equivalent is the Sv.

Table 13-2 Quality factor of radiation

Type of radiation	Quality factor Q	Type of radiation	Quality factor Q
X, β^+, β^-, γ-ray	1	Fast neutron, fast proton	10
Slow neutron	1-5	Recoil nucleon, α-ray	20

13.3.2 Protection to Radiation

Different kinds of radioactive nuclides and radiopharmaceuticals are widely used in medical investigations and treatments and other fields. Meanwhile individuals that have to contact with radioactive nuclides have become more and more. So it is important to take precautions for the radioactive rays. Now let's learn several concepts commonly used in the protection to radiation.

1. Maximum Permissible Dose

The radiation we all received continuously from natural background, occasionally from medical practices, and from some common commercial devices is part of our total radiation exposure. Regulatory agencies have set the allowable dose limit to the radiation accumulated during a period or received individually, which will not cause direct damage or harmful hereditary effect on the organism. This dose is called **maximum permissible dose**.

In our country the weekly limit for maximum permissible dose is 0.001 Sv, and the annual limit is 0.05 Sv.

2. Protection to the External Irradiation

The irradiation from the radioactive nuclides outside the body is called the **external irradiation**.

The dose of radiation received by a human body from the external irradiation is not only related to the distance between the body and the radioactive source, but also to the time of staying around the source. Thus, for the persons who have to contact with radioactive sources it is necessary to use some special kinds of tools which can operate in distance so as to avoid long staying near the sources. Meanwhile, the shielding between the radioactive source and the operator can reduce the dose of radioactivity. For α-rays, because of its low penetrating power and the short irradiating range, we can wear protective gloves for protection. For β-rays, besides the distance and the time protection, the shielding made of materials such as plexiglass, aluminum, and so on which are composed of atoms with the middle atomic numbers will be used, because inside the materials with high atomic numbers the bremsstrahlung takes place easily. For X-rays and γ-rays with strong penetrability, the substances with higher atomic numbers (such as lead, concrete, etc.) are usually used as their shielding materials. For neutrons' shielding, the principle is to slow down the fast neutrons by using materials such as iron, lead, and so on; in addition, materials containing boron or lithium can absorb these neutrons.

3. Protection to the Internal Irradiation

The irradiation from radioactive nuclides taken into the body and deposited inside the body is called the **internal irradiation**. For its strong ionization, the α-ray will cause more serious damages than those caused by the β-ray or γ-ray radiation inside the organism. it is necessary to avoid any kind of internal irradiation, so for the individuals who have to contact with radioactive nuclides it should be forbidden to take into radioactive materials through the inhalation, the ingestion, or the injury.

13.4 Applications of Radioactivity in Medicine

13.4.1 In Therapy

In therapy, the applications of the radioactivity make use of its biological effects or the fact that different cells have different sensitivities to ionizing radiations. Internal irradiation therapy, external irradiation therapy and near-surface radiotherapy are usually used.

(1) Open radioactive substances (radiopharmaceuticals) are used for the treatment of some diseases. Radiopharmaceuticals which carry some kind of radionuclide may localize in patient's body according to the metabolic properties. Therefore, cancer cells and the diseased tissues may be destroyed by the radiations. A typical example is the radioiodine therapy by using ^{131}I for the treatment of the thyrotoxicosis or the thyroid cancer.

(2) If the tumor is located deep inside the body, it will be irradiated from the outside with highly penetrating radiation (such as X-rays or high-energy particles) . This type of treatment is called external irradiation therapy. Cells which divide rapidly and have a high level of metabolic activity (such as those in malignant tumors) are more sensitive to radiations than those divide at a slower rate. Ionizing radiation, which is destructive to cells and tissues, can be used to treat tumors by killing tumor cells or controlling their growth. In hospitals, ^{60}Co is a commonly used material in radiotherapy. The powerful gamma rays produced by "cobalt bomb" can easily kill the cancer cells, which is mainly used in the treatment of deep tumors.

(3) Near-surface tumors can be treated with the radiation that does not penetrate deeply, such as the radiation of β-ray (close-range radiotherapy) . The healthy tissue lying deeper can be preserved. The contact irradiation uses sealed sources of beta radiation such as ^{32}P, ^{90}Sr. These substances are held near the tumor tissue for a period of minutes or hours until the required dose to treat the tumor is satisfied.

13.4.2 In Diagnosis

1. Radioactive Tracers

Radioactive tracers are radioactive substances added in minute amounts to the reacting elements or compounds in a chemical process and traced through the process by appropriate detection methods. Compounds containing tracers are often called to be tagged or labeled. This method is highly sensitive, even 10^{-18}-10^{-14} g of radioactive substances can be checked out.

Radioisotope renography is a form of kidney imaging involving radioisotopes. ^{131}I labeled OIH (Ortho Iodo Hippurate) is the most commonly used radiolabeled pharmaceutical. After injection into the venous system, the compounds are excreted by the kidneys and its progress through the renal system can be tracked with a gamma camera. Liver tumor can be detected by localized radioactivity with radioactive gold (^{198}Au) infusion. Colloidal ^{198}Au is retained in liver but not into the liver tumor and emits γ-radiation. Measurement of γ-radiation from outside can show the distribution of the marked colloidal ^{198}Au in the liver and give the determined size and location of the lesions.

2. Gamma Camera

Radiopharmaceuticals are taken internally, for example, intravenously or orally. Then, external detectors (gamma cameras) capture and form images from the γ-radiation emitted by the radiopharmaceuticals. These images give the distribution and metabolism of radioactive drugs in the body which is helpful for doctor's diagnosis.

Due to the computer technology, complex calculations perform quickly to convert the detected radiation into information, which is useful for radiologists. For example, a myocardial perfusion scan uses a few amount of a radioactive chemical to see how well blood can flow to the muscles of the heart. The gamma rays which are emitted from inside the body are detected by the gamma camera, are converted into an electrical signal, and sent to a computer. The computer forms an image by converting the differing intensities of radioactivity emitted into different colors or shades of grey. The images, created in a fraction of a second, allow doctors to follow the spread of the radioisotope throughout a patient's body in real time. This allows for early diagnosis of coronary heart disease, myocardial infarction, and for the evaluation of cardiac function.

3. Single Photon Emission Computed Tomography (SPECT)

SPECT imaging is performed by using a gamma camera to acquire multiple 2-D images; it is also called projections from multiple angles. A computer applies a tomographic reconstruction algorithm to the multiple projections and to yield a 3-D dataset. This dataset may then be manipulated to show thin slices along any chosen axis of the body. To acquire SPECT images, the gamma camera is rotated around the patient. Projections are acquired at defined points during the rotation. In most cases, a full 360-degree rotation is used to obtain an optimal reconstruction. SPECT imaging is the distribution of radioactive nuclide in the body tissues and organs, and is not related to the anatomical form.

4. Positron Emission Tomography (PET)

Positron Emission Tomography, or PET scanning, as its known, utilizes positrons as the following way. Certain radioactive isotopes decay by positron emission. Such isotopes can be injected into the body, inside the body they are collected at some specific sites. The positron emitted during the decay of the isotope will encounter an electron in the body tissue almost at once. This results in an annihilation of producing two γ-ray photons, which can be detected by devices mounted on a ring around the patient. The information from the numerous γ-ray photons then constitutes a computer-generated image that can be useful in diagnosing abnormalities at the sites where the radioactive isotope collected.

Nowadays, PET is widely used in the diagnosis of cardiovascular diseases, tumors and nerve diseases. The most commonly used imaging agents are labeled by ^{11}C, ^{13}N, ^{15}O or ^{18}F that are the isotopes of the basic elements of human tissues (C, N, O and F) . PET is a non-invasive method to detect the metabolism and physiology of the body. Positron detection has greatly improved the sensitivity. PET can create vastly superior images of metabolic activity, and make possible more accurate and detailed diagnoses.

13.5 Nuclear Magnetic Resonance

13.5.1 Basic Principles of Nuclear Magnetic Resonance

1. Theory of Quantum Mechanics

Besides the natures of the mass and the electric charge, a nucleus has also the character of spinning. The spin angular momentum of a nucleus is

$$L_I = \sqrt{I(I+1)}\frac{h}{2\pi} \tag{13-9}$$

where I is the **nuclear spin quantum number**. Table 13-3 lists some values of the nuclear spin quantum numbers for some nuclei. Table 13-3 shows the value of any nuclear spin quantum number is always an integer or a half-integer which is determined by the experiments. According to the general quantum regularity, the component of L_I in a given direction of magnetic field, the z-component L_{IZ} is

$$L_{IZ} = m_I\frac{h}{2\pi} \tag{13-10}$$

where m_I is the **nuclear spin magnetic quantum number,** m_I can be 0, ±1, …, ±I. Because the value of m_I can be any one the integers from $-I$ to $+I$, in an external magnetic field the nuclear spin angular momentum L_I, may have $2I$+1 different possible orientations.

Table 13-3 Nuclear Spin Quantum Number

Nuclide	Spin quantum number I	Lande factor g	Nuclide	Spin quantum number I	Lande factor g
$^{1}_{1}H$	1/2	5.5854	$^{16}_{8}O$	0	—
$^{13}_{6}C$	1/2	1.4048	$^{23}_{11}Na$	3/2	1.4783
$^{14}_{7}N$	1	0.4036	$^{127}_{53}I$	5/2	1.1238

Because a nucleus is positively charged and is keeping on spinning, it must have a **spin magnetic moment**. Suppose μ_I is the magnitude of the spin magnetic moment. The ratio of the μ_I to the magnitude of L_I is

$$\gamma = \frac{\mu_I}{L_I} = g\frac{e}{2m_P} \tag{13-11}$$

which is called the **gyromagnetic ratio**. g is **Lande factor**, determined by the experiments and shown in Table13-3, m_P is the mass of a proton, e is the quantity of charge of a proton. From Equation (13-11), we get

$$\mu_I = L_I\gamma = \sqrt{I(I+1)}g\frac{eh}{4\pi m_P} = \sqrt{I(I+1)}g\mu_N \tag{13-12}$$

where $\mu_N = \dfrac{eh}{4\pi m_P} = 5.050824 \times 10^{-27}\,\mathrm{A \cdot m^2}$ is called the **nuclear magneton**, as a common unit of magnetic moment.

The z-component of μ_N is

$$\mu_{IZ} = \gamma L_{IZ} = g\frac{e}{2m_P} \cdot m_I \frac{h}{2\pi} = m_I g \mu_N \tag{13-13}$$

Suppose the magnetic field $\boldsymbol{B}$ is directed along the +z-axis, as discussed previously, the energy E of the magnetic moment in the external magnetic field is

$$E = -\boldsymbol{\mu}_I \cdot \boldsymbol{B} = -\mu_I B \cos\theta$$

where θ is the angle between $\boldsymbol{\mu}_I$ and $\boldsymbol{B}$, $\mu_I \cos\theta = \mu_{IZ}$, so

$$E = -m_I g \mu_N B \tag{13-14}$$

Equation (13-14) shows, for the nucleus with the spin quantum number of I, its energy E may have $2I+1$ different possible values. This indicates that in the presence of an external magnetic field, the original nuclear energy level will be split into ($2I$+1) distinct energy levels. According to selection rules in quantum mechanics, for an allowed transition corresponding to $\Delta m_I = \pm 1$, the energy differences of these two levels is

$$\Delta E = -g\mu_N B\left[m_I - (m_I - 1)\right] = g\mu_N B \tag{13-15}$$

This shows, in an external magnetic field, the energy difference of two adjacent levels depends not only on the characteristics of the nucleus itself (Lande factor g) , but also on the value of the external magnetic field B. It is the feature of the nuclear magnetic energy levels.

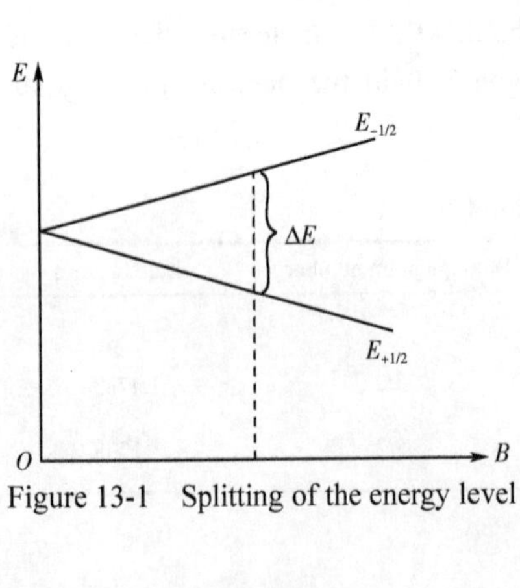

Figure 13-1 Splitting of the energy level

If the nuclear spin magnetic quantum number m_I of a nucleus is $\pm\frac{1}{2}$, we get $E = \pm\frac{1}{2}g\mu_N B$, so the energy difference of two energy levels is

$$\Delta E = g\mu_N B$$

This means that if the magnetic field B increases, so does ΔE , as shown in Figure 13-1.

In thermal equilibrium state, fewer atoms are in higher-energy levels than in lower-energy levels. If a weak high-frequency alternating magnetic field is added to the direction perpendicular to the static magnetic field $\boldsymbol{B}$, and the frequency satisfies the following equation:

$$h\nu = \Delta E = g\mu_N B$$

i.e.,

$$\nu = \frac{1}{h} g\mu_N B \tag{13-16}$$

The nuclei will absorb the energy of alternating magnetic field and jump to higher energy levels, the result is that there will be a macroscopic absorption of energy, which is called the **nuclear magnetic resonance**. If the number of atoms in lower-energy levels is much more than the number in higher-energy levels, the absorption is much more intense and resonance signal will be much stronger.

As soon as the high-frequency alternating magnetic field is added to the sample, transitions caused by absorptions begin to take place superiorly, but as the difference between the numbers of the atoms in respective the higher-energy levels and the lower-energy levels decreases the transitions slow down, until the transitions happen no longer, i.e., the so called saturation state is formed. In fact, another process will take place, in which some spinning nucleus may exchange energy with other spinning nuclei or particles around it. In this way, the nuclei in the higher-energy levels lose some of their energies and return to the lower-energy levels. This process is called the **relaxation process**. On one hand, some nuclei leap from lower-energy levels to the higher ones in the transitions caused by absorptions; on the other hand, some nuclei leap from higher-energy levels to the lower ones in the relaxation process. As these two processes keep on proceeding, the system is in a dynamic equilibrium state, so the nuclear magnetic resonance will go on and on.

2. Classical Theory

In an external magnetic field ***B***, the nucleus with the spin angular momentum of L and the magnetic moment of μ_I is acted by the magnetic torque ***M***. The magnetic moment μ_I precesses about the direction of the magnetic field ***B***. This precession is called **Larmor precession**. It is similar to the precession of a spinning gyroscope which is under the action of the gravity, as shown in Figure 13-2.

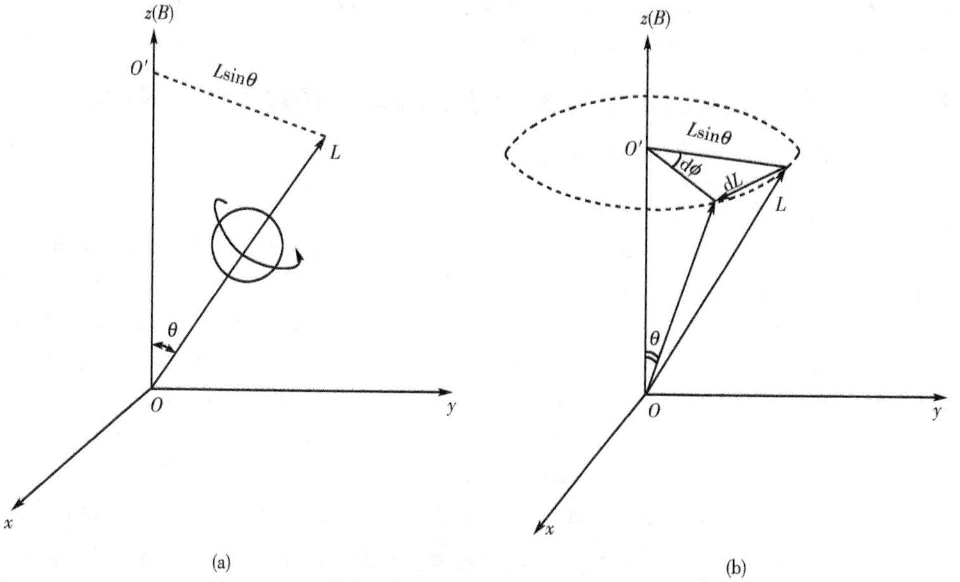

Figure 13-2 Larmor precession

As shown in Figure 13-2 (b), the relationship between dL and precession angle dϕ is d$L = L\sin$

$\theta d\phi$, thus

$$\frac{dL}{dt} = L\sin\theta\frac{d\phi}{dt} = L\sin\theta\omega_p$$

where ω_p is the **angular velocity of Larmor precession**. From the theorem of angular momentum, we have

$$dL = Mdt$$

The magnetic torque exerted on the spinning nucleus is $\boldsymbol{M} = \boldsymbol{\mu}_I \times \boldsymbol{B}$, so we get

$$M = \mu_I B\sin\theta = L\sin\theta\omega_p$$

$$\omega_p = \frac{\mu_I}{L}B = \gamma B$$

$$\gamma = \frac{\mu_I}{L} = g\frac{e}{2m_p}$$

Finally, we have the frequency of Larmor precession:

$$\nu = \frac{\omega_p}{2\pi} = \frac{\gamma}{2\pi}B = \frac{1}{h}g\mu_N B$$

It is just the same as the result got from quantum mechanics, expressed by Equation (13-16).

When the magnetic moment of a nucleus precesses about the direction of the external magnetic field, the angle between the directions of the axis of nuclear spin and the external magnetic field θ is fixed, meanwhile, the additional potential energy of the precessing nucleus is fixed too, and given by $E = -\mu_I B\cos\theta$. When an alternating magnetic field with the frequency of the Larmor precession is added in the direction perpendicular to the direction of the stable external magnetic field **B**, the nucleus will intensively absorb energy from the alternating magnetic field. Then the angle θ and the additional potential energy of the precessing nucleus E will be increased. It results in the phenomenon the nuclear magnetic resonance. This is the classical theoretic explanation to the nuclear magnetic resonance.

13.5.2 The Applications of Nuclear Magnetic Resonance in (NMR) Medicine

1. Structure and Principle of NMR

The structural diagram for the device of nuclear magnetic resonance is shown in Figure 13-3. The steady magnetic field generated by the electromagnet can be adjusted from 0.5 T to 2.5 T by the direct current. Place the sample inside a rotating tube and such kind of rotation can make the action exerted on the sample by the external magnetic field more uniform. The alternating magnetic field is generated by a small coil surrounding the sample and provided by the variable-frequency oscillator. There is another small coil surrounding the sample for detecting signals. The axis directions of the coils must be perpendicular to each other and to the direction of the constant magnetic field. When the nuclei in the sample meets the resonance condition of $h\nu = g\mu_N B$, the energy of the alternating magnetic field will be absorbed intensely by the nuclei in the lower-energy levels, and these nuclei will leap to the higher-energy levels. At the same time, the induced signal in the detecting coil can be detected and recorded by the recording system.

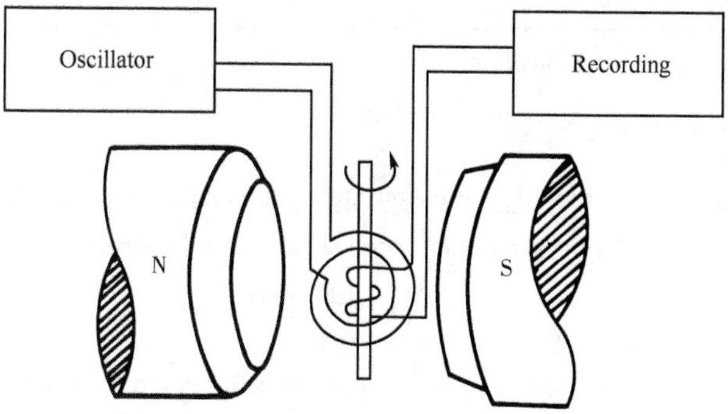

Figure 13-3 Sketch map for a NMR apparatus

2. Applications of NMR in Medicine

Nuclear Magnetic Resonance (NMR) spectroscopy is an analytical chemistry technique used in quality control and research for determining the contents and the purity of the organic compound as well as molecular structure. For example, NMR spectral libraries (atlases) for tens of thousands of organic compounds have been completed. For analyzing an unknown compound, we only need to detect its NMR spectrum first and then match it against the standard NMR spectral libraries to infer its basic structure and ingredients directly. Once the basic structure is known, NMR can be used for determining the molecular conformation in a solution as well as studying physical properties at the molecular level such as conformational exchange, phase changes, solubility, and diffusion.

NMR contains not only a great deal of qualitative information about the chemical compositions and chemical structures of samples of complex compounds, but also used as an important tool of quantitative analysis. ^{1}HNMR examination is the most common NMR examination. The amount of protons of each type in the spectrum of a pure sample can be determined directly from the integrals of each multiplet.

Another well-known application of NMR technology has been the Magnetic Resonance Imager (MRI), which is applied extensively in the medical radiology field to obtain image slices of soft tissues in the human body. MRI is a noninvasive imaging technique, which does not form artifacts like in CT, does not involve exposure to ionizing radiation and contrast injection. MR images of the soft-tissue structures of the body—such as the heart, liver and many other organs—are more likely to identify and accurately characterize diseases than other imaging methods in some instances. This detail makes MRI an invaluable tool in early diagnosis and evaluation of many focal lesions and tumors. MRI has been proven to be applicable in a broad diagnosing range of any conditions, including cancers, heart and vascular diseases, and muscular and bone abnormalities. MRI provides a noninvasive alternative to X-ray, angiography or CT for diagnosing problems of the heart and blood vessels.

A Brief Summarization of This Chapter

(1) Radioactivity and the law of decay: Radioactivity is the phenomenon that an unstable nucleus emits spontaneously some rays and becomes a new nucleus by itself.

1) Decay law: $N = N_0 e^{-\lambda t}$, where λ is the decay constant.

2) The relationship between mean life, decay constant and half-life: $\tau = \frac{1}{\lambda} = \frac{T_{1/2}}{\ln 2}$

3) The activity is defined as the number of nuclides decayed per second:

$$A = -\frac{dN}{dt} = A_0 e^{-\lambda t} = A_0 \left(\frac{1}{2}\right)^{t/T_{1/2}}$$

(2) Radiation dose and radiation protection:

1) Exposure (expressed by the symbol X) : $X = \frac{dQ}{dm}$

where dm is the mass of dry air and dQ is the quantity of the total charges (either positive or negative) .

2) Absorbed dose (expressed by the symbol D) is defined as energy absorbed per unit mass of material.

$$D = \frac{dE}{dm}$$

3) The dose equivalent (expressed by the symbol H) reflects the recognition of differences in the effectiveness of different radiations to inflict over all biological damages.

$$H = Q \cdot D$$

4) Radiation protections include external radiation protections and internal radiation protections.

(3) Nuclear magnetic resonance

1) The spin angular momentum of a nucleus: $L_I = \sqrt{I(I+1)}\frac{h}{2\pi}$

2) The z-component of the nuclear spin angular momentum: $L_{IZ} = m_I \frac{h}{2\pi}$

3) The spin magnetic moment of a nucleus: $\mu_I = \sqrt{I(I+1)}\frac{h}{2\pi}$

4) The z-component of the spin magnetic moment: $\mu_{IZ} = m_I g \mu_N$

5) The energy of the magnetic moment in the external magnetic field $\boldsymbol{B}$: $E = -m_I g \mu_N B$

Exercises 13

13-1. The half-life of ^{60}Co is 5.27 y. What is its mean life?

13-2. The half-life for ^{198}Au is 2.7 d. what is the ratio of the number of ^{198}Au atoms remained after 10 days' storage to the original number?

13-3. After 24 hours, the number of a certain radiopharmaceutical atoms remained is 1/8 of its original number. What is its half-life?

13-4. 25% of some nuclei have been decayed in 5min. What is the decay constant and the half-life?

13-5. The half-life of a sample is 30 a. What is the time t required for the activity to be decreased to 12.5% of the original value?

13-6. ^{226}Ra has a half-life of 1590 y. Find the activity of a 10 mg sample.

13-7. At 8: 00 pm on the 10th of a month, the activity of ^{131}I is 10 Ci. What is the activity of this sample at 8: 00 pm on the 22th of the same month? Here we know the half life of ^{131}I is 8 d.

13-8. The amount of potassium contained in human body is 0.2% of the body weight. In the natural potassium, the content percentage of radionuclide ^{40}K is 0.012%. What is the initial activity of ^{40}K in a human body with the body weight of 75 kg? Here we know the half life of ^{40}K is 1.3×10^9 d.

13-9. A small amount of solution of radioactive ^{24}Na with the half-life of 15 h is given intravenously to a patient. Initially, 12000 nuclei are detected to be decayed per minute. After 30 hours, the corresponding rate in 1 cm^3 blood is reduced to 0.5 per minute. Determine the total amount of blood in the patient's body.

13-10. The nuclear spin quantum number of ^{6}Li is $I = 1$. What are the spin angular momentum and its z-component? If the maximum component of spin magnetic moment is measured experimentally to be 0.8220 μ_N, try to determine its Lande factor g, the spin magnetic moment and its z-component.

13-11. The half-life periods of the two radioactive nuclides are 8 d and 6 h respectively. If these two kinds of nuclides have the same activity, what is the ratio of their mole numbers?